REIMAGINING MEDICAL EDUCATION

The FUTURE of HEALTH EQUITY and SOCIAL JUSTICE

The AMA MedEd Innovation Series

The AMA MedEd Innovation Series

REIMAGINING
MEDICAL EDUCATION
The FUTURE of HEALTH EQUITY and SOCIAL JUSTICE

The AMA MedEd Innovation Series

EDUARDO BONILLA-SILVA, PHD
James B. Duke Distinguished Professor of Sociology
Duke Trinity College of Arts and Sciences
Durham, NC, USA

EMILY A. HAOZOUS, RN, PHD
Research Scientist, Pacific Institute for Research and
Evaluation, Albuquerque, NM, USA

GERALD KAYINGO, MBA, PHD, PA-C
Executive Director, Assistant Dean and Professor
University of Maryland, Baltimore, MD, USA

WILLIAM MCDADE, MD, PHD
Chief Diversity and Inclusion Officer
Accreditation Council for Graduate Medical Education
Chicago, IL, USA

LISA M. MEEKS, PHD
Associate Professor of Family Medicine and Learning
Health Sciences, Meeks Research Group, University of
Michigan, Ann Arbor, MI, USA

ANA NÚÑEZ, MD
Vice Dean, Diversity, Equity and Inclusion, Professor of
Medicine, Division of General Internal Medicine
University of Minnesota Medical School
Minneapolis, MN, USA

TOYESE OYEYEMI, MPH, MCHES
Executive Director, Social Mission Alliance
Washington, DC, USA

JANET H. SOUTHERLAND, DDS, MPH, PHD
Vice Chancellor Academic Affairs and Chief Academic
Officer, LSU Health Sciences Center, New Orleans
New Orleans, LA, USA

JAVEED SUKHERA, MD, PHD
Chief of Psychiatry
Hartford Hospital, Hartford, CT, USA

ELSEVIER

Elsevier
1600 John F. Kennedy Blvd.
Ste 1800
Philadelphia, PA 19103-2899

REIMAGINING MEDICAL EDUCATION: THE FUTURE OF HEALTH EQUITY
AND SOCIAL JUSTICE   ISBN: 978-0-443-28671-1

Notice

Practitioners and researchers must always rely on their own experience and knowledge in evaluating and using any information, methods, compounds or experiments described herein. Because of rapid advances in the medical sciences, in particular, independent verification of diagnoses and drug dosages should be made. To the fullest extent of the law, no responsibility is assumed by Elsevier, authors, editors or contributors for any injury and/or damage to persons or property as a matter of products liability, negligence or otherwise, or from any use or operation of any methods, products, instructions, or ideas contained in the material herein.

Publisher: Elyse O'Grady
Senior Content Development Specialist: Erika Ninsin
Content Development Manager: Kathryn DeFrancesco
Publishing Services Manager: Deepthi Unni
Project Manager: Haritha Dharmarajan
Design Direction: Patrick Ferguson

Printed in the United States of America.

Last digit is the print number: 9 8 7 6 5 4 3 2 1

Working together
to grow libraries in
developing countries

www.elsevier.com • www.bookaid.org

CONTRIBUTORS

Eva M. Aagaard, MD
Washington University School of
Medicine
St. Louis, Missouri
Chapter 16

Scott J. Adams, MD, PhD
University of Saskatchewan
Saskatoon, SK, Canada
Chapter 2

Ora Batash, BA
Hackensack Meridian School of
Medicine
Nutley, New Jersey
Chapter 14

Kristin Berg, LSW, PhD
University of Illinois at Chicago
Chicago, Illinois
Chapter 6

Kimberly M. Birdsall, MPH
Health Coalition of Passaic County
Paterson, New Jersey
Chapter 14

Kelly E. Bowen, BS
Cleveland Clinic Lerner College of
Medicine
Cleveland, Ohio
Chapter 7

Justin L. Bullock, MD, MPH
University of Washington School of
Medicine
Seattle, Washington
Chapter 5

Amanda M. Caleb, PhD, MPH
Geisinger Commonwealth School of
Medicine
Scranton, Pennsylvania
Chapter 4

Kendall M. Campbell, MD
University of Texas Medical Branch
Galveston, Texas
Chapter 15

Nancy M. Chang, MD
Columbia University Vagelos College
of Physicians and Surgeons
New York, New York
Chapter 12

Youngjin Cho, MS, PhD
Geisinger Commonwealth School of
Medicine
Scranton, Pennsylvania
Chapter 4

**Jennifer Cleland, BSc (Hons), MSc,
D Clin Psychol, PhD**
Lee Kong Chian School of Medicine,
Nanyang Technological University
Singapore
Chapter 17

Grace C. Clifford, MAEd
David Geffen School of Medicine at
the University of California, Los
Angeles
Los Angeles, California
Chapter 3

Kendrick Davis, PhD
University of California, Riverside
Riverside, California
Chapter 10

Jennifer DeSantis, MAEd
Case Western Reserve University
Cleveland, Ohio
Chapter 3

Deborah Edberg, MD
Rush University, Oak Street Health
Chicago, Illinois
Chapter 13

Amarachi I. Erondu, MD, MS
David Geffen School of Medicine at
the University of California, Los
Angeles
Los Angeles, California
Chapter 9

Lucia A. Flores, BA
Partners In Health
Chicago, Illinois
Chapter 13

Jonathan Foo, PhD
Monash University
Frankston, VIC, Australia
Chapter 17

Priya S. Garg, MD
Boston University Chobanian and
Avedisian School of Medicine
Boston, Massachusetts
Chapter 16

**Anand Gourishankar, MBBS,
MRCP, MAS**
Children's National Hospital
The George Washington University
Washington, District of Columbia
Chapter 10

Vanessa Grubbs, MD, MPH
thenephrologist.com
Oakland, California
Chapter 1

Christoph Hanssmann, MPH, PhD
University of California, Davis
Davis, California
Chapter 1

Deana Herrman, PT, PhD
College of Health and Human Sciences,
Northern Illinois University
DeKalb, Illinois
Chapter 6

Erin Hickey, MD
University of Illinois at Chicago
Chicago, Illinois
Chapter 6

Daniel Z. Hodson, MD
Division of Internal Medicine –
    Pediatrics,
David Geffen School of Medicine at
    the University of California, Los
    Angeles
Los Angeles, California
Chapter 9

Miriam Hoffman, MD
Hackensack Meridian School of
    Medicine
New York, New York
Chapter 14

Maeve K. Hopkins, MD, MA
Cleveland Clinic
Cleveland, Ohio
Chapter 7

Abbas A. Hyderi, MD, MPH
Kaiser Permanente Bernard J. Tyson
    School of Medicine
Pasadena, California
Chapter 16

Sonoo Thadaney Israni, MBA
Stanford PRESENCE Center & the
    Program in Bedside Medicine
Racial Equity to Advance a
    Community of Health (REACH)
    Initiative
Restorative Justice Hub & Steering
    Committee
Stanford University
Palo Alto, California
Chapter 2

Sunam Jassar, JD
University of Saskatchewan
Saskatoon, SK, Canada
Chapter 2

Esther H. Kang, MD
David Geffen School of Medicine at
    the University of California, Los
    Angeles
Los Angeles, California
Chapter 9

Jennifer Karlin, MD, PhD
University of California, San Francisco
San Francisco, California
Chapter 1

Kristen S. Kurland, BA
Carnegie Mellon University
Pittsburgh, Pennsylvania
Chapter 10

Jason V. Lambrese, MD
Cleveland Clinic Lerner College of
    Medicine
Cleveland, Ohio
Chapter 7

Khanh-Van Le-Bucklin, MD, MEd
School of Medicine, University of
    California, Irvine
Irvine, California
Chapter 11

Candice Taylor Lucas, MD, MPH
School of Medicine, University of
    California, Irvine
Irvine, California
Chapter 11

Carol Major, MD
School of Medicine, University of
    California, Irvine
Irvine, California
Chapter 11

Akshara Malla, MD, MPH
University of California, Los Angeles
Los Angeles, California
Chapter 9

Stephen Maloney, PhD, eMBA
Monash University
Frankston, VIC, Australia
Chapter 17

Stephanie E. Mann, MD, HPEd
Methodist University/Cape Fear Valley
    Health School of Medicine
Fayetteville, North Carolina
Chapter 16

Ofelia Martinez, MD, MPH
Hackensack Meridian School of
    Medicine
Nutley, New Jersey
Chapter 14

Ryan McGraw, MS
Access Living
Chicago, Illinois
Chapter 6

Lisa M. Meeks, PhD, MA
DocsWithDisabilities Initiative
Meeks Research Group
University of Michigan Medical School
    Highland Heights, Ohio
Chapter 5

Charles P. Mouton, MD, MPH, MS
University of Texas Medical Branch
Galveston, Texas
Chapter 15

Mytien Nguyen, MS
Yale School of Medicine
New Haven, Connecticut
Chapter 5

Nataliya Pilipenko, PhD, ABPP
College of Physicians and Surgeons,
    Columbia University
New York, New York
Chapter 12

Charles G. Prober, MD
Stanford University School of Medicine
Stanford, California
Chapter 2

Carmela Rocchetti, MD
Hackensack Meridian School of
    Medicine
Nutley, New Jersey
Chapter 14

Nikita P. Rodrigues, PhD
Children's National Hospital
Washington, District of Columbia
Chapter 8

Steven K. Rothschild, MD
Rush University Medical Center
Chicago, Illinois
Chapter 13

Kate Rowland, MD, MS
Department of Family and Preventive
    Medicine, Rush University
Chicago, Illinois
Chapter 13

Janine Salameh, MPH
Illinois Leadership Education in
    Neurodevelopmental and Related
    Disabilities
Chicago, Illinois
Chapter 6

Lisa Sanchez-Johnsen, PhD
Medical College of Wisconsin
Milwaukee, Wisconsin
Chapter 13

Amanda Sharp, PT, DPT, PhD
Division of Physical Therapy and
    Rehabilitation Science, University
    of Minnesota
Minneapolis, Minnesota
Chapter 6

Zoie C. Sheets, MD, MPH
University of Chicago
Chicago, Illinois
Chapter 6

Jeffrey Shu, MSc
Cleveland Clinic Lerner College of
    Medicine
Cleveland, Ohio
Chapter 7

Avanté J. Smack, PhD
Children's National Hospital
George Washington University
Washington, District of Columbia
Chapter 8

**Janet H. Southerland, DDS, MPH,
PhD**
LSU Health Sciences Center, New
    Orleans
New Orleans, Louisiana
Chapter 15

Javeed Sukhera, MD, PhD
Hartford Hospital
Hartford, Connecticut
Chapter 5

Matthew A. Sullivan, PhD
School of Medicine, Washington
    University in St. Louis
St. Louis, Missouri
Chapter 3

BobbieJean Sweitzer, MD
Inova Health
University of Virginia
Fairfax, Virginia
Chapter 1

Anthony Tizzano, MD
Cleveland Clinic Lerner College of
    Medicine
Cleveland, Ohio
Chapter 7

Sarah E. Triano, MS, NCC, LPC
Geisinger Commonwealth School of
    Medicine
Scranton, Pennsylvania
Chapter 3

Charles Vega, MD
School of Medicine, University of
    California, Irvine
Santa Ana, California
Chapter 11

**Kieran Walsh, MB BCH, BAO,
DCH**
British Medical Journal
London, United Kingdom
Chapter 17

Ryan Weber, PhD
Geisinger Commonwealth School of
    Medicine
Scranton, Pennsylvania
Chapter 4

**Cara N. Whalen Smith, PT, DPT,
MPH, CHES**
Ohio Colleges of Medicine
    Government Resource Center
Columbus, Ohio
Chapter 6

**Michelle You You, BA, BEc,
MPA, PhD**
Peking University
Beijing, P.R. China
Chapter 17

Julie Youm, PhD
School of Medicine, University of
    California, Irvine
Irvine, California
Chapter 11

PREFACE

In 2021 the American Medical Association's (AMA) Council on Medical Education published a report calling for the AMA to work with appropriate stakeholders to commission and enact the recommendations of a forward-looking, cross-continuum, external study of 21st-century medical education. This externally commissioned study would focus on reimagining the future of health equity and racial justice in medical education, improving the diversity of the health workforce, and ameliorating inequitable outcomes among minoritized and marginalized patient populations.

After a thorough process to identify subject matter experts who could best represent reimagining the future of health equity and racial justice in medical education, the AMA convened a panel of nine expert editors for this project, who together recruited expert authors and selected content they saw most appropriate to fulfill the remit of this study. The editors of the book you have in your hands were selected in a collaborative process with the AMA's Center for Health Equity leadership. Specifically, we are experts who have been involved or experienced in medical/health professional education who were recommended both internally and by outside stakeholders and were considered against developed criteria.

We, the editors, focused on reimagining medical education, highlighting structures, systems, and practices that require intervention to improve social justice and equity. The approach we took looked to broaden the biomedical approach of education needed to train a 21st-century physician who meets the needs of all patients and not just a few.

It is very clear from previous iterations of medical school curricula that the social component did not have the platform it needed to address inequitable health outcomes, especially in populations that have been minoritized and marginalized. We hope that creating this book is transformative, although it needs to be matched with change to structures, systems, and practices.

One way would be to bring social components front and center and not let them stay where they tend to be, in the background. To do this we need to deliberately expand our focus from the biomedical sciences. The Flexnerian model training focused on biomedical sciences results in a prescription for how to do something or what needs to be done to fix something (usually by boiling it down to one person prescribing something). We have shifted the lens to look at the health system and the medical education system from different perspectives. That in itself may be transformative as it is not just one perspective but many. This hopefully can provide some breadth and depth of what could be.

We point out, however, that this book is a beginning. We hope it will inspire, through a lens of social justice and health equity, for others to join us and continue to look at health and health care from many different perspectives. We plant this seed for it to grow far beyond our initial work.

When we reflected on our process, we used the analogy of a photograph. Photographs capture a sense of certitude because they have so much detail and appear "complete." This book should not be viewed as a photograph. We see this book and our work as an impressionistic painting. The viewer (or in this case the reader) is not getting the future. You are not getting the change. You are just getting an "impression" of what could be, but even in this, we are just taking a snapshot of now as we think about the future.

The intersectionality of medicine, education, finance, regulation, clinical care, and health care delivery makes this a complex system to change. Education does not stand alone, and it is important to recognize that education is not the primary economic driver of this system. It is also important to recognize when putting the Bunsen burner of change under education that it may help change the system, but it alone is not going to change the whole system. We hope, coming from the space of formal education, that it can have a snowball effect to move us toward a better horizon.

Eduardo Bonilla-Silva, PhD
Emily A. Haozous, RN, PhD
Gerald Kayingo, MBA, PhD, PA-C
William McDade, MD, PhD
Lisa M. Meeks, PhD
Ana Núñez, MD
Toyese Oyeyemi, MPH, MCHES
Janet H. Southerland, DDS, MPH, PhD
Javeed Sukhera, MD, PhD

ACKNOWLEDGMENTS

The editors and authors of this book would like to thank Sarah Ayala of the American Medical Association (AMA) for her project management. Without her, this book would not exist. We would like to thank Olivia Westerbeck, also of the AMA, for her scheduling skills and project assistance. Victoria Stagg Elliott, AMA, gets our thanks for her copyediting and catching our misspellings and misused words. We give additional thanks to Joaquin Baca, PhD, AMA Medical Education Department's director of equity, diversity, and belonging, and David Henderson, MD, AMA Medical Education Department's vice president of equity, diversity, and belonging, for their vision for this book and ongoing support throughout the project.

CONTENTS

PART I

Understanding and Conceptualizing Transformative Ideas

1

Medicine and Medical Education Otherwise
Speculative Futures of the Healing Professions

Jennifer Karlin, Vanessa Grubbs, BobbieJean Sweitzer, and Christoph Hanssmann

SUMMARY

"It could have been otherwise."[1,2] According to scholars Woolgar and Lezaun, this statement characterizes a precis for the field of science and technology studies. In our chapter, we meditate on this phrase as a touchstone for reimagining medical education and clinical practice. What would have to be in place for medical care to be a site of vulnerability, exchange, and authenticity for physicians and patients alike? What would medicine look like were it not so profoundly shaped by structural racism, economic stratification, ableism, xenophobia, sexism, homophobia, and transphobia? Centering these questions, we reflect on how medicine could have been—and indeed, can still be—otherwise. In doing so, we draw on the creative tools of both autobiography and speculative fiction. Our chapter weaves together our own encounters as providers (and patients), our experiences in medical training, and historically documented histories of health activism to outline the structures necessary for a future of medicine that nurtures those who encounter it—patients and providers alike.

In our collective experience as patients, social scientists, and physicians with expertise in nephrology, gender-affirming care, anesthesiology, reproductive health, and primary care, each of us has encountered medical systems that have failed us as females, people of color, trans people, and nontraditional students. Despite these experiences—or maybe because of them—we have been driven to redefine medicine in our own practices and on our own terms. Some examples of this work include (1) envisioning the expansion of a disease-specific social needs–oriented health care system as seen in end-stage kidney disease (ESKD) and speculating what it might be like to apply a similar structure to preventive health and treatment; (2) incorporating integrative approaches to surgical care; (3) sharing our own vulnerabilities with students and foregrounding social and structural determinants of health in medical education; and (4) serving on admission and faculty search committees and documenting racial and economic inequities through our research, in attempts to diversify medical care and mitigate inequities.

While these individual commitments are small successes in cultivating sustainable and healing practices of care, we can no longer ignore the ways that structural problems continue to harm those who work or seek care within medicine. Ultimately, when we look with wistful nostalgia at some of the health activist projects that have attempted to imagine medicine as a site of support, equity, and healing, we see well-intentioned experiments that have rarely been given the space to flourish. Similarly, in all of our examples: (1) ESKD care was ultimately privatized and now perversely incentivizes dialysis profits over patient needs; (2) medical culture in which patients continue to be seen as organs and cases and not holistically; (3) doctors, lacking control over social services, are left incapacitated by the social needs of their patients; and (4) leadership in medicine remains mainly White and cis-male. As such, we turn to the techniques of speculative fiction to imagine what might have happened if our examples truly took root. Our chapter then concludes with a creative reflection about how comprehensive and transformative shifts might take shape in the healing professions and how we might achieve this more utopian outcome in the future. Linking health activist histories to future visions for medicine, we illustrate what the "otherwise" might look like in the phrase "it could have been otherwise" through speculative fiction that imagines a health care system not based on exceptionalism, hierarchy, and prejudices, but on our common humanness.

IT COULD HAVE BEEN OTHERWISE

"I'm sure you're all wondering why I've invited you here today," Diana said, looking at the social activists, physicians, scientists, and educators sitting around her dining room table. She had hand-picked each of them after watching their public responses in the aftermath of the recent protest. Each had been particularly outspoken and endured the backlash of going against those in power. These were her people.

Angel, a social justice activist, was the first to respond. "Given the secrecy and that we're meeting in your house, I'm assuming you have something controversial planned. And I'm here for it."

Samantha, a surgeon, nodded and took a sip of tea, "I hope it's to take action about this outrageous direction our health care system is going in. I'm just so ashamed of our profession sometimes. When I started my medical training, I was proud to be taking this path and endured what felt like unnecessary toxicity because I thought that I could help make things better. I knew it was going to be difficult, but the system seems beyond repair now. The more I learn…" she trailed off.

"Exactly. Since that White House protest against making pig kidney transplants available only to the 1%, I realized that we are at an inflection point. This way of thinking has got to stop. We missed an incredible opportunity with the passage of the Medicare ESKD legislation in 1972," said Diana. "We can't let that happen again."

"So, you're saying we *should* go down the path of pig kidneys for all?" scoffed Jaime, a member of the US Kidney Advocates, a patient advocacy group, and a kidney donor for her brother.

"No, I'm not saying that at all," Diana went on. "That would just be repeating what we did then. Now is the time to get *off* the path of focusing on disease and capitalization. I'm saying we go down a path of preventive health and healing."

"How so?" asked Jaime.

"Well, the ESKD program was the first…and still is the only disease-specific example of socialized medicine in the United States that was available to everyone with kidney

disease regardless of age, finances, or pregnancy status. But instead of generalizing the concept of taking care of everyone who has a medical need, dialysis treatment was corrupted into a multi-billion-dollar business—subsidized by taxpayer dollars, mind you… The same thing will happen if we double-down on investing in a technological fix of pig kidneys without considering the larger picture. I can already envision government-subsidized pig farms for parts to keep the wealthy alive and even more wealthy, while undocumented people do all the dirty work." Diana replied.

She paused to allow the collective groans and eye rolls to die down. "We can't solve this with technological fixes. We need a shift in our way of approaching our problems."

"Yeah, but what about the option for Medicare to help those over 65 or disabled and carve outs for pregnant people and children?" said Jaime.

"That's my point, Jaime," said Diana. "The carve outs. That's where we went wrong. Why do we only help some people with health care at only certain points in their lives? If we invested in a more robust…"

Just then, a figure breezed into the room. Two more followed. The strange trio sat on the sofa, gazing at the group. Usually unshakable, Diana stammered, "Who…Who are you?"

Angel rose to their feet. "You're going to have to leave," they ordered. "This is a closed meeting."

The first figure rose very slowly. Having caught their collective breath, the group noticed odd details about the interlopers. They all wore tailored shirts with thick rolled collars, fashioned from an exceptionally thin fabric. Beneath the right sleeve of one figure, a blue light pulsed dimly from within their inner wrist, like a heartbeat.

"My name is Joss," the blue-lit visitor said. "We haven't been invited, but we are here to ask you to help us with something very important." Joss looked at his two companions hesitantly. "Where should we begin?"

"We are from the future," interjected one of the other new arrivals. He had a scar across his cheek which he stroked tentatively. "Well, more specifically, we are all from different realities of the future. My name is Sandriz, and this is Paige." Sandriz gestured to a shorter individual who was shaking their leg nervously. "Paige and I approached Joss a few months ago because we are struggling. Think about the health care system you all are living with right now—with all its inequities for patients and health care professionals—that's the reality that Paige and I live in, but the problems are exponential. I know you all came together here because of that protest against the pig kidneys being developed to help with your limited number of organs for transplant, but it gets worse. In our reality," again, Sandriz gestured to Paige who was now actively nodding, "a third of the health care budget goes to subsidizing animal farms for organs, most of our population is uninsured, few are able to afford or even want to go to medical school, and the average lifespan has been decreasing every year."

Diana mirrored the wide-eyed stares of several around the table. If the moment and subject matter were not so dire, she would have bragged, *nailed it.*

"But I don't get it. How do you know what we are up to? *Why*, I mean, *how*, I mean, *what* are you doing here… I guess I should say, *now?*" Diana interjected instead.

"We are getting there." Joss continued with an imperceptible pause. "Paige and Sandriz approached us… By *us*, I mean my community—my reality. They came to us for help because we are the reality in your future that has been able to develop and live the most harmoniously and equitably. We have what can be best described as a healing system of care. Instead of focusing on technological fixes and pouring resources into innovations to save us from disease after we are already sick, we focus on prevention, community, and the collaborative. Whenever we run into a problem in our reality, we bring lots of different perspectives to the table— as many as we can think of. Power is shared. We all agree that no matter the ethnicity, race, sexuality, gender, ability of an individual, power corrupts. So, we all function from that perspective to make sure none of us are getting caught maximizing benefit only for ourselves as individuals. Our denominator is always the collective, so to speak. So, when Paige and Sandriz came to us and asked us to help them, we all came together—our teachers, social workers, healers, legislatures, artists, and cyborgs to try to come up with a solution for them. We thought of all kinds of interventions, but their system seemed too far afield; we couldn't figure out how it had gone so wrong."

"It seemed like it was too late for us," Paige said, with a trembling voice and tears welling in the corners of her eyes.

"We brainstormed about our paradigm of healing and prevention and realized the solution rested within that collective approach to health. We realized we needed to go back in time to a moment of inflection and see if we could understand what led us down a different path, and ultimately, an entirely different reality from theirs," said Joss, gesturing toward Paige and Sandriz. "So, we sent our cyborgs to work. Their artificial intelligence capabilities allow us to look back at history and highlight critical moments of change. They can seize on people's emotional tenor at the time when there is an inciting event that appears to have led to fundamental change."

All were hanging on Joss's every word.

"We noticed there were these distinct moments: the Civil Rights Movement in the 1960s in the US, the social protests and economic sanctions before the collapse of South African apartheid, the 2019 mosque mass shooting

in New Zealand before the banning of assault weapons, and many other examples large and small when big changes happened. I know you all are sickened by the gross health inequities among your racial groups and that, compared to other countries, you spend nearly twice that of countries of similar wealth.[3] We know you all are dealing with this after over 50 years of this being the case and not changing. We know you are beyond frustrated."

"That's exactly why I brought this group here to my house!" said Diana.

Angel followed Diana to her feet and shook a book in the air, flipping to a bookmarked page of *Body and Soul*.[4] "When I was reading this chapter, I kept thinking of the Ferguson uprisings in Missouri. I couldn't believe that editorial in *JAMA* that Nelson writes about[5]… I mean, I know it was the late sixties, but the doctors in that editorial are trying to convince others to look *away* from repression and poverty as contributing to violence. Those doctors argue we should focus on people being the source of poverty instead! If doctors who are supposed to focus on healing are contributing to the idea that some people are born more violent than others, no wonder we see cops and others frightened and killing Black people!"

Olivia looked up from her wheelchair with a sarcastic smile. "Yeah, and a half-century later, we have piles of research papers debating the existence of so-called 'violent brains' and still no national health system to speak of."

"Right," Angel inserted. "Because of White supremacy and racism."

The raised brows around the table prompted her to continue.

"I'm not making this up," she said. "There are books written that proposed to solve this so-called 'race problem' by denying health care to newly emancipated Black people so they would eventually die out. And that same attitude carried through each time groups like ours tried to reinvigorate the universal health care conversation. How do you think we ended up with Black people having the worst overall health outcomes in this country? It certainly ain't the 'genetic differences' the scientific community has been trying to prove since the 1700s to justify our enslavement and oppression."

"Wow, that's sinister. Like MLK said, 'Of all the forms of inequality, injustice in health is the most shocking and inhuman,'" said Olivia. "And, meanwhile, my primary care patients cannot get access to see specialists for their heart disease, cannot even walk into the door of an infertility clinic because it costs $2000 to even be seen in those clinics. Every day in my clinic, I can see how social economic status acts as another form of eugenics.[6] Even though I offer everything I can with testing. At the end of the day, the delays cost my patients their lives."

"Exactly. So, the question now is, can we move past this for the sake of us all? After all, when you make it hard for minorities to survive, only the rich can prosper," said Angel.

"Can we even imagine what that could look like?" said Olivia.

"Look, I know I am speaking to the converted here," Joss inserted after a long pause. "The converted and exhausted. The point is that we came here today because you are at one of those inflection points we mentioned. You all have the drive and vision about the kind of world you want to live in. You are willing to uproot old paradigms and patterns, and you have even brought together such a broad and unique group of perspectives. But, I can also see that you are all exhausted from the constant fight against exceptionalism and capitalism and racism—it may seem like nothing is ever going to change. Our artificial intelligence indicated that there is something about this meeting that causes the divergence between Paige and Sandriz's reality of extreme inequality and suffering and what has led to my harmonious reality."

"Maybe if you can tell us more about what your health care system is like, we can see and understand how you got on a different path," said Diana, turning to Joss. "Like, what exactly does *healing* look like?"

"It is a way of thinking, embedded in everything we do," said Joss, with eyebrows knitted not fully understanding the question. "We see ourselves as a collective, where we recognize everyone as contributors to…"

"We're going to need you to stop talking in platitudes. We need details," interrupted Diana.

"Perhaps I can better respond if you tell me what you do now. For example, how do you teach your people to be doctors in 2023?"

"Well, we pick people for medical school based on how well they performed on standardized tests and how much volunteer work they've done to prove how badly they want to be a doctor, when they are more of a measure of how rich of a family you came from," Samantha began.

"And then on the first day of medical school, we tell them to look to their left and right and tell them that one of their neighbors won't make it through the first 2 years of basic science lectures from PhD professors, much less the final 2 years of clinical rotations, where they are expected to answer esoteric questions to avoid embarrassment and stay in the hospital until a superior remembers to tell them they can go home," Olivia continued without taking a breath. "It used to be calling 'pimping,' which was a disgusting term to begin with, and finally went out of favor sometime after the #MeToo movement got some steam in the first decade of the millennium, but it still happens all the time."

Now Joss was the one to expand the vision of those assembled. "We do things very differently," they began. "We start by selecting everyone who has a desire to be a physician, paying careful attention to ensuring each medical school class mirrors our entire population from aspects of gender, racial and ethnic identity, sexuality, ability, socio-economic status, and we provide the support they need throughout medical school and residency training so that they all become doctors who partner with patients to make the clinical decisions to achieve the best possible health outcomes for all. As a result, our doctors aren't completely burnt out."

"How do you make sure that doctors 'have what it takes' to stay up all night and do a long surgery or think on their feet effectively after hours of work?" Samantha asked.

"Ha! That is just like a surgeon to ask that," smiled Olivia.

"Now I can see how my reality came to be. Even the best of you is brainwashed!" Paige said, cutting her off, unable to contain his outrage at what he was hearing. "Look, in Joss's reality, they don't base their judgements on exceptionalism. *Everyone* has individual talents that they bring toward their desire to support healing, and the education system is there to help make sure everyone is competent. It is *assumed* that everyone can be competent, rather than assuming that some people are better than others because they do well on standardized tests. There is less competition because the salary compensation for doing procedures and intellectual medicine is the same.[7] And, salaries are not based on volumes but on outcomes and patient satisfaction. Every medical school, every residency trains toward competence. And, once competence is achieved for all, excellence is thought to be those special characteristics in personality and style that we all have but are different for everyone as an individual. If you don't do that, then you think of doctors as a limited resource. And that gets us to a place like our future in which we don't have enough people to take care of our population and we keep having to limit the number and time spent with health care professionals."

Sandriz nodded in complete agreement.

"Right, but I worked really hard to get into a prestigious program for residency and fellowship, so I could do lots of kidney transplants so that I could be excellent at it, attain prestige and power, and be compensated handsomely," Samantha winked.

"Samantha," now it was Olivia's turn to explain, "I think what Paige is trying to say is that if we get rid of the concept of exceptionalism in medical education and training and make sure that all programs have the ability to train to competency, to excellence, then you would have chosen to go to a residency program that was near your family in the Midwest. Because *that* program would be just as prestigious and excellent as the one you went to because we would not have these inquities in the care we offer. We wouldn't be competing to get into the so-called best residency programs. We could make choices based on lifestyle choices and the kinds of problems we want to work with patients to solve."

Samantha stared off into space. Then she smiled and said, "Yeah, and maybe trainees and physicians could pay attention to their own health and well-being? I was thinking of that nephrology fellow who requested the accommodation. Do you remember that? It was all over social media at the time. That fellow was seen as 'weak' for not being able to work nights because of his health needs and people were discrediting him for asking for accommodations!"

"That same thing happened a few months ago where, I mean *when* I live, but with a very different outcome," started Joss. At the hospital where I work, we received a compliment card for one of our doctors who had previously asked for accommodation. Dr. Hal lives with his bipolar diagnosis, and it is not ideal for him to work nights. So, of course, he received the medical accommodation he asked for, and guess what? The next day when he worked, Hal was able to diagnose a patient presenting with mania. And, not only was he able to diagnose the patient effectively just like anyone with his training would, but Hal shared his real-life experiences. This patient was so grateful for both the technical and real-life *personal* information, that he wrote to thank Hal."

"Wow. That's such a different response. I remember being in fellowship and doing I think my three-hundredth transplant, and I started dripping blood down my leg. I was having my second miscarriage. But I couldn't leave the operating room. I was scared I would be seen as weak or that my co-fellow who was a man would get the job that was opening for one of us. I didn't want the program to know I was even trying to get pregnant since I would be a solo parent…" she paused and began to weep silently.

"It sounds like training is really challenging, but hopefully all that competition during training corresponds to better patient satisfaction and better outcomes. Is that the idea?" asked Paige.

"Not exactly," replied Olivia. "Because primary care is reimbursed at a lower rate, it means that my clinic makes me see patients every 15 minutes so that we can keep our doors open. I don't mean to toot my own horn, but I have figured out how to communicate well to show my patients that I am interested in them, as human beings, while also trying to address all their concerns. But the real problem is that I need to make all these referrals to specialists. I don't really need to use the specialists because I know how to manage most of the basics. I would say there are probably 10% of indications for which I would need a specialist. But I don't have the kind of time like they do. They get an hour to talk about one issue, and I get 15 minutes to talk about everything! Anyway, my patients end up feeling like

a conglomeration of multiple organs rather than a person simply because I end up having to send them to so many specialists. Again, this is because reimbursement rates prioritize hyperspecialization and procedures."

"Yeah, we talk about this all the time at the US Kidney Advocates!" piped in Jaime. "Why don't we have meditation, cooking classes, or yoga at a dialysis center? Or showing videos on the benefits of transplantation? Instead, we just see people plugged into machines watching TV three times a week. Or, what about doing primary care when someone shows up to be checked in before surgery?[8] Why are we only now creating holistic care for patients prior to surgery? These centers are few and far between. I've tried to help people find supportive integrative care, and it's almost impossible! There are just no financial incentives to corporations or to biotechnology or pharmaceutical companies. They make money off novel proprietary drugs and technological fixes."

"We do not think of technology as saving us," Joss mused. "We still have innovation and technology—that has not changed. Our artificial intelligence that got us here today is also helping us bring new molecules to market, and some of them have certainly been lifesaving and had previously eluded even our most astute scientists. What we don't have, however, is a profit-driven culture. Since AI has data from all previous trials and all our trials enroll diverse populations who will benefit from the innovations, ours is a collective endeavor. We apply the collective mentality to individuals and to corporations—none of this innovation is as effective unless we realize it is all based on our collective intelligence, data, and sharing of resources. We are successful so everyone buys into this paradigm. What we don't know is how we got to this point. That's partly why we are back here with you all today."

"That's a lot of pressure to put on our little tea party." Diana winked.

"Diana, earlier you mentioned we missed the opportunity to do things right with the Medicare ESKD program," said Olivia. "Say more about what you think we should have done back then to reshape medical education and health care. Maybe that can help us figure out how to pivot now."

"Yeah, good idea," echoed Angel.

"Well, if you all recall, when dialysis first became a reality, there was limited capacity so they created a group that became known as 'The God Committee' to decide who could have this new life-saving technology," started Diana.

"Yes, I read about this! It was a group of people appointed by a medical society in Seattle, to decide who was 'worthy' of this scarce resource," said Olivia.

"Right. In 1961, Seattle was the birthplace of maintenance dialysis for people with irreversible kidney failure. It should come as no surprise to anyone here that everybody on that committee was White, nor that the first few thousand people who were 'chosen' were 91% White, 91% under age 55, and 75% men. It wasn't until young White men who were considered 'worthy' started dying because there weren't enough dialysis machines available that prompted passage of legislation to extend Medicare benefits to provide dialysis treatment to essentially every citizen if a nephrologist said it was indicated."

"Interesting how that word 'citizen' was specified so that later it could be used to deny dialysis for undocumented immigrants," said Angel.

"Exactly. But within 6 years of the legislation, the dialysis population looked a lot more like those who actually had kidney failure—nearly half over age 55, half women, and a third Black."

"But Black people are only 13% of the US population *and* half as likely to get a transplant as White people, right?" said Angel.

"Yep, which is emblematic of the point you raised earlier. The system couldn't justify denying Black people dialysis outright without backlash, but they could certainly put rules in place to make it so they stayed on the treatment with the highest mortality without having to specify race. I mean, when race is built into our algorithms, we don't see that it's even part of the calculation that results in making it more difficult for Black patients to receive treatments, like getting on the transplant list.[9] The race-based correction built into the algorithm itself makes them look like their kidneys are doing better than they are!"

"I hate it here," sighed Angel. "I think about how I was told that I had less of a chance to successfully have a vaginal birth after my C-section. I looked up the calculation afterward … only because I always think that there is something behind all the so-called objective measures, and I found out that the only reason I was given a less than 50% chance of success[9] was because I am Black! I remember saying to my partner when it got difficult during labor that I just couldn't do it anymore because they had already told me that I was less likely to succeed. Ended up with another C-section."

"Sis, same," said Diana. "That article *Hidden in Plain Sight*[10] was so great for highlighting these race-based algorithms and how they get naturalized and seen as something objective but are really based on social constructs. They highlight how Black race is built into pulmonary function tests, choosing blood pressure agents, estimating kidney function, and on and on."

"I loved that article too, but did you know that even though the authors were talking about race-based calculations, they did not ask anyone who was Black or Latino/a who worked on those original studies to coauthor with them?" Olivia's voice started rising in volume. "These prejudices even end up affecting those with the best intentions.

It's insidious! Again, a fancy editorial in the prestigious *New England Journal of Medicine*, based on the work of scientists of color, ends up publishing and giving those in power all the credit.[10] It's not the science itself that is affected by categories, but also about authorship, exceptionalism, patriarchy, and capitalism. We need a different paradigm,[11] a new intellectual foundation, to medical care. I just don't know how we tackle all of that."

"This all feels so big," Samantha sighed. She was exhausted.

"We have been making some incremental changes," Diana said tentatively, "Like, remember how medical students forced the major kidney associations to stop using 'if Black race' in the equations to estimate glomerular filtration rate, or GFR? It was a tough fight, I remember. But they did it."

"I don't think I understand why people would put up such a fight once the problem was made clear," Sandriz murmured to Paige.

"I do," Angel said, overhearing. "White supremacy. And the GFR with the race-based calculation was in place for 20 years without anyone even questioning the baseless assertion that Black people had different kidney function than others."

"I know," echoed Samantha, "And to think all of those assertions started from scientists trying to justify chattel slavery and prove Black people were 'inferior.' That it took years of a diverse group of medical students refusing to be ignored to right a wrong when a race-free measure was already available is a travesty. And it was just a drop in the bucket toward eliminating race inequities in access to nephrology specialty care and kidney transplantation."

"Agree, but it is an amazing story of how people's minds were changed by a few folks who were not even in positions of power who spoke out," Diana responded. "And it highlights that we need a way to uplift the voices of those most affected. But you are right, Samantha, it took a lot of effort and risk, and it was just a small change. How do we make sure we don't just keep making incremental changes which keep the same paradigm and system of leadership in place?"

Everyone around the table leaned in a little more, as if it was choreographed.

"I guess you are looking at me to answer my rhetorical question," Diana went on. "Well, in the example that brought us here today, why don't we, instead of doubling-down on accessibility of life-saving treatment for end-stage disease, turn our attention to the prevention of the *need* for dialysis? Of course, this means so much more than universal health coverage. As we all know, health care accounts for only about 10% of health outcomes.[12] Other sectors must address the social determinants of health simultaneously—housing, social work, food processing—but we can lead the way for health care."

"So, what are you suggesting happens to the people with end-stage disease?" asked Jaime.

"We take care of our sick," said Diana. "But, within the context of the larger community, and not just what the individual or their family might want."

"I couldn't agree more," said Jaime. "I read that 10% of all our health care dollars goes toward end-of-life care. Like we're literally spending billions of dollars every year to maintain people in vegetative states because the family 'wants everything' while 10% of the population is uninsured."

"Right," said Diana. "And we keep paying even more for emergency room care for problems that could be prevented or managed in an outpatient setting for a fraction of the cost."

"It's insanity!" said Jaime.

"But if we're going to change the paradigm, we have to change *all* of it," said Olivia. "Including how we train physicians. Not just how we pick them."

"Go on," said Diana, excited to hear others engaging.

"Well, like I was saying earlier," Olivia went on, "instead of having a bunch of PhD professors giving basic science lectures to medical students in a void because they wrote a dissertation on a topic, we could have real educators who know how to teach and patients with real lived experiences engage in helping students understand why what they are learning matters. You know, like shifting the focus to people instead of rote disease-based memorization."

"Yes!" said Samantha. "The same could be said for residency training. Imagine how much healing we could engender if training stressed the *person* living with disease as much as we stressed lab data and medication orders."

Joss, Paige, and Sandriz watched in satisfied silence as the group continued to toss around ideas.

It wasn't until the room started darkening that anyone seemed to be aware of how much time had passed. Diana stood to turn on the overhead light, then turned back to the group, smiling. There was so much energy in the room. "Let's make this happen!"

"If we're going to avoid the dystopian reality Jaime describes," Olivia hesitated, "we are going to have to convince the powers that be—those who are predominantly cisgender, heterosexual, able-bodied, supposedly Christian White men—to move past that."

"That means we have to change the powers that be," said Diana. "Look around this table. There's nobody here who fits that description, Olivia. That was on purpose. They and the White women who raised them are the reason why we're in this place staring down the barrel of a cannon that will blast us into that dystopia."

"And you think those in power are just going to relinquish it?" questioned Olivia.

"Well, if the rest of us stop allowing them to drive wedges between us with nonsense rhetoric like 'model minority,' then they won't have a choice," said Angel.

"True. You make an excellent point," said Jaime. "I'm reminded of how they murdered Fred Hampton from the Black Panthers Party because he was making major strides in convincing poor White and Latino folks to join forces with the Black Panthers."

"Exactly," said Angel. "It's only those at the bottom of this hierarchy that whiteness created who can really lead us all to true equity. And that's Black women."

A silence fell over the group as heads nodded. After a beat, Samantha drew in a quick breath and tightened her lips. "Well," she said, "I can't really argue with that, but I guess I wonder if there's more."

"What do you mean?" Angel said, her eyes locking with Samantha's.

"Well," replied Samantha haltingly, "I don't know if Condoleezza Rice is going to sail us to liberation on her oil tanker, for one. I'm not trying to say that Black women shouldn't be at the heart of leadership, or even question what I think is our shared value that people who are most targeted by systemic harms should be the ones pointing us in better directions."

Joss, Sandriz, and Paige leaned in, looking a bit confused with some of the nuances of historical references.

Samantha took a breath, surveying the faces that studied hers. "I guess I'm saying that I think power works in a lot of ways, and some of them are sneaky. For example, I got invited to take part in this diversity initiative at the hospital where I work. I was one of two women—two out of ten people! It seemed like the things I said just got ignored. But the other woman who was there—she's someone I've butted heads with before—she would say things like, 'Well, unlike the extreme feminist position that *some* people here are taking, I think that maternal leave is actually really generous here.' And then the administrators would smile and turn around and say that a woman on the diversity committee agrees that our lousy leave policy is just terrific."

Angel said, "Hmm, it's a good point. I know intellectually that experiencing racism doesn't necessarily mean having a clear view of what causes it or how to fight it. And yeah, maybe it's too simple to think about specific groups of people being in possession of power. Though there's plenty of times that feels true enough!"

Samantha said, "Yeah. I mean, I'm not trying to say I think you all are wrong—I don't think that at all. It's just that I think it's complicated. How can we figure out how to change things if we don't even have a clear sense of how power works, and how people who are marginalized sometimes end up perpetuating marginalization? It makes me feel a little at a loss, to be honest with you."

Once again, the room fell silent, and people nodded.

"Basically, what we're saying is that we have to really see past our differences so we can understand that we *are* all in this together and if you win, I win," summed up Olivia.

"But *how*?" said Samantha. "It all feels so hopeless. Like, what has to happen to change the power dynamics?"

"Right. Sandy Hook, George Floyd, and a global pandemic weren't enough to incite lasting change. What will?"

Aisha hesitantly leaned forward into the light. "We've been working on something for a while that I think can help."

All eyes turn to face Aisha. Until that moment, they had been sitting quietly rocking and appearing inattentive.

"Who is this *we*?" said Diana, curious.

"My scientist colleagues within The Neurodivergent Society," they said. "We have invented and tested an implantable device."

"I thought we said we can't rely on a 'technological fix' to solve this problem," said Samantha.

"This is different," said Aisha. "It doesn't alter one's brain chemistry or DNA. It simply glows blue when the wearer comes from a place of true integrity and humanism. Like a mood ring that allows collective-minded people to find one another. Because when collective-minded people can find each other, they build movements rather than struggle alone in silos. And, movements can develop bolder solutions instead of just tinkering with what's already not working. We are hoping it will help us all recognize who is ready for this bolder change and keep us aware of those who are afraid or resistant."

The others looked at one another, slowly nodding, feeling the immensity of Aisha's words.

"You mean an implantable device like this?" said Joss, stepping forward once again. This time he extended his right wrist so that the sleeve withdrew and revealed the dim blue light pulsing beneath his skin.

All eyes turned to Joss, then to Aisha, and then back to one another, widened with the possibilities before them.

TAKE-HOME POINTS

1. To shift medical education and caregiving systems in the United States, fundamental changes in the ways in which we approach one another as humans are needed.
2. A change in the medical paradigm requires a broad coalition including patients, doctors, regulators, and trainees.
3. Revamping medical education to create a culture of caring, inclusion, and support for trainees demands restructuring the power dynamics.

4. Broadening opportunities to train more diverse physicians will foster systems to care for diverse populations of patients.

QUESTIONS FOR FURTHER THOUGHT

1. Why did the authors choose to write this as speculative fiction? What possibilities does this allow, and what is challenging about approaching the topic from that genre?
2. Can you name five specific changes that the characters in this story mention about medical education and resident training?
3. What is the theory of change and power underlying the discussion among the characters in this essay?
4. The essay concludes with a technological device that allows like-minded people committed to changing the medical paradigm to find one another more easily. How might we create similar connectivity without a technological device?
5. Can you identify the key qualities of the meeting that enable the development of a shared mission to fundamentally change an approach to health care?
6. What aspects of this meeting can be employed on a larger scale to build a coalition that might be able to make fundamental changes in our collective approach to health care? What are the current barriers standing in the way of these shifts in thought and action?

REFERENCES

1. Woolgar S, Lezaun J. The wrong bin bag: a turn to ontology in science and technology studies? *Social Stud Sci*. 2013;43(3):321–340. https://doi.org/10.1177/0306312713488820.
2. Woolgar S. Struggles with representation: could it be otherwise?. In: Coopmans C, ed. *Representation in Scientific Practice Revisited*. MIT Press; 2014:329–332.
3. Blitz J, Swisher J, Sweitzer B. Special considerations related to race, sex, gender, and socioeconomic status in the preoperative evaluation. Part 1: Race, history of incarceration and health literacy. *Anesthesiol Clin*. 2020;38(2):247–261. https://doi.org/10.1016/j.anclin.2020.01.005.
4. Nelson A. *Body and Soul*. University of Minnesota Press; 2011.
5. Mark VH. Role of brain disease in riots and urban violence. *JAMA*. 1967;201(11):895. https://doi.org/10.1001/jama.1967.03130110121050.
6. Swisher J, Blitz J, Sweitzer BJ. Special considerations related to race, sex, gender, and socioeconomic status in the preoperative evaluation. Part 2: Sex considerations and homeless patients. *Anesthesiol Clin*. 2020;38(2):263–278. https://doi.org/10.1016/j.anclin.2020.02.001.

7. Gottlieb JD, Polyakova M, Rinz K, Shiplett H, Udalova V. *Who Values Human Capitalists' Human Capital? The Earnings and Labor Supply of U.S. Physicians*. In: NBER Working Paper Series. National Bureau of Economic Research; 2023:1 p. https://www.nber.org/system/files/working_papers/w31469/w31469.pdf.

8. Benesch C, Glance LG, Derdeyn CP, et al. Perioperative neurological evaluation and management to lower the risk of acute stroke in patients undergoing noncardiac, nonneurological surgery: a scientific statement from the American Heart Association/American Stroke Association. *Circulation*. 2021;143(19):e923–e946. https://doi.org/10.1161/cir.0000000000000968.

9. Faulkner S, Haas M, Wang D, et al. 746 The effects of removing race from the VBAC calculator: implications for counseling. *Am J Obstet Gynecol*. 2021;224(2):S467–S468. https://doi.org/10.1016/j.ajog.2020.12.769.

10. Vyas DA, Eisenstein LG, Jones DS. Hidden in plain sight — reconsidering the use of race correction in clinical algorithms. *N Engl J Med*. 2020;383:874–882. https://doi.org/10.1056/nejmms2004740.

11. Kuhn TS. *The Structure of Scientific Revolutions*. University of Chicago Press; 1962.

12. Karlin J. Sam's story: the financial and human costs of disjointed logics of care. *Ann Fam Med*. 2022;20(1):84–87. https://doi.org/10.1370/afm.2763.

A Precision Medical Education Approach to Achieving Justice, Equity, Diversity, and Inclusion

Sunam Jassar, Sonoo Thadaney Israni, Charles G. Prober, and Scott J. Adams

OUTLINE

SUMMARY

In this chapter, we present a vision for how the concept of precision medical education can help achieve a future medical education system that addresses longstanding issues that have resulted in suboptimal diversity, inclusivity, and equality of learners impacted by historical injustice. Our proposed approach borrows from the concept of precision health, which analyzes large amounts of multimodal digital health data to predict, prevent, diagnose, and inform the treatment of disease using artificial intelligence (AI). We discuss how precision medical education may be equitably designed with relevant critical collaborators and implemented across the medical education continuum to reduce inequities and injustices in medical education. The chapter describes the potential for precision medical education to leverage big data and AI, along with **design thinking** and **restorative justice frameworks**, to surface harms, needs, and stakeholder obligations. Our goal is to address historic inequalities in access to medical education while improving on more personalized teaching and curricular delivery, learner assessment, and student services. While a substantial body of literature has described bias in AI algorithms, we present more recent approaches to using AI to address human bias. The chapter discusses how a precision education approach combined with restorative justice and design thinking frameworks can transform medical education to make it more learner-centered, equitable, and effective, delivering **justice, equity, diversity, and inclusion (JEDI)**. We discuss how this approach may reduce health inequities on a population scale, with health care practitioners who are better prepared across the competencies that society needs to achieve health equity and social justice within health systems.

INTRODUCTION

In an era marked by advances in health care and technology, the realm of medicine is undergoing a shift, transitioning from the traditional "one-size-fits-most" approach to an individualized model. Precision health centers on tailoring preventive, diagnostic, and therapeutic approaches based on individual patient characteristics. Precision approaches hinge on the use of AI to analyze large amounts of health data with the goal to optimize prevention, personalization, and precision of medical care.[1]

Applying precision approaches to medical education yields a new framework termed precision medical education. Precision medical education is an extension of precision medicine, a subset of precision health, with a similar approach of tailoring learning, assessment, and coaching to individual learners.[2] Precision medical education has recently been defined as "a systematic approach that integrates longitudinal data and analytics to drive precise educational interventions that address each individual learner's needs and goals in a continuous, timely, and cyclical fashion."[2] The goal of precision medical education is to optimize training for medical learners, enabling them to provide more effective and equitable care for their future patients. Precision medical education transcends the conventional boundaries of medical training with the aim of improving educational, clinical, and system outcomes in medicine.[2]

Our focus in this chapter is to explore the concept of precision medical education to help achieve a future medical education system that addresses longstanding issues that have resulted in suboptimal diversity, inclusion, and equality of learners impacted by historical injustice. The persistent inequities and disparities inherent in medical schools and health care systems have been extensively studied.[3] However, further action is required to address inequities that have been deeply ingrained over time and continue to undermine JEDI. These inequities and disparities manifest in multiple ways throughout the course of medical education, beginning with medical school admissions, curriculum design, and assessment of students. Prominent issues include the underrepresentation of minoritized people, prejudice, bias, and stereotyping. Disparities, which are often influenced by factors such as race, ethnicity, gender, sex, socioeconomic status, and other aspects of historical privilege, have far-reaching consequences on medical education and the health care delivery system.

This chapter discusses how a precision medical education approach, combined with restorative justice and design thinking frameworks, can transform medical education to make it more learner centered, while prioritizing JEDI. We discuss how this approach may reduce health inequities on a population scale, with physicians who are better prepared across the competencies that society needs to achieve health equity and social justice within health systems.

BUILDING INCLUSIVE PRECISION MEDICAL EDUCATION SYSTEMS

AI is the engine for precision medical education, with big data as the fuel. AI can be used to facilitate learner-centered curricula delivery that focuses on the needs of individual learners, dismantling a one-size-fits-all approach to medical education. Using AI to achieve precision medical education overcomes challenges related to the volume and complexity of data and allows for timely insights. These insights are subsequently used to promote learner outcomes and learner success.[2] With increased potential to effectively and efficiently respond to the diverse needs of learners, AI powers the potential of precision medical education to help achieve JEDI in medical education.

Examination of Bias in Precision Medical Education

AI has the potential to promote diversity and overcome biases if designed with principles of fairness and commitment to inclusivity from stakeholders.[4] Stakeholders play a key role in developing AI systems that incorporate justice, inclusivity, and diversity by defining the trade-offs, outcomes, and processes related to AI algorithms; using appropriate datasets to train AI algorithms; and collaboratively addressing biases and usability challenges that may disproportionately affect marginalized groups.[4] A known and pressing challenge of AI is the presence of bias rooted in historical processes, assumptions, and definitions of success. Due to the key role AI plays in ensuring the success of precision medical education, it is essential to examine and understand where these biases exist.

Bias and discrimination can exist within the datasets upon which AI algorithms are trained, and AI is limited by the quality of data it uses for training.[5] AI systems trained on biased data can perpetuate and amplify societal prejudices, leading to discriminatory outcomes. Examples of bias in datasets include sex, gender, race, age, and socioeconomic status. Biased data can have significant implications where AI data are relied upon. For example, there is a high error rate for identifying dark-skinned females compared to light-skinned males in commercially available facial recognition systems.[4] Historical artifacts of bias are dominant in AI datasets. One AI system, trained on online news texts, associated the word "woman" with homemaker and "man" with computer programmer and attributed "father" with doctor and "mother" with nurse.[6] This stems from historical datasets that are predominantly based on White male majorities, along with heteronormative and ableist assumptions. In medical education, similar biases could emerge among specialties dominated by specific demographics. This highlights the importance of using diverse and inclusive datasets with better representation of all identities for training AI systems, with the potential need for manual engineering to overcome biases within datasets.

Another source of algorithmic bias can result from the people building the algorithms.[7] Bias can inadvertently and unintentionally arise from the limited perspective of algorithm creators. Females and minoritized groups are often underrepresented in the tech industry, leading to oversights when creating certain AI algorithms.[4] An example of such bias is Apple's health app, which was initially released without a menstrual period tracker.[7] While algorithm developers may be committed to inclusivity and diversity, the needs of minoritized groups may not be entirely understood in the absence of direct representation. Unless relevant stakeholders, who have been historically excluded from tables of power, are included, historical injustice will be cemented into existing systems, continuing to exacerbate inequities. Diversity in the teams that build the algorithms is essential to reducing bias.

To successfully use precision medical education to reduce inequities and injustices in medical education, AI tools need large datasets representing diverse backgrounds. Biases skew AI results and create negative downstream effects. Biases can emerge from biased assumptions of algorithm creators, historical data imbalances, cultural differences, and biases among those implementing AI tools. A comprehensive examination of the AI algorithms used in precision medical education is crucial. This involves conducting thorough audits of stakeholder power differences, representing the decision-makers, and training data, identifying potential sources of bias, and evaluating the impact of biased decisions. By acknowledging and understanding bias, developers can take proactive steps to mitigate its influence and build AI models that promote JEDI.

Approaches to Using Precision Medical Education to Surface and Overcome Bias

While AI has been implicated in perpetuating biases, it has recently been shown to address and overcome human biases. When used strategically with appropriate datasets, AI technologies can help reduce the risk of bias.

AI is now being used as a tool to mitigate discrimination, particularly in human resources departments.[8] In human resources, AI can successfully eradicate bias by requiring organizations to use appropriate AI solutions throughout the entire recruitment process and by educating recruiters on how to use AI solutions to promote diversity in the workplace.[8] AI tools have also been used to help companies identify biases in their past hiring decisions by detecting patterns in their data and uncovering evidence of hidden preferences.[4] Extending this concept to precision medical education, AI can be an effective tool to counteract bias

and foster a JEDI-anchored education system, beginning with the medical school admissions process. Analyzing the data about students accepted to medical school or residency programs with the use of AI can surface patterns of bias, including unconscious bias. Researchers developed a machine learning-based decision support tool in one study to identify candidates for residency interview offers.[9] The machine learning model identified desirable candidates that may have otherwise been overlooked due to human or metric biases.[9] Program directors used the decision support tool to select 20 applicants to interview who had previously been screened out during the human review process.[9] This highlights the use of AI to achieve a fairer assessment of candidates and overcome biases that exist in the traditional selection process.

Developers can create AI systems that detect and flag biased patterns in data, highlighting potential areas of concern in real time. For example, AI is used to alert clinicians about disparities in documentation in real time and to review possibly inappropriate opioid prescriptions at the end of the clinic day when decisions are particularly prone to bias.[5] Algorithms are designed to learn from these corrections and feedback, progressively reducing bias over time. Employing adversarial training, resampling, and debiasing algorithms, AI systems can be trained to make impartial decisions, ensuring fair treatment across various demographic groups.

Other steps to mitigate bias involve addressing the overt or underlying biases held by algorithm creators. Incorporating diverse teams and stakeholders in the development and validation of AI algorithms allows for relevant and representative perspectives to be considered and works to reduce the risk of perpetuating unconscious and historical biases.

Design Thinking and Restorative Justice Frameworks

Precision medical education presents an opportunity for JEDI by addressing the experiences and needs of all individuals. However, without careful attention to the structure and design of AI tools, benefits may be limited to select groups, further exacerbating existing inequities.[10] Design thinking and restorative justice frameworks provide an approach for how precision medical education tools may be developed and implemented in medical education to achieve JEDI-anchored learner outcomes.

Design thinking is a user-centered approach that emphasizes problem-solving and collaboration. It is often based on the IDEO model which uses a five-stage design thinking approach.[11] The stages, in order, are empathize, define, ideate, prototype, and test.[11] The IDEO process can be further expanded to be used as a tool for equity and social justice.[11] Incorporating additional stages to reflect, contextualize, and democratize creates a model that works toward comprehensively addressing issues of social justice.[11] The first step requires reflecting on one's own personal biases and positionality.[11] Reflecting is a continuous process with the goal of promoting dialogue about privilege and oppression.[11] This promotes the potential for building inclusion and understanding among individuals. The second step of contextualizing requires designers to examine the problem in the context of ongoing "struggles for identity, culture, place, and power."[11] Contextualizing the problem with an understanding of the individual's social and economic realities provides a greater opportunity to tailor solutions that will work in the long term.[11] The next step, democratizing, values all participants and their community expertise and creativity.[11] This allows individuals to learn from each other and collaborate on problem-solving. Entwining relevant stakeholders within each step of design thinking has the promise to deliver impactful JEDI.

Restorative justice frameworks focus on addressing harms and strengthening relationships through collaborative decision-making.[12] In medical education, restorative justice presents a way to sustain learning communities and address harm when it occurs. Having a framework in place to address harm is essential to promote principles of social justice among learners. Medical schools can use a continuum of restorative justice practices that incorporate three tiers.[12] The first tier focuses on building and strengthening relationships by developing interpersonal communication skills and mutual understanding.[12] Tier two involves responding to conflict and harm. The last tier focuses on the reintegration process using support reentry and accountability principles.[12] There are many opportunities to apply these restorative justice practices within the medical education system to create a culture of inclusion. Restorative justice practices have been used in the past to mitigate the mistreatment of faculty and learners and proactively identify mistreatment.[12] Programs can use the restorative justice framework as a guide for the effective development and implementation of precision medical education and the creation of a pathway for social justice.[12]

IMPLEMENTATION OF PRECISION MEDICAL EDUCATION ACROSS THE MEDICAL EDUCATION CONTINUUM

Integrating Precision Medical Education Across Medical Education Activities

Medical education is currently undergoing transformation but is still largely based on a standard uniform system that is not optimally designed to advance JEDI. The standard approach includes a uniform curriculum with limited elements of personalized learning in the form of individualized feedback or learning plans.[2,13] There is a need to adopt a system centered on the learner that improves individual outcomes. A precision approach to education delivery compared to the standard "one-size-fits-all" model is more likely to result in superior learner outcomes while enhancing JEDI in medical schools.[13] Precision medical education focuses on the needs of individual students to improve their personal learning experience. Precision medical education can be implemented at different stages across the continuum to enhance learning and improve learning outcomes. Medical education encompasses admissions, curriculum development, teaching, curricular delivery, and learner assessment across undergraduate, graduate, and continuing medical education. Precision medical education can be applied to each of these domains to optimize learning for students and identify and mitigate barriers for those underrepresented in medicine (Table 2.1).

Several approaches to precision education are described.[13] The approach to precision education explored by Cook et al. aims to move beyond the traditional question of "did an intervention work?" to "what intervention worked for whom and how did it work?" This approach focuses on applying personalized interventions tailored to individual students to enhance outcomes. Using this approach, precision education incorporates four structural components. The first component is problem analysis, which identifies the individual student's needs.[13] These needs can include the presence of maladaptive behaviors, the absence of adaptive skills, or the existence of adverse environmental factors.[13] Once the student's needs are identified, the second component focuses on developing corresponding adaptive interventions. These interventions encompass strategies tailored to meet the needs identified in the first component. The third component of precision education under this framework involves monitoring the individual's progress over time. This allows for any modifications to be made depending on the individual's response and progress. The last component corresponds to collaboration. The goal of this component is to have relevant team members regularly meet to review progress and plan for the next steps. These components are continuous until the desired outcomes are achieved. Systems are built to coach and mentor educators to assist in questioning unintended historical biases in creating curricula, giving feedback, and prioritizing JEDI principles in all aspects of teaching and training.

A precision approach to teaching and learning in medical education can be realized through the use of AI and intelligent tutoring systems. The goal of intelligent tutoring systems is to provide individualized instruction through computer programs that model learners' psychological states.[14] Psychological states incorporate an

TABLE 2.1 JEDI-Anchored Precision Medical Education

Domains	Standard Approach	Precision Medical Education Approach
Admissions	• Potential for inter- or intraobserver variability among interviewers • Potential for implicit bias from interviewers	• Using AI to screen applicants and reduce variability among interviewers • Providing AI algorithms with only the necessary information required to screen applications to minimize bias and foster equity, diversity, and inclusion
Learning	• Uniform curriculum for all students • Standard learning resources provided to all students regardless of personal progress or areas of weakness • Inconsistencies in clinical training due to varying types of exposure to patient presentations	• AI-curated learning resources specific to each student's needs • Use of AI to track progress and exposure to specific patient presentations during clinical training • Flag areas where competency is not yet achieved • Use of intelligent tutoring systems to create learner-specific teaching modules
Student support	• Often provided too late, at the stage when the student is already struggling	• Using AI to recognize students who may require additional support early on
Assessment	• Uniform assessment forms and evaluations • Potential for bias based on race or gender	• Using AI to neutralize variables of race and gender • Tailored based on individual learning goals and progress
Coaching and planning	• Based on standard processes of progression and evaluations	• Data-driven coaching • Tailored to students based on cycles of insight

individual's subject matter knowledge, learning strategies, motivations, or emotions.[14] Intelligent tutoring systems offer a technological foundation for implementing precision medical education and have been shown to be more effective when compared to outcomes of teacher-led large-group instruction, nonintelligent tutoring system computer–based instruction, and textbooks or workbooks.[14] Similar systems are built to inform educators on JEDI prioritization, self-assessment, regulation, and improved decision fitness.

The use of AI and intelligent coaching and tutoring systems at various stages in the medical education curriculum can facilitate personalized learning, enhance competencies, and promote success for all learners in a program, helping to overcome individual and systemic barriers and facilitating JEDI. Leveraging big data and AI to understand student backgrounds better can enable medical schools to intervene and assist students. Machine learning can be used to identify students at risk of declining academic performance.[15] A case study in Taiwan looked at the use of machine learning to predict the probability of university students dropping out based on student academic performance, loan applications, number of absences from schools, and the number of flagged subjects.[15] They could predict the probability of dropping out with an 80% accuracy rate.[15] Similar principles can be applied in medical school to predict clinical performance and professionalism and to ultimately identify students who may benefit from targeted and individual assistance. Readily identifying and mitigating barriers, with the help of AI, for those underrepresented in medicine may allow medical schools to offer support early to improve learner outcomes and enhance learner experience throughout medical training and contribute to training future physicians representative of and able to serve their community's diverse population needs.

AI can be used to facilitate greater learning during the clinical years of medical education by taking into account unique individual needs. Clerkship and residency are based on learning in the workplace. Workplace-based learning or situational learning occurs when students apply their knowledge and skills to real workplace settings under supervision.[16] This form of learning primarily occurs in hospitals, clinics, and community settings. Workplace-based learning is considered to be one of the most effective forms of learning in the medical context.[16] However, many barriers and limitations can accompany this form of learning. Workplace-based learning relies on the physical learning environment and exposure to patients to optimize the breadth of learning.[16] Precision medical education and AI can be applied to this setting to overcome these barriers and inconsistencies in learning.

Radiology education is an example of incorporating AI to achieve precision education in workplace-based learning. Radiology education is largely dictated by the number and types of cases encountered, which means there are inconsistencies in learning across students.[17] Students will have different skill levels and varying exposures to imaging, making it difficult to teach and learn with a standardized curriculum. With the use of AI, specific cases can be assigned to learners based on interests and missing competencies.[17] AI-curated teaching files can support the curriculum and be delivered at optimally relevant times based on individual progress.[17] The content of the teaching files can also be adapted to individual performance to enhance learning outcomes.[17] Through intelligent tutoring systems, individualized modules are created for students where learning style and performance are tracked.[17]

The use of AI and intelligent tutoring systems allows for both individualized learning and reduced inconsistencies in the radiology curriculum. This can be extended to other aspects of clinical learning to ensure students obtain exposure to key aspects of medicine and that they are modified according to the progress of individual students. Clinical workplace-based learning has inconsistencies in teaching as it depends on the availability of patients and preceptors. For example, a student may not encounter a vaccine-hesitant patient and therefore may not have the opportunity to achieve the associated competency relating to difficult patient discussions. Integrating AI into the curriculum can help overcome these inconsistencies by tracking student exposure and flagging missing competencies. This will transcend the rigid bounds of a standardized curriculum and make it more learner centered.

Approaches to Reducing Inequities and Injustices in Medical Education

The medical education system is unfortunately not exempt from institutional racism or inequities for particular groups based on race, gender, class, and other social identities.[3] There is a long history of racially exclusionary practices within medical schools.[18] Students of color are underrepresented in the medical education system and disadvantaged by the traditional curriculum and evaluation methods.[3] Inequities and injustices exist at every stage of medical training, from the application process to residency.[18] Race-neutral processes in accordance with individual biases and interpersonal discrimination perpetuate racial inequality among medical learners.[18] The inequities and disadvantages faced by people of color and groups underrepresented in medicine may further contribute to trainees pursuing less competitive specialties and attrition from academic careers.[18] There is a critical need to dismantle racism and address inequities in the medical education system. Reducing inequities and injustices in medical education can be achieved through a precision education approach. Precision education focuses on the unique needs and challenges of individual learners and can highlight the needs of diverse student populations.

For example, the medical school admission process heavily focuses on the Medical College Admission Test (MCAT) score, undergraduate grades, extracurricular activities, and interview performance. While medical schools use categories such as MCAT scores and grades to standardize parts of the admissions process, there remains significant inter- and intraobserver variability among evaluators.[6] There is potential for bias and interpersonal discrimination in the medical school admission process, particularly during the interview portion.[18] Bias can arise from racial or demographic information, applicant gender, ethnicity, appearance, and regional or institutional bias.[6] AI can be used to screen applicants and reduce the chance of biases and interviewer variability that may influence admissions decisions. By inputting only the necessary information required to screen applicants into AI algorithms, inter- and intraobserver variability may be reduced and a fair standard can be applied across applicants while also maintaining nuances as part of the traditional screening process.[6]

Another area within the medical education system that is prone to bias and can perpetuate inequities is learner assessment. Unbiased assessment of medical learners is essential to ensure fair and equal monitoring of progression throughout various stages of training. Learner assessment can have important implications on success in the residency match process and future career paths. Unfortunately, there is potential for discrimination of learners based on race, orientation, ethnicity, and gender. All medical students have equal expectations on paper; however, students of color and students underrepresented in medicine face additional discrimination.[18] Discrimination and lack of inclusivity in the clinical learning environment contribute to stereotype threat.[18] This leads to grading disparities;

students underrepresented in medicine are less likely to receive honors compared to their peers, regardless of their academic performance on a rotation.[18] Gender bias is another factor that impacts medical learner assessment and poses a potential threat to the validity and integrity of the assessment process.[19] Implicit gender bias is pervasive in medical training and drives gender inequities in medicine. Women continue to remain underrepresented in the medical profession, particularly in leadership roles. As opposed to their male counterparts, females are seen as less likely to be career oriented and are more often described as "compassionate" or "sensitive" on evaluations.

Precision medical education can be used to mitigate these issues and address the resulting inequities. The term "amplification cascade" has been coined to describe the cumulative unequal impact on underrepresented students in medicine where slight initial differences compound into significant differences in long-term outcomes.[18] Neutralizing these factors by forcing greater transparency, reflection, questioning, and training through the use of AI could mitigate these biases to achieve more equitable learner assessment. AI could make the assessment process fairer by removing or neutralizing variables such as race and gender, whereby potential for bias exists. AI algorithms based on unbiased and diverse datasets will be required to reduce inequity in the medical learner assessment process and bring equity to medical education.

Similarly, precision medical education could bring greater visibility across nationwide systems to facilitate a fairer assessment process by adding granularity for variables such as race/ethnicity, ableism, gender, and other variables where the potential for bias exists. Precision medical education can also be used to identify learners requiring unique and/or additional support to foster successful outcomes.

The literature is rich in describing the discrimination in the current medical education system, with particular attention to bias in the medical admissions process and learner assessment. Precision medical education provides a solution to reduce the inequities and injustices inherent in the education system by leveraging AI to reduce unconscious and overt bias and to support students.

Aligning Precision Education With Competency-Based Medical Education

Competency-based medical education (CBME) is gaining traction as the new paradigm in graduate medical education and is increasingly implemented in undergraduate and continuing medical education. CBME, like precision education, is based on the premise that learners are unique, with different areas of strengths and levels of progression. CBME uses entrustable professional activities (EPAs) to assess learner competencies and determine whether milestones are met at different stages of training. CBME focuses on individual observations as the basis for assessing and determining if competencies are met.

The majority of residency training programs across the United States and Canada have adopted CBME. CBME has thus far been successful in that it allows flexibility in the medical training curriculum and provides personalized assessments and feedback.[2] A challenge of CBME, however, is trying to utilize the assessment data to establish insights. An increasing amount of assessment data has resulted from the individual feedback and EPAs provided to learners. A large amount of data were collected on trainees with corresponding issues of data and assessment overload.[2] Under the CBME model, however, there is an absence of resources and tools to deliver timely data insights to learners and programs.[2]

Precision medical education and the use of AI provide a solution to analyze and integrate the data collected from CBME.[2] The data from CBME are integrated and assessed by AI to provide insights at the individual learner level.[2] The data are used to inform educational decision support tools and automated suggestions for individual learners.[2] After multiple cycles of analysis over time, an optimized learning system is created based on increased data and outcomes from diverse learners.[2]

Integrating precision medical education into the CBME curriculum and leveraging AI tools to analyze data creates an optimal and efficient educational framework. Precision medical education can be used to solve the challenges and limitations of CBME to further improve outcomes for learners.

Potential Barriers and Pitfalls to Implementation

Precision medical education presents a new approach to reducing inequity and injustices in the medical education system. However, it is not immune to barriers and challenges to widespread implementation. Barriers to implementation largely correspond to the use of big data and AI as a method of achieving precision medical education.

The first barrier to implementation is the required use of resources. Precision medical education hinges on the concept of tailoring learning to individual student needs. Diverse educational pathways and catering to specific learner needs introduce a new element of complexity for medical school programs.[2] Training and faculty development efforts will be necessary to help modulate this complexity.[2] This will be resource intensive. To provide personalized learner support under the precision medical education framework, there may be implications on the duration of education, tuition, and curricular planning.[2] The insights gained from the data-driven precision medical education approach will be required to inform academic planning and implementation of this new framework.[2] Additional resources and staff will be required to leverage big data and AI to obtain timely insights.

The second barrier to the implementation of precision medical education focuses on the challenges that come with the use of AI. AI is at the core of precision medical education and is the key to ensure the successful implementation of precision medical education. AI, however, has its own vulnerabilities that can impact the success of precision medical education and its ability to achieve social justice. AI is vulnerable to biases in the datasets used. The quality of input data influences its accuracy and outcomes. It is therefore imperative that AI datasets are unbiased and represent diversity. Students historically underrepresented in medicine are underrepresented in AI datasets.[2] With the emergence of CBME and increased data collection, there is the potential to increase diversity in the datasets relied upon for training AI. AI also relies on a large amount of data from various sources. A large and diverse dataset will optimize precision medical education. However, there are challenges in trying to assure privacy and confidentiality to access the data. While high-quality datasets exist for training in certain aspects of precision education, they are not easily accessible.[17] Barriers to implementation also exist in understanding the various regulatory and policy barriers across different institutions and regulatory bodies.

Precision medical education is an emerging paradigm, and there will be challenges and barriers to implementation in the initial stages. There will be a significant learning curve for institutions, teachers, and students alike. Some of these challenges can be predicted and mitigated prior to implementation, such as understanding the impact of historical privilege and power, authentically engaging and empowering those who lack privilege, ensuring unbiased datasets, and putting additional resources in place to facilitate delivery. Other challenges will become evident throughout the implementation process.

POTENTIAL IMPACT OF PRECISION MEDICAL EDUCATION ON POPULATION-SCALE HEALTH INEQUITIES

Precision medical education not only can impact the medical education system but can also play a role in improving population-wide health inequities. Medical students represent the future of health care, and it is imperative that JEDI is promoted at the medical school level. The use of precision medical education to address health inequity and injustices in medical education can also have a subsequent impact on how students tailor their future practices and approach health inequities. Promoting diversity and addressing

biases throughout medical training enhances medical education and has lasting implications for society. There is evidence that increased medical school diversity has a positive impact on minoritized trainees' experiences and outcomes as well as on White trainees and their likelihood of serving underserved communities.[18] A survey of medical students found that contact and interactions with diverse peers enhance educational experiences for all students.[6] It has been shown that underrepresented minoritized physicians are more likely to serve their communities compared to their majority counterparts.[6] Promoting diversity at the medical school level has the potential to support the expansion of health care to traditionally underserved communities.[6] Minoritized people are more likely to choose physicians of their own race.[6] Historical injustices have fostered an environment with suboptimal diversity and inequity in medical training, which hampers the overarching goal of contributing to health equity. Supporting a JEDI learning environment with the use of AI driving precision medical education allows for greater diversity reflected in the physician workforce. Precision medical education, with the aid of AI, can start with mitigating biases at the medical school admissions level to increase the diversity of students. It can further support students underrepresented in medicine throughout medical education training by providing learner-focused assistance.

Precision medical education provides programs with the tools and insights required to address the unique needs of individual learners and achieve greater equity in medical education.[2] Transforming medical education to make it more learner centered and equitable allows students to succeed and be better prepared across the competencies required of them. Establishing a physician workforce that has been built on the foundation of an equitable system with a focus on individual progress will play an impactful role in society. Precision medical education can be used to reduce bias, promote diversity, and establish effective learning strategies. Precision medical education creates a foundation to comprehensively train the next generation of physicians to work toward recognizing and improving health inequities. Addressing historical inequities beginning at the medical school level through the implementation of precision medical education can help equip future physicians with the skills required to address health inequities at the societal level.

CONCLUSION

Precision medical education, when combined with restorative justice and design thinking frameworks, holds tremendous potential to address historical harms and exclusion within medical education and health care systems. It offers a transformative approach using big data and AI to reduce inequities and injustices in medical education while providing more personalized teaching, curricular delivery, learner assessment, and student services. A precision medical education approach recognizes that learners are unique, and there is great utility in personalizing medical education. Adopting a precision medical education strategy, guided by design thinking and restorative justice frameworks, promotes learner-centered, equitable, and effective medical education while addressing issues of historical injustice. This is possible through recent advancements in AI that enable new opportunities for medical educators to leverage big data and derive actionable education insights that can improve learning outcomes and reduce bias. The successful implementation of a precision medical education strategy can equip medical learners with the competencies required as future health care practitioners to recognize and address health equities and issues of social injustice within health systems.

REFERENCES

1. Mesko B. The role of artificial intelligence in precision medicine. *Expert Rev Precis.* 2017;2(5):239–241. https://doi.org/10.1080/23808993.2017.1380516.
2. Triola MM, Burk-Rafel J. Precision medical education. *Acad Med.* 2023;98(7):775–781. https://doi.org/10.1097/ACM.0000000000005227.
3. Hess L, Palermo AG, Muller D. Addressing and undoing racism and bias in the medical school learning and work environment. *Acad Med.* 2020;95(12):44–50. https://doi.org/10.1097/ACM.0000000000003706.
4. Daugherty PR, James Wilson H, Chowdhury R. Using artificial intelligence to promote diversity. *MIT Manage Rev.* 2018. https://sloanreview.mit.edu/article/using-artificial-intelligence-to-promote-diversity/.
5. Parikh RB, Teeple S, Navathe AS. Addressing bias in artificial intelligence in health care. *JAMA.* 2019;322(24):2377–2378. https://doi.org/10.1001/jama.2019.18058.
6. Keir G, Hu W, Filippi CG, Ellenbogen L, Woldenberg R. Using artificial intelligence in medical school admissions screening to decrease inter-and intra-observer variability. *JAMIA Open.* 2023;6(1):1–8. https://doi.org/10.1093/jamiaopen/ooad011.
7. Stinson C. Algorithms are not neutral. *AI Ethics.* 2022;2:763–770. https://doi.org/10.1007/s43681-022-00136-w.
8. Lewis N. *Will AI Remove Hiring Bias?* 2018. https://www.shrm.org/resourcesandtools/hr-topics/talent-acquisition/pages/will-ai-remove-hiring-bias-hr-technology.aspx.
9. Burk-Rafel J, Reinstein I, Feng J, et al. Development and validation of a machine learning-based decision support tool for residency applicant screening and review. *Acad Med.* 2021;96(11):54–61. https://doi.org/10.1097/ACM.0000000000004317.
10. Cohn EG, Henderson GE, Appelbaum PS. Distributive justice, diversity, and inclusion in precision medicine: what will success look like? *Genet Med.* 2017;19:157–159. https://doi.org/10.1038/gim.2016.92.
11. Miller K. Chapter 7: What is design thinking and what does it have to do with equity? In: *Introduction to Design Equity.* 2018. https://open.lib.umn.edu/designequity/chapter/chapter-7-what-is-design-thinking-and-what-does-it-have-to-do-with-equity/.
12. Acosta D, Karp D. Restorative justice as the Rx for mistreatment in academic medicine: Applications to consider for learners, faculty and staff. *Acad Med.* 2018;93(3):354–356. https://doi.org/10.1097/ACM.0000000000002037.
13. Cook CR, Kilgus SP, Burns MK. Advancing the science and practice of precision education to enhance student outcomes. *J Sch Psychol.* 2018;66:4–10. https://doi.org/10.1016/j.jsp.2017.11.004.
14. Ma W, Adesope O, Nesbit JC, Liu Q. Intelligent tutoring systems and learning outcomes: A meta-analysis. *J Educ Psychol.* 2018;106(4):901–918. https://doi.org/10.1037/a0037123.
15. Tsai SC, Chen CH, Shiao YT, Ciou JS, Wu TN. Precision education with statistical learning and deep learning: a case study in Taiwan. *Int J Educ.* 2020;1712 https://doi.org/10.1186/s41239-020-00186-2.
16. Sajjad M, Mahboob U. Improving workplace-based learning for undergraduate medical. *Pak J Med Sci.* 2015;31(5):1272–1274. https://doi.org/10.12669/pjms.315.7687.
17. Duong MT, Rauschecker AM, Rudie JD, et al. Artificial intelligence for precision education in radiology. *Brit J Radiol.* 2019;92(1103). https://doi.org/10.1259/bjr.20190389.
18. Klein R, Julian KA, Snyder ED, et al. Gender bias in resident assessment in graduate medical education: review of the literature. *JGIM.* 2019;34(5):712–719. https://doi.org/10.1007/s11606-019-04884-0.
19. Hui K, Sukhera J, Vigod S, Taylor VH, Zaheer J. Recognizing and addressing implicit gender bias in medicine. *CMAJ.* 2020;192(42):1269–1270. https://doi.org/10.1503/cmaj.200286.

PART II

From Surface to Structures

Creating a More Equitable Medical School Experience

Fostering Well-Being and Inclusivity in Medical Education Through Varied Curricular Timelines

Grace C. Clifford, Jennifer DeSantis, Matthew A. Sullivan, and Sarah E. Triano

OUTLINE

SUMMARY

As the medical education system continuously strives to meet the dynamic and fluid needs of matriculating medical students, the system and those who run it must learn to navigate uncertainty and actively embrace change. Throughout this chapter, we explore the critical importance of normalizing varied curricular timelines; emphasize the need to incorporate high-touch, holistic support systems that prioritize the mental health and overall well-being of medical students; and advocate for a paradigm shift to further incorporate universally designed approaches to assessment and evaluation in undergraduate medical education (UME). In doing so, medical schools can create a future where medical education embraces the diverse identities of its students, ensuring equitable opportunities for every aspiring physician.

INTRODUCTION

In 2017 the AMA released a publication titled, "Creating a Community of Innovation," which included an outline of notable initiatives developed by medical institutions throughout the country *and* a charge to continually progress and improve the landscape of medical education in the United States.[1] More than 5 years later, we must revisit that charge. Due to an increasing physician shortage, institutions have looked to shortening curricular timelines, exploring the possibility of a 3-year model, which has proved effective for some medical students with an aptitude for expeditious degree completion. The standard 4-year medical school model, while effective for many students pursuing a traditional path to the profession, has proved challenging and compressed for some students, offering limited time to engage with necessary support. When academic failure or unexpected life events occur and a fifth year is required, students struggle with the stigma of being left behind by classmates, incurring added educational costs, and having to explain the additional time in residency applications and interviews.

These considerations often overshadow the benefits of a decompressed curriculum, including additional time to learn and master material, time to engage with necessary mental health and medical supports, and time to address acute life events. The reality of these proposed structures is that each offers opportunities to best support a varied subpopulation of medical students. As such, medical schools need to embrace such opportunities to meet students where they are to matriculate, retain, and graduate diverse and highly skilled future physicians.

Within this chapter, we advocate for a more flexible, equitable, and inclusive medical education experience. We encourage institutions to construct and destigmatize varied educational timelines that allow students to take advantage of dedicated medical school mental health and wellness supports. Furthermore, while examining and implementing alternate forms of assessment, we must acknowledge and address long-standing systemic barriers that continue to unjustly impact students with diverse backgrounds and needs. By analyzing current structures, we feel medical schools can create a transformational educational experience, rather than a transactional educational delivery—one that matches the compassion of the educators within the system and allows students to engage in the support necessary to remain healthy and present, regardless of their path to program completion.

UNDERSTANDING THE FOUNDATION OF OUR CURRENT MEDICAL EDUCATION SYSTEM

At the beginning of the 1900s the AMA (along with other prominent medical associations) began adopting minimum standards for medical education, which included the formalization of a standard 4-year medical curriculum, a framework for medical education that has remained relatively unchanged since.[2] Shortly thereafter, Abraham Flexner, a philosopher by training, conducted a comprehensive analysis of American medical training programs in 1910. The analysis, which would come to be known as the Flexner report, analyzed the strength of hospital-medical school partnerships, admissions standards, physical facilities, laboratories and associated resources, quality of instruction, exposure to clinical material, faculty credentials, and the overall quality of medical education.[3]

Within his report, Flexner categorized medical schools into three separate classifications: (1) well-established medical training programs—associated medical practices—inclusive of updated facilities, cutting-edge technologies/equipment, and top educational scholars—with admissions standards requiring advanced study in science-based courses; (2) institutions in need of development, but also displayed potential to improve, typically included lower admissions standards only requiring a high school diploma; and (3) institutions that were beyond saving due to financial instability, minimal admission requirements (many trainees attending with less than a high school-level education), low educational standards, and high attrition rates.[3] Unfortunately, a third of American medical schools of that time fell within the last category. Flexner used his findings to advocate that a systematic dismantling of the existing medical education structures was required. Somewhat nearsighted, yet well-intentioned, Flexner stated, "This solution deals only with the present and the near future—a generation, at most. In the course of the next thirty years, needs will develop of which we here take no account."[3] A century later, this is the basis of our current medical education system.

The realization that our current framework for medical education has remained largely unchanged since its creation in the early 1900s should give us pause for thought. However, the realization that our system is built upon a report that had a devastating impact on the historically Black medical schools of the time should be even more concerning. In the report, Flexner directly criticized the seven "medical schools for Negroes," stating, "five are at this moment in no position to make any contribution of value to the solution of the problem." These five schools included Flint Medical College, Leonard Medical School, Knoxville Medical College, Medical Department of the University of West Tennessee, and National Medical College.[3] Following the release of Flexner's report, only Flint Medical College in New Orleans survived the initial closures. It eventually closed in 1983. Howard University College of Medicine and Meharry Medical College were the only two Black medical schools at the time not recommended for closure. This historical background is essential in understanding how our current system is haunted by biased interpretations of how medical education should look and who should become a physician. To move forward, we must address the destructive ramifications of the Flexner report and acknowledge that the current restrictive curricular formats continue to perpetuate privilege while creating unnecessary and pernicious barriers for underrepresented, underresourced, and minoritized student populations.

THE CHANGING CURRICULUM

Typically, UME programs consist of preclinical, basic science curriculum, and clinically based learning over 4 years. Although the general sequencing may vary, phase 1 (year 1/2) generally is foundational curricular content intertwined with clinical observation and exposure. Phase 2 (year 2/3) progresses into clerkship rotations, active experiential learning, and career exploration. Phase 3 (year 3/4) culminates in specialty elective clerkships, sub-internships, and residency interviews.

Four-Year Model

A traditional 4-year approach to medical education has remained an effective and appropriate path to physicianship for many students, allowing learners to engage in the curriculum while providing the necessary flexibility for institutions to create adjustments as required. While effective, this model can still feel as if too much is being asked for in too little time. Medical schools require students to be fully present in their clinical rotations, which can require 8- to 14-hour shifts, 5 to 6 days a week, while also expecting them to actively prepare for and pass National Board of Medical Examiners (NBME) Subject examinations and the US Medical Licensing Examination (USMLE) Step examinations. This may contribute to the fact that the 4-year graduation rate has remained relatively stagnant throughout the 21st century at approximately 84%,[4] while the mental health crises among medical students are on the rise.[5]

Three-Year Model

Three-year medical programs have existed for quite some time and have become an increasingly attractive option for students aiming for early entry into the field with reduced student loan debt; for the field, this approach offers a potential method for addressing the increasing shortage of physicians.[6] Certainly, accelerated 3-year medical education programs are necessary pathways to the profession and have been found to maintain educational quality, instill residency preparedness, and, as previously mentioned, reduce debt among some medical trainees.[7] By design, 3-year medical programs cater to a specific type of learner with a strong propensity to absorb, retain, and demonstrate understanding of complex material at an accelerated rate.[8]

While we recognize some students might be able to make the transition to an accelerated 3-year training program with ease and appreciate a reduced timeline to income generation with less debt, we must also consider the potential ramifications related to diversity, equity, and inclusion if the flexibility to shift from a 3- to 4-year program after matriculation is not permitted due to rigid curricular formats.

Inflexibility within this model may unintentionally result in students self-selecting out of such programs due to the "unknowns" that can exist for students who experience unexpected acute life events, have disabilities, or are parents. This approach also requires students to engage in early decision-making regarding specialties, which can limit opportunities for exploration. Although there are some positives to this approach for some students, it begs the question—is there a place in medical education for learners who require more time to observe, absorb, process, and experiment?

EMBRACING 5-YEAR CURRICULAR TIMELINES

It is common practice for medical schools to scaffold educational opportunities and clinical experiences in a manner that reflects the profession—long hours, demanding patient loads, and making life-and-death decisions quickly. Instead of maintaining the status quo, what if medical schools became the catalyst for change by acknowledging the **depressogenic**[9] nature of our current medical school structure? This nature is created, in part, by the current inflexible and condensed curricular structures, which can have profound negative impacts on student well-being. By reassessing and reworking these structures to provide opportunities to decompress the curriculum, either intentionally from the onset or when required due to unexpected life events, medical schools can meet the needs of varied student populations.

To address the multifaceted and layered reasonings associated with a growing physician shortage,[10] an equally multifaceted and layered approach is required. In addition to offering opportunities to engage in a condensed curriculum, programs similarly need to normalize and destigmatize a decompressed option to address burnout and attrition among medical students. As mentioned previously, the 4-year graduation rate has stagnated at approximately 84%, whereas the 5-year graduation rate of medical students has been maintained at approximately 95%.[4]

While some might consider an intentionally designed extended curriculum superfluous, we need to recognize that many paths can lead to the same destination and, for some learners, a fifth year is critical to their success as a medical practitioner. The notion of medical school decompression is not revolutionary and has existed for decades. For example, the University of Illinois at Urbana-Champaign has offered decompression of the M-1 year in response to underperformance and found that students decompressing their educational journey positively outperformed those who failed and repeated the curriculum.[11] Another decompressed option is offered by the University of North Carolina School of Medicine, which delivers a deceleration of the first 2 years for voluntary or involuntary reasons (e.g., poor performance or personal emergency).[12]

While poor performance is one reason students take additional time to complete the degree, it is not the sole reason. Some use the time to enhance their fount of knowledge by focusing on research opportunities, participating in additional elective rotations, or expanding credentials for a more competitive residency application. Others may engage in a fifth year out of necessity to reengage with material not fully mastered or related to other progressional pauses (e.g., standard and/or medical leaves due to personal or disability-related reasons).[13] When the latter applies, it is important to consider whether it is the student who must rethink their approaches to learning the material or the institution's rigid approach to curricular timelines that must change. One example of such change is a proactively designed decompressed curriculum similar to that of Western Michigan University Homer Stryker M.D. School of Medicine's "CLEAR Curriculum."[14]

It is well known that students matriculating to medical schools have much more complex needs and higher rates of mental illness than the general population,[15-17] and a solution aligned with these needs is critical. Yet, our approach to medical education has predominantly focused on fitting in more content and experiences over a standard (or even shorter) period of time. Instead of an increasingly more compressed curriculum, we advocate for normalizing the option of a decompressed experience, such as a 5-year path to graduation. By offering and promoting this extended timeline option as an intentional path to degree completion, we reduce stigma and reframe decompressions as a proactive measure of student support, rather than a punitive action.

Associated Considerations for a 5-Year Structure

To destigmatize decompressed curricula as a viable pathway to the profession, medical schools must promote the option while actively addressing the most poignant student concerns:

- How will this impact my ability to match?
- Will residency programs see a fifth year as a "red flag"?
- How much additional student debt will I incur by taking advantage of this option?

We do not have definitive answers to these questions, but if we hope to matriculate, retain, and graduate qualified and diverse candidates (and address the physician shortage by actively addressing burnout), it is our job to develop responses to these important questions. It is on us as medical schools to lead the charge by communicating the need for and benefits of varied curricular formats. Just as medical schools have investigated methods for adopting a 3-year medical program to provide an expedited pathway to the profession to decrease debt accrual, we must avoid penalizing students for taking the required time to master material by developing financial support for those who require a fifth year. It should also be emphasized that a candidate's selection of a 3-, 4-, or 5-year timeline should not be considered a reflection of their caliber or fitness for any particular specialty to residency programs. By avoiding the development of a "traditional" or "preferred" educational timeline while reconstructing curricular formats, we can communicate to our students that individuals learn at different paces and in nonlinear ways and normalize alternate educational timelines. We propose that by offering and normalizing the option of a 5-year curricular model, we would attract and retain a separate pool of equally qualified and talented medical trainees.

DEVELOPING AND MAINTAINING DEDICATED HOLISTIC, HIGH-TOUCH STUDENT SUPPORTS

Understanding the intensity of medical education and the impact that it has on students, the Liaison Committee on Medication Education (LCME) developed requirements that call for "an effective system that promotes well-being and facilitates adjustment to the physical and emotional demands of medical education."[18] However, we continue to witness students forgoing regular medical and mental health appointments to avoid losing study time or having to request time off during their clinical rotations. By creating intentional, flexible curricular timelines as described above, medical schools create the necessary space, time, and culture for students to actively engage in ongoing self-care.[19-21] Furthermore, we create opportunities to retain and graduate diverse student populations through dedicated holistic, high-touch supports that can address the increases in stress, anxiety, and exhaustion among medical students.[22]

Mental Health and Wellness Services

As many staff can attest, medical students regularly struggle to identify time outside of class, educational requirements, and studying to attend required meetings and complete activities of daily living, such as laundry, cleaning, and grocery shopping. Once a medical student enters the clinical portion of their program, it can feel impossible to identify time for self-care and active disability management amid the long shifts and ongoing Shelf examinations and Step preparation. This can make the added burden of identifying a physician or other health care professional who accepts their insurance, is local (or provides telehealth services), offers hours that match a student's schedule, and is a good fit therapeutically seem insurmountable to many students. Not surprisingly, such cumbersome processes can actively deter students from seeking necessary mental health and medical support essential to retaining and graduating future physicians. Research has demonstrated that, post COVID-19 pandemic crisis, many college students meet the clinical criteria for a mental illness. Although similar rates of mental health concerns are identified among all races, we know students from historically underresourced backgrounds are far less likely to seek treatment, adding additional barriers to diversifying the profession.[23] The ability to select a curricular timeline that best meets their needs would allow students to finally engage in necessary supports; however, appropriate infrastructure and scaffolding will be required to avoid overloading current student support systems.

At present, most school-based counseling services are not equipped to provide regular (weekly or biweekly) appointments due to the sheer volume of requests. Furthermore, these offices are struggling to retain staff post pandemic[24] as many psychiatrists, psychologists, and mental health professionals are experiencing high rates of burnout and are exiting the field seeking better pay and work-life balance.[25] If we are to increase access and reduce the staff turnover that can impact continuity of care, continued therapeutic engagement, ability to obtain critical letters of support for the USMLE accommodation request processes, and overall well-being of medical students, it is essential for medical school-specific mental health and wellness supports to become a funding and resource priority.

With the appropriate funding and resources, we can go beyond the "compliance" approach to the LCME student well-being requirement and truly meet the needs of our students.[26] Specifically, we can move toward a system that increases resources for medical school counseling departments to allow for a minimum of biweekly appointments without overloading provider caseloads. This is especially important as medical school mental health providers may be the best people to document disabilities for the USMLE Step accommodation request process, which requires detailed information.[27] Similarly, resources and funding should be created to ensure access to free or low-cost neuropsychological assessments for students with limited resources.[28] This is necessary to ensure students with

undocumented disabilities or without adequate, updated documentation are appropriately supported and have strong documentation for accommodation requests (both institutionally and for the USMLE Step examinations).[29,30] Such supports are particularly needed for underresourced and minoritized medical students, who statistically are far less likely to have their disabilities identified earlier in life. These delays can further compound historical marginalization when pursuing accommodations on licensure examinations, leading to low or failing Step scores and a negative impact on a student's ability to progress, graduate, and ultimately match into residency.[30] Therefore we recommend integrating clinical professionals from diverse backgrounds who can understand and address the complexities related to help-seeking behavior.[31] By providing these services at no or low cost, we reduce the privilege-based barriers to equitable access too commonly experienced by groups that have been socially or economically marginalized.

Integration of Occupational Therapy Services

Another recommended approach to increasing access to mental health and wellness supports while reducing strain on counseling center caseloads is to incorporate occupational therapy (OT) into a medical school's student wellness offerings.[32] By offering free or low-cost OT services, students would have access to disability management support, as well as **executive functioning** and stress management coaching.[33] This is especially needed as the hectic clinical schedules paired with ongoing Step examination preparation often result in an exacerbation of disability symptoms and burnout among medical students.

Development of a Targeted Diverse Mentorship Program

The need for enhanced support extends beyond the baseline provision of counseling and mental health care. Integrated mentorship from practicing physicians with shared identity backgrounds is necessary if we wish to destigmatize varied curricular timelines. Many historically minoritized and underresourced students, including students with disabilities, struggle with **impostor syndrome**[34] and **stereotype threat**. Impostor syndrome refers to an individual's difficulty or inability to accept their success as deserved, real, or the result of their own skills, abilities, or efforts, and is common among medical professionals.[35] Stereotype threat is the fear or risk of affirming negative stereotypes related to the individual's ethnic, racial, cultural group, or gender, which can lead to impaired academic focus or performance.[35,36] To combat these experiences, there is a need for physician mentors who are representative of the increasingly diverse student population.[37] These relationships serve to provide guidance and support to students while avoiding perpetuating myths and misconceptions regarding paths to the profession or who can and should become a physician. By providing this, we not only diversify the physician workforce but also enhance a sense of belonging among our students and increase the likelihood of persistence, retention, match, and graduation.[31] While representation and engagement through mentoring are crucial in establishing a sense of belonging, the need for support extends beyond community building.[26]

Dedicated Medical School Case Management

As acute situations arise that create stress and anxiety for medical students but do not squarely fall within counseling or student affairs purview or bandwidth, we must consider options for providing high-touch guidance and support. The integration of a dedicated medical school case manager, familiar with available curricular structures, timelines, requirements, and campus resources, can guide students in crisis through stressful situations and assist in making informed decisions during difficult times. This is especially important as medical students often fear "getting off track" with USMLE Step examination timelines, residency applications and interviews, and program completion, as well as the implications these have for their finances and ability to match. Normalizing and destigmatizing transitions from one curricular format to another will be critical, but providing support to determine whether such changes are required and what financial resources exist to support the shift is necessary. In addition to assisting with curricular transitions, a dedicated case manager within the medical school can provide short-term case management services for various complex situations without adding burden to the student or existing administration.[38] Examples of emergent or acute needs requiring enhanced support include, but are not limited to:

- Assisting students in identifying and acquiring health insurance (including short-term disability insurance) and locating providers within their network
- Connecting students to outside health providers/specialists
- Connecting students to intensive outpatient programs and identifying insurance/funding options
- Checking in with students following medical hospitalizations and procedures
- Checking in with students following a personal emergency (e.g., family health crises, death in the family, victim of crime)
- Assisting students in navigating leaves of absences[39]
- Addressing financial insecurities or barriers
- Addressing home insecurity
- Addressing transportation barriers

- Visa complications/concerns
- Pregnancy and parenting needs

In addition to the above reactive supports, a designated case manager can provide proactive mental health and well-being workshops to further promote self-care and increase awareness of available on-campus resources while destigmatizing help-seeking behavior.[40] Programming can be provided synchronously or asynchronously and cover essential topics such as executive functioning,[41,42] **mindfulness**,[43] and suicide prevention.[44]

Designated Medical School Disability Resource Provider

Research has demonstrated that the number of medical students with disabilities is steadily increasing.[21] As such, the addition of a designated, highly knowledgeable **disability resource provider (DRP)** familiar with the nuanced needs of medical education reduces the risk of miscommunications/misunderstandings related to accommodations and compliance for students and faculty alike.[45] The medical school DRP can provide proactive guidance regarding available supports, as well as common didactic and clinical accommodations, while reviewing options for maintaining medical and disability management supports during medical education (including curricular timeline options). Additionally, the DRP can educate faculty on the reality of equal access in medical education within the didactic and clinical spaces. This includes providing proactive training to clinical faculty and residents on common clinical accommodations,[46] integrating available assistive and adaptive technologies,[47,48] and navigating the logistics related to the implementation of accommodations. These supports will reduce unnecessary faculty pushback due to the "fear of the unknown," misconceptions regarding ability to meet technical standards or maintain patient safety, or frustrations with "added responsibilities" associated with ensuring students receive equitable access within the clinical environment.

Equally important is the ability for consistent and knowledgeable support related to the complex process of requesting accommodations on the USMLE Step examinations.[28] As research suggests, the process to request accommodations on the USMLE examinations is time consuming and, without support, often results in a disproportionately low approval rate for reasonable accommodations, short-term leaves of absence after falling "off track" waiting for request responses, extended timelines to degree completion, and the overall attrition of medical students with disabilities.[30] By adding a medical school DRP to the administrative team, medical schools are more likely to maintain student-desired timelines, improve ability to match by ensuring equitable access to licensure examinations, and retain and graduate students with disabilities. By doing so, we also convey an importance beyond compliance by emphasizing disability as a valued and important aspect of our greater justice, equity, diversity, and inclusion (JEDI) mission.

Funding and Advocacy Considerations

It is important to note that creating the resources above alone would be insufficient to provide continued enhanced, holistic student support if the infrastructure does not increase with the need and level of student engagement. As such, we recommend monitoring caseload numbers for counseling, OT, mentors, case management, and disability resource providers. If we fail to do so, we are likely to overwhelm these systems, which can result in limited access and therefore recreate privilege and barriers to vital resources.

We recognize that the recommendations mentioned above require time, staffing, resources, training, and, most importantly, funding. As the cost to attend and complete medical school, including the costly registration fees for the USMLE Step examinations, already serve as a barrier for many students, it is important to avoid funding structures that include increased tuition and student fees. If we are to extend beyond "student wellness" as a buzzword and establish student health and well-being as institutional priorities, advocacy for student mental and health wellness resources must be reflected in strategic planning efforts and funding structures. By doing this, we meet our greater JEDI goals of retaining and graduating a more diverse population of students while addressing the physician shortage and actively diversifying the profession.

REIMAGINING ASSESSMENT AND EVALUATION

Rethinking curricular timelines provides not only a unique opportunity to increase the breadth and depth of comprehensive support services but also allows us the necessary time to diversify our means of assessment. In the realm of UME, the imperative for a comprehensive systematic overhaul of evaluation and assessment practices has become increasingly evident. The conventional reliance on standardized examinations as the primary means of ranking and residency planning has raised concerns regarding accuracy in gauging a student's true potential and competency within a dynamic health care landscape.[49] If we take advantage of the flexibility provided by varied curricular timelines, we can advocate for a paradigm shift toward a more comprehensive and insightful approach to evaluation to ensure that we do not sacrifice diversity in the name of expediency. We argue the ability to reimagine assessment and evaluation in UME by shedding light on the limitations and inherent bias of standardized examinations, amplifying

the concept of *competency-based education* (CBE) in all coursework, advocating for the integration of meaningful formative assessments and diverse evaluation methods, and exploring the prospects of a universally designed testing protocol that ensures equitable evaluation opportunities for all aspiring medical professionals.

HISTORY AND PITFALLS OF STANDARDIZED TESTING

The use of standardized testing as a cornerstone of evaluation and hierarchical rankings in UME warrants critical examination due to its historical and contemporary biases that disproportionately disadvantage historically marginalized groups, including Black and Hispanic students, as well as females and students with disabilities.[50] The lineage of bias embedded within standardized tests traces back to their early origins, marked by the discriminatory underpinnings of early IQ tests, the dark shadows of eugenics, and the segregationist policies during the Jim Crow era. Furthermore, bias within test content becomes evident when analyzing data and research highlighting how high-stake examinations have favored White individuals and males, perpetuating an inequitable representation within medical education.[51] The concept of stereotype threat further compounds this issue, as the psychological burden of conforming to negative stereotypes adversely impacts the performance of historically disenfranchised individuals in such examinations.[52] The inequitable access to test preparation resources also creates an uneven playing field, further exacerbating the existing inequity. To retain and graduate a diverse population of medical students, we must actively reflect on the current systems that contribute to attrition. Are we misinterpreting test performance as an effective measurement of competency? In efforts to prepare students for standardized examinations, are we unintentionally sacrificing justice, equity, diversity, and inclusion? Are we actively reassessing our evaluation methods to more accurately and equitably determine student mastery of material and skill development?

In addition to the historical pitfalls and marginalization of historically disadvantaged students, female students, and disabled students, UME's typical reliance on standardized testing disadvantages many students by overemphasizing test scores as indicators of overall excellence and promise. This approach, paired with expeditious curricular timelines that create systems prioritizing standardized test scores, fail to provide equitable pathways to success or the socially constructed definition of excellence that focuses on standardized examination performance. Overemphasis on class ranks, tiered honor systems, and examination performance-based selection criteria for medical honor societies further perpetuate the exclusion of many students who historically have not been served by standardized examinations and/or require alternate timelines to have equal access.

SHIFT TOWARD COMPLETELY COMPETENCY-BASED EDUCATION

Dr. Ronald M. Epstein and his colleague Dr. Edward M. Humbert eloquently defined CBE as "the habitual and judicious use of communication, knowledge, technical skills, clinical reasoning, emotions, values, and reflection in daily practice for the benefit of the individuals and communities being served."[53] This definition encapsulates the spirit of competency as multifaceted, holistic, contextual, ongoing, and developmental.

CBE constitutes a progressive educational approach that centers on the mastery of specific skills and knowledge, focusing less on the completion of specific courses in a set period of time. At its core, CBE embodies a paradigm shift in learning, emphasizing the attainment of demonstrable competencies that align with real-world applications and professional demands. Most importantly, CBE allows programs to ensure a high-quality foundation for its graduates based on the necessary skills within the field.[54]

Several fundamental principles underpin this approach, as CBE is designed to:

1. Prioritize the learner, recognizing the diversity of learners' backgrounds, paces, abilities, and learning styles while enabling them to progress upon mastery rather than adhere to rigid timelines.
2. Emphasize clearly defined and measurable learning outcomes, ensuring transparency and consistency in assessing competence attainment.
3. Promote personalized learning experiences, allowing students to engage deeply with areas that require more attention and accelerate through familiar content. CBE encourages active learning, focusing on practical application, problem-solving, and critical thinking.
4. Incorporate ongoing formative assessment, providing continuous feedback and opportunities for improvement, thus fostering a growth mindset and enhancing the educational journey.

Competency-based education embodies a dynamic and learner-centered approach that aligns education with the skills and proficiencies demanded by today's ever-evolving professional landscape.

Implementing Competency-Based Education in Undergraduate Medical Education

The adoption of varied curricular timelines and the integration of dedicated support within medical programs would set the stage for the implementation of more inclusive forms of assessment. CBE has found some footing in UME as programs move toward a pass/fail curriculum. The benefit of this is mandating a "floor," or the minimum knowledge required measured through written examinations, as well as dynamic means of evaluation, such as clinical simulation, video-based assessment, direct observation, and learning portfolios. Ideally, all these methods are utilized in synergy as both formative (providing feedback, reassurance, and opportunity for reflection) and summative assessments (assurance of minimum competency and readiness to progress to the next level of training).[49,55]

The movement away from tiered ranking systems within UME clerkships should also be considered if we are to foster a more fair and truly equitable learning environment that promotes growth, collaboration, holistic skill development, and a leveling of the playing fields for diverse learners. The traditional tiered ranking system creates a hierarchical atmosphere, fostering competition among students rather than nurturing a cooperative and supportive atmosphere for learning. Furthermore, it places the emphasis on the destination rather than the journey within medical education—perpetuating stigma in the event an alternate path is required. By removing tiered rankings, medical students are encouraged to focus on their individual growth and development rather than being preoccupied with comparisons to their peers. This shift enables students to engage more fully in the learning process, taking risks, exploring various medical specialties, and embracing a comprehensive understanding of patient care. The absence of tiered rankings encourages students to seek out and accept a broader range of clinical experiences, fostering a more diverse skill set and well-rounded medical education. The differentiation of students (e.g., honors, high pass, pass, fail) is enticing as it allows program directors and residency programs to filter students in or out; however, it is typically based primarily on standardized examinations, such as NBME Subject examinations, which feeds back into the besmirched marginalization of diverse learners. Utilizing a tiered ranking system based on examination performance also leaves room for inaccurately associating a medical trainee's ability to perform well on standardized examinations with their potential effectiveness as a medical provider. While medical knowledge is essential, its utility is diminished without other key skills, such as social context/understanding of health inequities, communication skills, teamwork, commitment to lifelong learning, ethics, professionalism, and problem-solving.[56]

One way to move toward CBE in medicine from a grading perspective is to embrace a shift toward pass/fail standardized assessments (e.g., USMLE Step examinations, COMLEX Level examinations, and NBME/COMAT

Subject examinations). While we recognize the need for high-stakes board examinations to ensure students achieve a fixed threshold of medical knowledge required to advance to the next level of training and achieve required licensure, we are concerned about perpetuating bias and barriers for diverse learners. Although there are undoubtedly benefits to multiple-choice testing, which we will explore shortly, it can unintentionally act as a gatekeeper that undermines the comprehensive nature of health care.

MULTIPLE MEANS OF ASSESSMENT

The concept of multiple means of assessment and evaluation is not new; in fact, it is foundational in applying universal design in education. Still, some of the most emphasized components of a residency application are scores on USMLE Step examinations, clerkship grades, and honor society status, which is in part determined by standardized test scores.

Written Examinations

The use of multiple-choice tests to ensure competence and assess foundational levels of knowledge is a widely employed method in education. These tests offer several advantages, including efficient administration and grading, which is particularly valuable for faculty when assessing a large number of students. The structured format of multiple-choice questions allows for evaluating a broad spectrum of topics, ensuring a comprehensive assessment of the curriculum's core concepts. Additionally, well-designed multiple-choice questions can test factual recall and higher-order thinking skills, such as critical analysis and problem-solving, providing a more nuanced evaluation of a student's understanding. However, it is essential to acknowledge that while multiple-choice tests have their merits, they should be part of a comprehensive assessment strategy that includes other methods to assess skills, application, and real-world context, ensuring a well-rounded evaluation of a learner's competency. Additionally, multiple-choice tests contain limitations, such as reliance on cueing or shortcuts wherein students do not actively reach a differential diagnosis before choosing the next-order solution.[57-59]

For examinations that must be delivered in a controlled/proctored environment, universally designed testing locations are paramount to ensure equitable access and inclusivity in assessment. Centralized testing centers would create a consistent experience for students with disabilities or with varied needs, minimizing inequities. Furthermore, offering testing windows provides learners the opportunity to engage with the material on a day and time that best fits their needs—allowing programs to more accurately assess the student's fount of knowledge.

Practical-Based Learning: Clinical Simulation, Video-Based Assessment, and Direct Observation

Clinical simulations have become pivotal for evaluating medical students' aptitude and preparedness in diverse health care scenarios.[60] These simulations involve realistic scenarios or virtual environments that mimic clinical settings, providing students with hands-on experiences without patient risk. Such simulations enable the assessment of critical thinking, decision-making, and procedural skills in a controlled, educational context. Educators can measure students' clinical judgment, adaptability, and teamwork through simulations, comprehensively evaluating their competency and readiness for real-world medical practice.[61]

Video-based assessment has become valuable for evaluating medical students' clinical skills and communication abilities. This approach involves recording student-patient interactions, procedures, or simulations, allowing for detailed review and analysis. Video assessments offer objectivity, enabling educators to evaluate performances consistently and mitigate bias. Moreover, students benefit from self-reflection by reviewing their videos, identifying areas for improvement, and enhancing their overall competence and patient-centered care.[62,63]

Direct observation is crucial in medical education to evaluate students' clinical skills and competencies. Skilled faculty, physicians, or preceptors observe students engaging with patients, performing procedures, and providing care. This approach provides insights into clinical performance, communication, professionalism, and practical application of medical knowledge.[64] Direct observation evaluates patient interactions, diagnoses, and treatment plans, offering benefits like identifying strengths and improvement areas and assessing both technical and soft skills like empathy. Feedback follows observation, guiding students' growth and connecting theory with practice. This method is adaptable to diverse clinical settings, aiding in assessing proficiency across specialties and promoting well-rounded, compassionate medical professionals' development.[65-67]

Learning Portfolios

Learning portfolios, a curated collection of diverse artifacts, such as case presentations, reflective essays, research projects, and clinical experiences, provide a holistic view of a student's progression and competence. The use of learning portfolios in medical education varies across institutions and programs. Though not a new concept, portfolios have yet to rise to the relevance of other modes of assessment. Still, learning portfolios are increasingly recognized as valuable tools for promoting reflective learning, self-assessment, and holistic skill development in medical students.[68]

Portfolios serve as a comprehensive and dynamic assessment tool for medical students, allowing them to showcase their growth, achievements, and reflections throughout their educational journey. Learning portfolios enable students to engage in self-assessment actively, set personalized learning goals, and document their evolving skills and knowledge.[69] Additionally, educators gain insights into a student's development trajectory, facilitating tailored feedback and fostering a deeper understanding of the student's strengths and areas for improvement. The use of portfolios as an assessment strategy encourages metacognition and emphasizes lifelong learning and self-directed development, aligning with the multifaceted demands of modern medical practice. Further, learning portfolios can serve as a meaningful tool in the residency application process (particularly in lieu of class rankings or high-stakes licensure examinations).[70] Regardless of the timeline to completion, the use of learning portfolios allows learners to display their wealth of knowledge throughout their medical school experience.

TAKE-HOME POINTS

By embracing these recommendations, institutions can foster a transformative shift toward a more flexible, inclusive, socially just, and overall, more compassionate undergraduate medical experience. Furthermore, we create a future where medical education embraces the diverse identities of its students, ensuring equal access and robust opportunities to thrive in medical education for every aspiring physician.

1. Varied curricular timelines: Develop destigmatized varied curricular timelines for all students and create flexibility to shift from 3 to 4 years or 4 to 5 years as required.
2. Dedicated and holistic mental health supports: Prioritize funding for dedicated medical school mental health and wellness supports to retain and graduate an increasingly diverse population of medical students.
3. Reimagined assessment practices: Proactively and deliberately reevaluate assessment methods, incorporating comprehensive and equitable approaches that accurately reflect the diverse learner population.

CONCLUSION

As we navigate the landscape of medical education, it becomes evident that the charge to innovate should not fail to consider the needs of all learners. When analyzing methods for addressing the physician shortage, we must recognize that abbreviating the timeline to graduation is not the only solution. We equally need to examine the causes of medical student burnout and attrition to appropriately develop effective mechanisms to reduce these phenomena.

Throughout this chapter, we have advocated for a transformative shift in UME, urging institutions to embrace recommendations that foster flexibility, inclusivity, and compassion.

By remaining vigilant of the key takeaways, institutions can create an inclusive and socially just environment where students from diverse backgrounds can excel and realize their full potential while maintaining their health and sense of identity. The flexibility in curricular timelines, enhanced mental health and wellness services, and the integration of other dedicated medical student supports are all vital steps in this journey. Additionally, the adoption of competency-based education, a shift toward pass/fail assessments, and the promotion of multiple means of assessment will further support the holistic development of future physicians. Collectively, these recommendations propel us toward a brighter future where medical education aligns with the principles of equality, diversity, and inclusion, empowering all aspiring physicians to thrive in their educational journey.

REFERENCES

1. American Medical Association. *Creating a Community of Innovation.* American Medical Association; 2017. https://www.ama-assn.org/sites/ama-assn.org/files/corp/media-browser/public/about-ama/ace-monograph-interactive_0.pdf.
2. American Medical Association (AMA). *House of Delegates Proceedings, Annual Session.* 1905. https://ama.nmtvault.com/jsp/PsImageViewer.jsp?doc_id=1ee24daa-2768-4bff-b792-e4859988fe94%2Fama_arch%2FHOD00003%2F00000023.
3. Flexner A. *Medical Education in the United States and Canada: A Report to the Carnegie Foundation for the Advancement of Teaching.* Science and Health Publications, Inc; 1910. http://archive.carnegiefoundation.org/publications/pdfs/elibrary/Carnegie_Flexner_Report.pdf.
4. Association of American Medical Colleges (AAMC). *Graduation Rates and Attrition Rates of U.S. Medical Students.* 2022. https://www.aamc.org/media/48526/download.
5. Meeks L. *The Future of Medicine is at Risk: Medical Students and Suicide.* LinkedIn; 2016. https://www.linkedin.com/pulse/future-medicine-risk-medical-students-suicide-lisa-meeks-phd.
6. Abramson SB, Jacob D, Rosenfeld M, et al. A 3-year M.D.—accelerating careers, diminishing debt. *N Engl J Med.* 2013;369:1085–1087. https://doi.org/10.1056/NEJMp1304681.
7. Leong SL, Gillespie C, Jones B, et al. Accelerated 3-year MD pathway programs: graduates' perspectives on education quality, the learning environment, residency readiness, debt, burnout, and career plans. *Acad Med.* 2022;97(2):254–261. https://doi.org/10.1097/ACM.0000000000004332.
8. Raymond Sr JR, Kerschner JE, Hueston WJ, Maurana CA. The merits and challenges of three-year medical school curricula: time for an evidence-based discussion. *Acad*

Med. 2015;90(10):1318–1323. https://doi.org/10.1097/ACM.0000000000000862.

9. Pelzer A, Sapalidis A, Rabkow N, Pukas L, Günther N, Watzke S. Does medical school cause depression or do medical students already begin their studies depressed? A longitudinal study over the first semester about depression and influencing factors. *GMS J Med Educ.* 2022;39(5): https://doi.org/10.3205/zma001579. Doc58. Published 2022 Aug 4.

10. HIS Markit Ltd. *The Complexities of Physician Supply and Demand: Projections From 2019-2034.* AAMC; 2021. https://www.aamc.org/media/54681/download?attachment.

11. Kies SM, Freund GG. Medical students who decompress during the M-1 year outperform those who fail and repeat it: a study of M-1 students at the University of Illinois College of Medicine at Urbana-Champaign 1988–2000. *BMC Med Educ.* 2005;5:18. https://doi.org/10.1186/1472-6920-5-18.

12. Offices of Medical Student Education Office of the Registrar. *Deceleration.* UNC School of Medicine. https://www.med.unc.edu/ome/registrar/deceleration/.

13. Kosarek C. 5 Reasons for Completing Medical School in 5 Years. *U.S. News & World Report.* November 5, 2019. https://www.usnews.com/education/blogs/medical-school-admissions-doctor/articles/2019-11-05/5-reasons-to-consider-completing-medical-school-in-5-years.

14. Western Michigan University Homer Stryker M.D. School of Medicine. *Decompressed Curriculum at WMED Provides Students With Balance and Flexibility in Their Medical Education.* WMed; 2020. https://wmed.edu/node/2324.

15. Rotenstein LS, Ramos MA, Torre M, et al. Prevalence of depression, depressive symptoms, and suicidal ideation among medical students: a systematic review and meta-analysis. *JAMA.* 2016;316(21):2214–2236. https://doi.org/10.1001/jama.2016.17324.

16. McKerrow I, Carney PA, Caretta-Weyer H, Furnari M, Miller Juve A. Trends in medical students' stress, physical, and emotional health throughout training. *Med Educ Online.* 2020;25(1):1709278.

17. Berkowitz C., Council on Medical Education. *Study of Medical Student, Resident, and Physician Suicide (Resolution 959-I-18). CME Report 6-A-19.* American Medical Association; 2019. https://www.ama-assn.org/system/files/2019-07/a19-cme-6.pdf.

18. Liaison Committee on Medical Education (LCME). Functions and Structure of a Medical School: Standards for Accreditation of Medical Education Programs Leading to the MD Degree. *LCME: Standards, Publications, and Notifications.* 2023. https://lcme.org/publications/.

19. Yancy CW, Bauchner H. Diversity in medical schools—need for a new bold approach. *JAMA.* 2021;325(1):31–32. https://doi.org/10.1001/jama.2020.23601.

20. Aysola J, Ibrahim S. Promoting access to medical school and physician workforce diversity. *JAMA Health Forum.* 2023;4(4):e230251. https://doi.org/10.1001/jamahealthforum.2023.0251.

21. Pereira-Lima K, Plegue MA, Case B, et al. Prevalence of disability and use of accommodation among US allopathic medical school students before and during the COVID-19 pandemic. *JAMA Netw Open.* 2023;6(6):e2318310. https://doi.org/10.1001/jamanetworkopen.2023.18310.

22. Jupina M, Sidle MW, Rehmeyer Caudill CJ. Medical student mental health during the COVID-19 pandemic. *Clin Teach.* 2022;19(5):e13518. https://doi.org/10.1111/tct.13518.

23. Wilkinson E. Medical students face high levels of mental health problems but stigma stops them getting help. *BMJ.* 2023;81:933. https://doi.org/10.1136/bmj.p933.

24. Komer L. COVID-19 amongst the pandemic of medical student mental health. *Int J Med Stud.* 2020;8(1):56–57. https://doi.org/10.5195/ijms.2020.501.

25. Son C, Hegde S, Smith A, Wang X, Sasangohar F. Effects of COVID-19 on college students' mental health in the United States: interview survey study. *J Med Internet Res.* 2020;22(9):e21279. https://doi.org/10.2196/21279.

26. Hale EW, Davis RA. Supporting the future of medicine: student mental health services in medical school. *Front Health Serv.* 2023;3:1032317. https://doi.org/10.3389/frhs.2023.1032317.

27. Clifford G. Disability access in higher education: documenting as university health service providers. In: Vaughn J, Viera A, eds. *Principles and Practice of College Health.* Springer International Publishing; 2021.

28. Jain NR, Meeks LM, Lewis C. Requesting accommodations on certification, licensing, and board exams: assisting students through the application. In: Meeks LM, Jain NR, Laird EP, eds. *Equal Access for Students With Disabilities: The Guide for Health Science and Professional Education.* 2nd Ed. Springer Publishing; 2020.

29. Schneider H, Eisenberg D. Who receives a diagnosis of attention-deficit/hyperactivity disorder in the United States elementary school population? *Pediatrics.* 2006;117(2):601–609. https://doi.org/10.1542/peds.2005-1308.

30. Petersen KH, Jain NR, Case B, Jain S, Meeks LM. Impact of USMLE Step-1 accommodation denial on US medical schools: a national survey. *PLoS One.* 2022;17(4):e0266685. https://doi.org/10.1371/journal.pone.0266685.

31. Bonifacino E, Ufomata EO, Farkas AH, Turner R, Corbelli JA. Mentorship of underrepresented physicians and trainees in academic medicine: a systematic review. *J Gen Intern Med.* 2021;36(4):1023–1034. https://doi.org/10.1007/s11606-020-06478-7.

32. Keptner KM, McCarthy K. Disruption of academic occupations during COVID-19: impact on mental health and the role of occupational therapy in tertiary education. *World Fed Occup Ther Bull.* 2020;76(2):78–81. https://doi.org/10.1080/14473828.2020.1822575.

33. Keptner KM, Harris AL, Mellyn JC, Neff NR, Rassie N, Thompson KM. Occupational therapy services to promote occupational performance, performance satisfaction, and quality of life in university freshmen: a pilot study. *Occup Ther Ment Health.* 2016;32(2):185–202. https://doi.org/10.1080/0164212X.2015.1100319.

34. Franchi T, Russell-Sewell N. Medical students and the impostor phenomenon: a coexistence precipitated and perpetuated by the educational environment? *Med Sci Educ.* 2022;33(1):27–38. https://doi.org/10.1007/s40670-022-01675-x.

35. Rice J, Rosario-Williams B, Williams F, et al. Imposter syndrome among minority medical students who are underrepresented in medicine. *J Natl Med Assoc.* 2023;115(2):191–198. https://doi.org/10.1016/j.jnma.2023.01.012.

36. Bullock JL, Lockspeiser T, Del Pino-Jones A, Richards R, Teherani A, Hauer KE. They don't see a lot of people my color: a mixed methods study of racial/ethnic stereotype threat among medical students on core clerkships. *Acad Med.* 2020;95:S58–S66. https://doi.org/10.1097/ACM.0000000000003628. (11S Association of American Medical Colleges Learn Serve Lead: Proceedings of the 59th Annual Research in Medical Education Presentations).

37. Farkas AH, Allenbaugh J, Bonifacino E, Turner R, Corbelli JA. Mentorship of US medical students: a systematic review. *J Gen Intern Med.* 2019;34(11):2602–2609. https://doi.org/10.1007/s11606-019-05256-4.

38. Molnar J, Falter B, Dugo M. Summary and analysis of case management in higher education. *J Campus Behav Interv.* 2017;5:66–74.

39. Meeks LM, Murray JF. Leaves of absence in health science programs: not a catch-all solution. *Disabil Compliance High Educ.* 2019;25(5):6–7. https://doi.org/10.1002/dhe.30754.

40. Higher Education Case Managers Association (HECMA). Mission & Vision. HECMA website. https://hecma.org. Accessed September 1, 2023.

41. Blair C. Educating executive function. *Wiley Interdiscip Rev Cogn Sci.* 2017;8(1–2): https://doi.org/10.1002/wcs.1403. 10.1002/wcs.1403.

42. Solanto MV. *Cognitive-Behavioral Therapy for Adult ADHD: Targeting Executive Dysfunction.* The Guilford Press; 2011.

43. Daya Z, Hearn JH. Mindfulness interventions in medical education: a systematic review of their impact on medical student stress, depression, fatigue, and burnout. *Med Teach.* 2018;40(2):146–153. https://doi.org/10.1080/0142159X.2017.1394999.

44. American Foundation for Suicide Prevention. *Struggling in Silence: Physician Depression and Suicide.* State of the Art, Inc; 2002.

45. Murphy B. *AMA Seeks More Help For Medical Students, Residents With Disabilities.* American Medical Association; 2021. https://www.ama-assn.org/education/medical-school-diversity/ama-seeks-more-help-medical-students-residents-disabilities. Accessed January 26, 2024.

46. Meeks L, Serrantino J, Jain N, et al. Accommodations in didactic, lab, and clinical settings. In: Meeks L, Jain N, Laird E, eds. *Equal Access for Students with Disabilities: The Guide for Health Science and Professional Education.* 2nd ed. Springer; 2020.

47. Kenney M, Sullivan L, Clifford G, Jain N. Learning in a digital age: assistive technology and electronic access. In: Meeks L, Jain N, Laird E, eds. *Equal Access for Students with Disabilities: The Guide for Health Science and Professional Education.* 2nd ed. Springer; 2020.

48. Moreland CJ, Fausone M, Cooke J, McCulloh C, Hillier M, Clifford GC, Meeks LM. Clinical accommodations and simulation. In: Meeks LM, Neal-Boylan L, eds. *Disability as Diversity.* Springer; 2020:213–260.

49. Carraccio C, Wolfsthal SD, Englander R, Ferentz K, Martin C. Shifting paradigms: from Flexner to competencies. *Acad Med.* 2016;91(5):663–667. https://doi.org/10.1097/00001888-200205000-00003.

50. Association of American Medical Colleges. *Altering the Course: Black Males in Medicine.* AAMC; 2015. https://store.aamc.org/altering-the-course-black-males-in-medicine.html.

51. Hacker A. Standardized tests are the new glass ceiling. *The Nation.* March 21, 2016. https://www.thenation.com/article/archive/standardized-tests-are-a-new-glass-ceiling/.

52. Nguemeni Tiako MJ, Ray V, South EC. Medical schools as racialized organizations: how race-neutral structures sustain racial inequality in medical education—a narrative review. *J Gen Intern Med.* 2022;37(9):2259–2266. https://doi.org/10.1007/s11606-022-07500-w.

53. Epstein RM. Assessment in medical education. *N Engl J Med.* 2007;356:387–396. https://doi.org/10.1056/NEJMra054784.

54. Frank JR, Snell LS, Cate OT, et al. Competency-based medical education: Theory to practice. *Med Teach.* 2010;32(8):638–645. https://doi.org/10.3109/0142159X.2010.501190.

55. Holmboe ES, Sherbino J, Long DM, Swing SR, Frank JR. The role of assessment in competency-based medical education. *Med Teach.* 2017;39(6):609–615. https://doi.org/10.3109/0142159X.2010.500704.

56. Brokaw JJ, Torbeck LJ, Bell MA, Deal DW. Impact of a competency-based curriculum on medical student advancement: a ten-year analysis. *Teach Learn Med.* 2011;23(3):207–214. https://doi.org/10.1080/10401334.2011.586910. PMID: 21745054.

57. Roediger HL, Marsh EJ. The positive and negative consequences of multiple-choice testing. *J Exp Psychol Learn Mem Cogn.* 2005;31(5):1155–1159. https://doi.org/10.1037/0278-7393.31.5.1155.

58. Couch BA, Hubbard JK, Brassil CE. Multiple–true–false questions reveal the limits of the multiple–choice format for detecting students with incomplete understandings. *BioScience.* 2018;68(6):455–463. https://doi.org/10.1093/biosci/biy037ne.

59. Rear D. One size fits all? The limitations of standardized assessment in critical thinking,. *Assess Eval High Educ.* 2019;44(5):664–675. https://doi.org/10.1080/02602938.2018.1526255.

60. Okuda Y, Bryson EO, DeMaria S, et al. The utility of simulation in medical education: what is the evidence? *Mt Sinai J Med.* 2009;76(4):330–343. https://doi.org/10.1002/msj.20127.

61. Issenberg SB, McGaghie WC, Hart IR, et al. Simulation-based medical education in clinical skills laboratory. *Med Teach.* 1999;21(6):581–585. https://doi.org/10.2152/jmi.59.28.

62. Pattni C, Scaffidi M, Li J, et al. Video-based interventions to improve self-assessment accuracy among physicians: a systematic review. *PLoS One.* 2023;18(7):e0288474. https://doi.org/10.1371/journal.pone.0288474.

63. Yeates P, Moult A, Lefroy J, et al. Understanding and developing procedures for video-based assessment in

medical education. *Med Teach.* 2020;42(11):1250–1260. https://doi.org/10.1080/0142159X.2020.1801997.

64. Lörwald AC, Lahner FM, Nouns ZM, et al. The educational impact of Mini-Clinical Evaluation Exercise (Mini-CEX) and Direct Observation of Procedural Skills (DOPS) and its association with implementation: a systematic review and meta-analysis. *PLoS One.* 2018;13(6):e0198009. https://doi.org/10.1371/journal.pone.0198009.

65. Ramani S, Krackov SK. Twelve tips for giving feedback effectively in the clinical environment. *Med Teach.* 2012;34:787–791. https://doi.org/10.3109/01421 59X.2012.684916.

66. Hattie J, Timperley H. The power of feedback. *Rev Educ Res.* 2007;77(1):81–112. https://doi.org/10.3102/003465430298487.

67. Johnson CE, Keating JL, Boud DJ, et al. Identifying educator behaviours for high quality verbal feedback in health professions education: literature review and expert refinement. *BMC Med Educ.* 2016;16:96. https://doi.org/10.1186/s12909-016-0613-5.

68. Snadden D, Thomas M. The use of portfolio learning in medical education. *Med Teach.* 1998;20(3):192–199. https://doi.org/10.1080/01421599880904.

69. Van Tartwijk J, Driessen EW. Portfolios for assessment and learning: AMEE Guide no. 45. *Med Teach.* 2009;31(9):790–801. https://doi.org/10.1080/01421590903139201.

70. Buckley S, Coleman J, Davison I, Khan K, Zamora J, Malick S, Morley D. The educational effects of portfolios on undergraduate student learning: a Best Evidence Medical Education (BEME) systematic review. BEME Guide No. 11. *Med Teach.* 2009;30(6):535–551. https://doi.org/10.1080/01421590902889897.

4

From Empathy to Epistemic Justice
Reconceptualizing Disability in Medical Education Using the 4R Model

Ryan Weber, Amanda M. Caleb, and Youngjin Cho

SUMMARY

Medical school curricula have long conceptualized disability as a problem in need of a solution, which has perpetuated **epistemic injustice** for people with disabilities and their families. Compounding this problem is a growing body of evidence indicating that clinicians often lack the comfort, knowledge, and experience needed to engage with people with disabilities, which has resulted in barriers to equitable health care and even increased levels of harm. As a boundary-crossing solution for these issues, we propose a transdisciplinary 4R model for improving educational practices grounded in epistemic justice that achieves many of the Core Competencies on **Disability** for Health Care Education published by the Alliance for Disability in Health Care Education. This longitudinal, transformative approach is informed by integration of the humanities into medical education and entails four parts: reflecting, reframing, revoicing, and revisiting. We begin by outlining strategies for teaching students to reflect on their assumptions surrounding disability and on the lived experiences of people with disabilities. From individualized approaches to **empathy**, in the first section we turn to a critical examination of models of care to problematize the classifications that have been used to create pathologies. By combining **reflection** with awareness of the historical processes and contemporary social forces that have been used to inaccurately assess the quality of life of disabled people, we then in the second section offer methods to reframe bodies using personal experience as narrative evidence for care, shifting the evidence paradigm. In turn, the third section examines avenues for revoicing the lived experiences of disabled patients. Finally, this chapter concludes by examining the process of revisiting the effectiveness of this dynamic process for continuing education. Collectively, the 4R model fosters disability **humility**, enabling medical students and trainees to uncouple the category of disability from the damaging processes of pathologization, to challenge the structures of **ableism** that permeate medical discourse, and to reconceptualize disability as a path for possibilities.

INTRODUCTION

The prevailing paradigm of disability within medical education is to approach this heterogeneous category as a deviation from a perceived standard of **normality**, making disability a pathology in need of cure rather than a dimension of human diversity. This concept is deeply rooted in the history of medicine and reinforces ableism—a pervasive system of beliefs that equates disability with deficiency and devalues people with physical, intellectual, or psychiatric disabilities. As a result, students lack adequate awareness and training about the lived experiences and needs of people with disabilities (PWD) and may perpetuate negative attitudes and assumptions without ever recognizing their own biases. These structural issues ultimately lead to persistent barriers to access to health care for PWD.

Therefore, in this chapter, we propose a 4R model as a transformative longitudinal approach to medical education grounded in epistemic justice. Our understanding of epistemic justice is based on the observations of Galasiński et al.[1] who note, "Epistemic justice is often viewed in reverse and called epistemic injustice. The term refers to how we communicate in ways that may be judged to be unjust." Such practices silence an individual by dismissing or distorting their lived experiences, which are realized through institutionalized hegemonic epistemologies.[2] At the same time, we recognize that although disability is a contested category, the definition proposed by Leonardi

et al. provides the most applicable framework for our study. They note, "Disability is a difficulty in functioning at the body, person, or societal levels, in one or more life domains, as experienced by an individual with a health condition in interaction with contextual factors."[3] Collectively, we aim to uncouple concepts of disability from the flawed **pathologization** of ableism and reconceptualize disability as a path for possibilities. Furthermore, we recognize the rich diversity of lived experiences that encompass the myriad constructions of disability. As Joel Michael Reynolds and Christine Wieseler have noted, "there is no consensus... concerning the term 'disabled people' vs. 'people with disabilities,' etc."[4] For these reasons, we adopt various nomenclatures that reflect these multiple perspectives.

The Current State of Disability in Medical Education

The current state of the disability curriculum in medical education is problematic in both approach and scope. In a 2017 review of disability curricula in US medical schools, researchers estimated that fewer than 25% of medical schools offered a disability awareness curriculum. Of those limited offerings, many were found to contain inconsistent pedagogies and content.[5] Most were exposure-based awareness sessions, often coupled with didactic pedagogies in single courses. The objectives of over 90% of those curricula were developed primarily by physicians without disabilities, not PWDs. Disability training modules for the clerkship are mostly confined to electives and not integrated into the rest of the curriculum, with a narrow focus on so-called medical aspects of disability. To address these issues, in 2019, The Alliance for Disability in Health Care Education published Core Competencies on Disability for Health Care Education in an effort to establish a standard for disability curriculum content and integration.[6] However, a follow-up study in 2020 revealed that little has changed in that the majority of medical schools continue to have limited opportunities for disability education.[7] There are scarce learning opportunities in medical curricula that foster a sustained level of engagement with communities of PWD. Moreover, there are persistently low rates of matriculating medical students and practicing physicians who identify as disabled.[8,9] This lack of representation further limits opportunities for interpersonal disability education. Consequently, we are in a morally unacceptable position where over 80% of physicians wrongly assign a lower quality of life for PWD than people without, and only 41% of physicians are confident in their ability to provide the same level of care to PWD as those without.[10] Medical schools, however, continue to permit graduates to enter practice without sufficient knowledge of the day-to-day experiences of disabled lives and with little to no exposure to disability cultures, activism, and perspectives.

Barriers to Epistemic Justice in Medical Education

Further exacerbating these obstacles to inclusion are several barriers that contribute to the continued deprioritization, marginalization, and misrepresentation of disability in medical education. While our list is not exhaustive, we address several key problems in this chapter. The first of these barriers is the pathologization of deviance—a perspective that views disabilities solely as deviations from a presumed norm. Second, the imbalance of authority, which first emerged during the professionalization of medicine in the 19th century, has led to what is often referred to as a diagnostic regime. When combined with the pathologization of deviance, this system reduces complex human experiences to oversimplified categories of observable biological deficiencies. Even today, diagnosis and categorization are often presented as neutral, apolitical tools without acknowledging the constructed nature of the concept of "normal" nor the contested classifications that fall under the expansive category of "pathology."

Third, medical education curricula rarely unpack the tangled history of medicine and the unstable notions of disability. The resultant lack of historical awareness permits students and trainees to accept the socially constructed nature of concepts like health and normality as biological inevitabilities. This oversight leads to the fourth barrier, which is the dualistic conception of health and disease. The **medical model of disability** often presents health/normality and disease/disability as binary opposites, wrongly casting disability as the absence of health. This rigid framework ignores the reality that health and disability can intersect in complex ways for PWD and reinforces the belief that disabilities are inherently undesirable. Following from these flawed associations is a fifth barrier, which is the conflation of disability with pain and suffering. This conflation has contributed to the widespread presence of the so-called disability paradox, which refers to the fact that many PWD report a higher quality of life than that which health care providers ascribe to disabled lives. Indeed, some studies had yielded the astonishing finding that over 80% of physicians assign a lower quality of life to PWD.[10]

Lastly, throughout this chapter, we explore ways in which internalized ableism causes negative self-perception for PWD, making it difficult to disclose disabilities and seek adequate care or accommodations. We also examine how internalized ableism in health care professionals can extend outward, leading to negative stereotyping, attitudes, and behaviors toward PWD. Collectively, we recognize that these paths create a dynamic feedback loop in which deleterious associations are both internally rationalized and externally justified. In sum, without a critical evaluation of the power dynamics and structural inequities that have shaped current assumptions of disability, learners are seldom given the opportunity to challenge ableist notions of health and belonging.

The 4R Model for Reconceptualizing Disability

In order to remove these barriers to epistemic justice and address lingering sources of exclusion in medical education, we outline a four-part, dynamic model and apply it to various scenarios using techniques adapted from esthetic approaches to inclusion. The first section focuses on critical reflection as a way of engaging learners with uncomfortable knowledge using Mezirow's theory of **transformational learning**.[11] We then develop a matrix of reflection and apply this tool to the circuits of **normalization** that have denied agency and even sentience to disabled people. The second section focuses on reframing categories of exclusion by embracing lived experiences of disabled people. In it, we outline six layers necessary for reframing disability as a valuable source of culture and way of being in the world: temporality, space, **epistemology**, certainty, categorization, and authority. We then offer suggestions for applying techniques employed by modernist artists to each of these domains across the medical education curriculum.

The third section explores the concept of revoicing as a mode of advocacy. We begin by briefly discussing epistemic injustice and its impact, framing it alongside modes of humility that respond to forms of epistemic injustice. This process serves as the foundation for developing methods of revoicing within medical education that work toward a model of epistemic justice and coadvocacy. In turn, the final section is dedicated to revisiting lingering assumptions by emphasizing the need for lifelong personal and professional reflection, which we position within both theories of **professional identity formation** and practices of humility outlined in the fourth section. Taken together, the interlocking methods of reflecting, reframing, revoicing, and revisiting may serve as a powerful tool for incorporating transdisciplinary perspectives of disability across the medical education curriculum and addressing both Accreditation Council for Graduate Medical Education (ACGME) competencies and the Core Competencies on Disability for Health Care Education (Fig. 4.1). Doing so, we argue, enables students to transform exclusionary discourses and practices into inclusive paradigms of belonging.

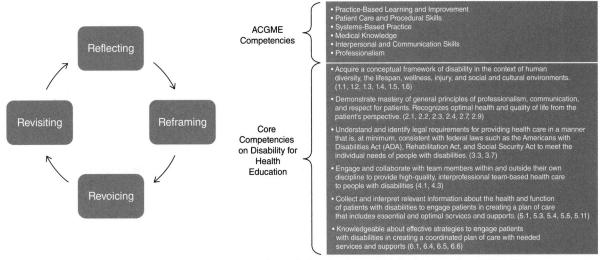

Fig. 4.1 The 4R Model Mapped to Accreditation Council for Graduate Medical Education (ACGME) competencies and the Core Competencies on Disability for Health Care Education. On the left, the figure shows the 4R model as a continuous and reinforcing process. On the right, we have represented how the model, aligns with ACGME competencies and many of the Core Competencies on Disability for Health Care Education, indicating which subcompetencies are met through the deployment of the 4R model. As certain competencies may map more explicitly to certain steps of the 4R model, we emphasize that it is implementation of the dynamic model as a whole that achieves these competencies and even encourages further reflection on the opportunities and limitations of these competencies.

REFLECTING ON HISTORICAL AND PERSONAL ASSUMPTIONS: TRANSDISCIPLINARY APPROACHES TO CULTIVATING AWARENESS

This section addresses the pivotal role of critical reflection in engaging medical students with "uncomfortable knowledge" that underscores transformative learning.[11] We employ the term "uncomfortable knowledge" to refer not just to complex topics such as death and disease that are addressed in the traditional curriculum but also to the ways in which some forms of care can contribute to the marginalization and even harm of disabled people.[12] In this chapter, we place particular emphasis on the practices of labeling and classifying as two of the many deleterious processes that arise from an imbalance of power. This section is arranged according to three key principles adapted from Mezirow's foundational theory of **transformational learning**, which are summarized in Fig. 4.2.[11,13] Listed adjacent to these principles are three key functions of **esthetics** in medical education, which have been adapted from Elliot Eisner's seminal work. His research has illustrated that the separation of the arts from epistemological matters is a product of a positivist tradition that is grounded in false assumptions; namely, that the arts are confined to the emotional domain and thus have little to offer knowledge systems. On the contrary, he argues, when unmoored from traditional approaches to scientific knowledge, students are empowered to embrace the values conferred by ambiguity, uncertainty, and the "deliteralization of knowledge," which "opens the door for multiple forms of knowing."[14] For these reasons, we demonstrate that, by embedding esthetics into the curriculum, educators can utilize "multiple forms of knowing"[14] to rupture the circuits of normalization that have long occupied biomedicine, resist oppressive structures of ableism, and embrace liminality as a foundation for epistemic justice. In sum, by synthesizing these principles and applying them to medical education, esthetics can serve as the key to unlocking new ways of knowing and a catalyst for personal identity transformation.

Categorizing Bodies, Assigning Meaning: Patterns of Thought and the Power to Classify

In their eponymous study on health, health care, and health education, Stewart Mennin et al. note, "We perceive the world as dynamic patterns. They are everywhere, and they

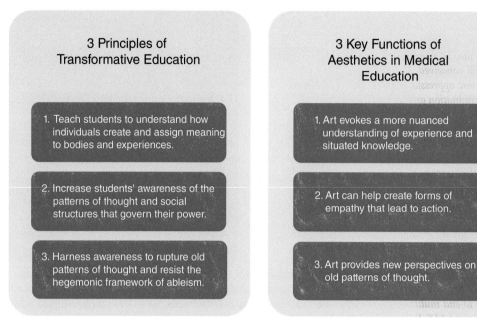

Fig. 4.2 Principles of transformative education and the functions of esthetics in medical education. (Adapted from Mezirow J. Transformative learning theory. In: Illeris K, ed. *Contemporary Theories of Learning: Learning Theorists in their Own Words.* 2nd ed. Routledge; 2018: 114–128; Eisner E. *Handbook of the Arts in Qualitative Research: Perspectives, Methodologies, Examples, and Issues.* 2008 2023/10/11. SAGE Publications, Inc.)

come in all shapes and sizes."[15] The authors further explain that patterns enable understanding because "prediction, replication, control, and reliability depend on clear measurable boundaries: differences and similarities with relatively strong stable connections."[15] Yet, from the moment students enter medical school, they are faced with conflicts between the patterns that have shaped their past ways of knowing and those created by their socialization into medicine. They learn about life through death, as in the dissection of cadavers. They prepare for a career in "the clinic" via the classroom, which creates discontinuities between theory and practice. In addition, they are expected to demonstrate confidence and acumen across a host of different environments while often feeling insecure in their skills and professional identity. Even more, they are trained to employ evidence-based paradigms in their decision-making while being plunged into uncertainty. The methods of biomedicine commonly address these tensions by encouraging students to sort people and perceived pathologies into binary categories. Either one is healthy or unhealthy, mentally fit or unfit, normal or abnormal, able-bodied or disabled. Even more, these binaries have been entrenched in cultural scripts by applying a hierarchy that privileges desired (and thus limited) forms of **personhood.** Further complicating this process is the reliance on

standardized measures to determine the course of care or, in some cases, the denial of treatment.[16]

All these practices attempt to impose borders between the known/unknown and acceptable/unacceptable (categories that Mennin et al. subsequently critique).[15] Consequently, the prevalence of either/or paradigms in biomedicine requires one to employ fixed, predetermined categories that establish not only the significance of biological conditions but also the perceived social value and status of apparent "disorders." This means that another type of (often implicit) categorization transpires simultaneously to the sorting of symptoms; it is the labeling, grouping, and classifying of types of people.[17] Thus, by conflating identity with impairment as part of a deficit-based paradigm, caregivers frequently exacerbate the imbalance of power that occurs between the one who holds the authority to assign the label and the one charged with passively receiving it. Joel Michael Reynolds has explored the effects of "clinicians' power to name disabilities," observing,

Through the creation, maintenance, and revision of diagnostic categories, health care in general and the practice of physicians in particular play distinctive roles in both establishing and responding to that which is named a disability or as disabling. Clinician misunderstanding

concerning the meaning of disability and the resultant miscommunication between clinicians and people with disabilities can lead not only to negative health outcomes but also to much larger social consequences, ranging from ill-conceived state and federal policies that result in systemic oppression to various forms of interpersonal discrimination and stigmatization.[18]

His analysis points to the fact that, behind the veneer of objectivity, lies an equally pervasive process of subjectively choosing and un-choosing. The poet and activist Eli Clare speaks to this fantasy of control in his book *Brilliant Imperfection*, lamenting,

We un-choose disability in hundreds of ways. We condone genetic testing for pregnant people and rarely question the ethics of disability-selective abortion... We accept as a matter of course that sperm banks screen out donors with a whole host of body–mind conditions considered undesirable... We walk to end breast cancer, run to end diabetes, bike to end multiple sclerosis, dump ice water on our heads to end ALS. We want to control how, when, and if disability and death appear in our lives.[19]

Clare's personal narrative sheds light on the pervasive problem of ableism entrenched in biomedicine since the rise of the medical model of disability in the 19th century. Correspondingly, many recent studies have exposed the structurally embedded forms of exclusion that contribute to ableism as well as the resulting health inequities.[10,20,21] And despite the many practices that contribute to its insidious circulation, there is one common factor: the "belief that impairment or disability (irrespective of 'type') is inherently negative and should the opportunity present itself, be ameliorated, cured, or indeed eliminated."[22] Clare also speaks to this objective, noting, "The desire for eradication runs so deep. It is revealed in specific moments, places, and histories... But the desire for eradication is also a pattern reaching across time and space. The un-choosing of disability fits into this pattern, one force among many, threatening to create a human monoculture."[19] Thus, because systems of oppression are sustained through patterns of thought, we must guide students in cultivating an awareness of the historical and personal assumptions that have allowed ableism to proliferate unabated.[23]

Cultivating Awareness Through Critical Reflection

Creating awareness of the patterns of thought and social structures that govern one's power can only be achieved through a critical mode of reflection that leads to personal transformation. Fig. 4.3 illustrates a matrix of the dimensions of discourse and zones of reflection that are involved in this process. The inner circle represents the four dimensions, including the exterior-facing forces (cultural scripts, social patterns, shared narratives, and structural systems of oppression) and interior-facing factors (personal narratives, beliefs, values, and biases) as well as the past and present

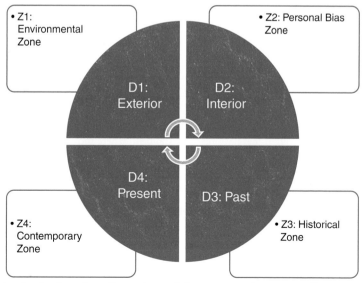

Fig. 4.3 Matrix of reflection: four dimensions of discourse and corresponding zones of reflection.

TABLE 4.1 Application of the Matrix of Reflection to Sample Reflection Questions

Three Themes for Critical Disability Studies	Example Reflection Questions	Representative Dimensions and Zones
Question of the Human	1. In what ways have assistive technologies shaped the boundaries of our bodies? 2. How have normative ways of thinking shaped your understanding of **autonomy?**	Z1/D1 Z2/D2 Z4/D4
Bodies that Matter	1. What labels have you used or observed in medical school that categorize bodily differences as deficits? 2. How does ableism in medicine place a higher value on non-disabled bodies?	Z1/D1 Z2/D2 Z4/ D4
Global Biopolitics of Dis/ability	1. How have Western notions of individualism denied justice to disabled persons? 2. In what ways do the classifications of intellectual disabilities in the Global North differ from the labels employed in the Global South? How can cultural concepts from the Global South help to improve patient- and family-centered care?	Z1/D1 Z3/D3 Z4/D4

Adapted from *Goodley D. Disability Studies: An Interdisciplinary Introduction.* SAGE Publications; 2017.

temporal dimensions. The outer flanking boxes illustrate the corresponding zones of reflection that should be used to explore each level of discourse. Moreover, the sections of the circle are separated to indicate the liminal spaces that, as we discuss next, are crucial to granting epistemic justice to those who occupy those spaces.[24] Furthermore, because disability is a concept that cuts across measurable boundaries, it is important that this matrix is employed in a manner that complements relevant competencies, thereby engaging students with contradictions and preparing them for dealing with uncertainty. Table 4.1 illustrates a set of sample reflection questions applied, in this case, to the three themes of critical disability studies outlined by Dan Goodley, which are listed in the first column on the left.[25] The center column lists the corresponding dimensions and zones from the Matrix of Reflection (Fig. 4.3). Collectively, these can be useful tools for expanding the aims of other established methods that similarly seek to break the patterns of thought that have sustained the institutionalization of ableism.[20,21,23,26,27]

Toward Rupture and Resistance: Using Critical Awareness to Dismantle the Medical Model of Disability

Assisting students in developing the skills necessary to dismantle the circuits of **normalization** that have occupied biomedical science requires inverting traditional perspectives. Fig. 4.4 illustrates how the "cure/kill paradigm"—a key feature of the medical model of disability, has often been the key driver of misleading and oppressive narratives surrounding disability.[28] These narratives have led to false assumptions and dangerous conflations across society in general and in biomedical circles in particular. For instance, many studies have demonstrated that health care professionals frequently ascribe a lower quality of life to disabled people than what those same people have reported.[16,29–31] The cure/kill paradigm has also generated a series of dangerous assumptions, including what Joel Michael Reynolds has termed the "ableist conflation." This perspective uncritically collapses the distinction between disability on one hand and pain and suffering on the other. Reynolds also illustrates how medical education has been a driving force in perpetuating these false narratives. As a result, agency, sentience, and personhood have been denied to people with disabilities. This is especially true in the case of cognitive or intellectual disabilities, "where those lacking the intrinsic cognitive capacities that mark personhood have the reduced moral status of non-human animals with comparable intrinsic properties."[32]

Yet "to combat the ableist conflation," Reynolds contends, "it is not enough to claim that experiences of disability and pain are separate—it also requires reflection in a rigorous and not reflexive manner."[33] Therefore, we propose inverting traditional paradigms by starting with the integration of critical reflection that embraces all dimensions and zones of the Matrix of Reflection. This will reverse these circuits of normalization and replace them

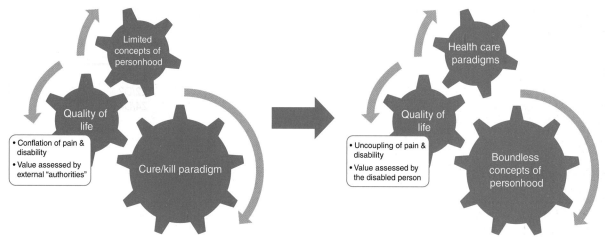

Fig. 4.4 Transforming circuits of normalization into mechanisms of liminality. This figure shows the shift from the medical model of disability to the social model of disability facilitated by the 4R model. On the left, the cure/kill paradigm is the prime driver of change, which controls assumptions of quality of life that limit concepts of personhood. On the right, this process has been inverted so that boundless concepts of personhood become the catalyst for overturning flawed assumptions about the quality of life, which shape inclusive health care paradigms.

with mechanisms of liminality, thereby shifting "from a rhetoric of classification… to a rhetoric of identification."[34] In this paradigm, boundless concepts of personhood become not the endpoint, but the starting point. Students learn to displace the narrative of curing and fixing, or even overcoming, which Clare refers to as "cure's backup plan," and instead embrace disability as an aspect of diversity (a point we return to below).[19] By replacing "deficit-oriented assumptions"[27] with the notion that personhood is expansive and devoid of thresholds that one must meet, learners can begin the process of uncoupling pain and disability and (re)valuing disabled lives through deeper reflection. Only then can we shut off those long-running circuits that have led to internalized ableism and "acknowledge disabled people's history of oppression and their individual and collective trauma stemming from such experiences." [35]

What is needed most to achieve these aims is rupture and resistance—the very qualities medical education has minimized through a reliance on standardized systems of measurement and either/or categorizations that flatten out difference while reducing the possibilities of personhood. Achieving the type of rigorous reflection that we are suggesting can be challenging in any context. For this reason, we advocate the use of "critical esthetic pedagogy"[36] to help build what Jain refer to as a "restless reflexive" stance. It is an approach that "allows us to question the known and familiar ways of working to imagine how new approaches to inclusion might be possible with our work ever in progress."[27] But, as Alan Bleakley has observed, "in medical education, aesthetics is a

lost or unknown territory."[37] This is due to another paradox medical students face, which occurs between the anesthetizing strategies that dull the senses and sensitizing approaches like empathy that seek to awaken them.[37] To this end, while the arts have played a significant role in assessing the body's value throughout history, they also have a key part to play in reassessing it. Thus, after engaging students in uncomfortable knowledge, we can enable them to reframe the medical model with the social model of disability. In the following sections, we offer a closer look at possible strategies as a form of praxis or theory-in-action.[37]

REFRAMING CATEGORIES OF EXCLUSION: STRATEGIES FOR EMBRACING LIVED EXPERIENCE

Throughout this section, we explore the six interrelated layers necessary for reframing the medical model with the tenets of the social model of disability, which are summarized in Table 4.2. We conclude by offering a framework for viewing disability as a source of culture and a valuable site of meaning-making before outlining strategies for teaching students to embrace liminal states of being through esthetics.

Reframing the Time and Space of Disability

Neo-liberalism in the West has long contributed to the commodification of the body. The roots of this oppression

TABLE 4.2   Six Layers of Reframing Disability

Temporality	Space	Knowledge (Epistemology)	Certainty	Categorization and Classification	Authority
• Eschew neoliberal emphasis on efficiency and progress • Embrace "crip time" & the complexity of disabled experiences	• Place disability at the core of the curriculum • Disabled experiences become "dwelling spaces"	• Cripistemology that resists compulsory able-bodiedness • Rupture historical models that have led to disability oppression	• Embrace liminality • Value cognitive and affective dissonance • Recognize limits of biomedical methodologies • Rethink narratives of "fixing" and "curing"	• Replace binary categorization of health, functionality, and value with spectra in which disability is fully embedded • Employ esthetics to develop new meanings	• Coconstruct narratives of inclusion • Decentered sharing • Patients are experts in the shared decision-making process

can be traced back to the 19th century. Sarah Rose has demonstrated that the concept of disability emerged as a category of social exclusion after the Civil War in the United States. Prior to this time, "the lives of people with disabilities were as diverse as the terms used to describe them."[38] She points to three factors that converted heterogeneous individuals into a homogeneous group of "unproductive citizens": the transition to industrial capitalism, the rise of mechanized factory labor as a central part of the economy, and, paradoxically, the development of public policies intended to prevent public dependency.[38] When combined with the narrowing of the concept of "normal,"[39] the spectrum of ability that once dominated the cultural imagination all but vanished, turning disability into a problem in need of a solution. The vectors of exclusion extended into the 20th century, when disability became "fundamentally linked to the needs of capital accumulation."[40] As a result, capitalism enacted "dramatic changes in the ideological classification and treatment of disabled people,"[40] locking them out of the workforce and denying them basic human rights. The residue of the pressure to instill "progress," "efficiency," and "productivity" remains with us to this day, contributing to allostatic forms of stress for disabled people.[41] The temporal domain, then, affords two possibilities for reframing this unstable category. The first requires students to grapple with the historical contingency of the various taxonomies of exclusion. The second requires the incorporation of "crip time" into our contemporary practices and pedagogies. Ljuslinder et al. define crip time as "the way disability disrupts normative understandings of time and the life course as their focus."[42] Drawing on the work of Petra Kuppers, they explain,

> "Crip time challenges ableist normativity and recognizes diverse bodies and minds by redefining time. This challenge to normativity facilitates a social approach to disability whereby the environment must be changed, not the body. Kafer defines crip time as a shift in mindset: 'rather than bend the bodies and minds to meet the clock, crip time bends the clock to meet disabled bodies and minds.'[43] Petra Kuppers describes crip time as a recognition that people move, think, and speak at a different pace to the normate, embracing this is a form of 'disability culture politics.'"[44]

Following the modification of time is the need to reconceive both the limiting and liberating properties of space. Rosemarie Garland-Thomson's seminal work *Extraordinary Bodies* reveals the many ways in which disabled bodies have been subjugated in the public sphere. In it, she illustrates how ideologies of self-reliance, autonomy, progress, and work flourished alongside the medicalization of disabled bodies to give rise to discriminatory social practices.[45] Correspondingly, Schweik's rigorous scholarship has shed light on the many ways disabled bodies have been policed through so-called ugly laws.[46] Further complicating these damaging practices are the myriad ways in which public spaces have been designed using an ableist lens, leading to the physical annexation of disabled people. For these reasons, we must go beyond the principles of universal design and place disability at the core of not just our societies and public spaces, but also the curriculum.[20] This goal demands considering the figurative space of the disabled body alongside the physical space it cohabits. Quoting Heidegger, Nicole Piemonte has observed, "Physical space is always more than just space; it is not simply the measurable area containing materials objects, but the 'wherein [that] I live,' the space where we dwell."[47] This is a powerful metaphor for reconceiving disability in medical education. By conceptualizing disability as a dwelling place, we can facilitate a deeper understanding of the lived experience of disability and the near-infinite ways it is embodied, and use this knowledge to reimagine an entirely new spirit of social change.[48] Neera Jain has similarly argued that the "potential of a transformative approach hinges on a new ethos, one that fosters cooperation, interdependence, and collective benefit rather than individual success, assumptions of independence, and competition as driving principles. A radically new image of health education and practice, one that centers on justice while ensuring high standards of patient care, is necessary."[27] In this paradigm, certainty becomes subordinate to the uncertainty disability affords disabled people in their daily lives.

From Cripistemologies to Reframing Authority: Integrating Lived Experience Into Evidence-Based Practices

Integrating these six layers also requires reframing accepted ways of knowing. So-called **cripistemologies** recognize disabled experiences as a form of knowledge by critiquing the concept of normalcy and resisting the compulsion to be able-bodied.[49] Most recently, Susanne Hamascha has offered an examination of the "knowledge borne by disabled bodies"[50] by tracing notions of failure that emanate from the "relation between bodies, minds, and the expectations placed upon them by their environments." Using the writing of breast cancer veterans, she forms resistance to measuring disabled experiences according to ableist standards by "placing the knowledge produced by and through disability closer to the center of cultural visibility."[50] Such cripistemologies also require us to reframe the central place given to certainty in biomedical spheres and replace it with an embrace of liminality. This position turns contradiction into a resource for new meaning-making by inverting the values of traditional medical education and placing value on cognitive and affective dissonance.[51] But embracing contradiction, uncertainty, and liminality means first altering the alignment of the concepts of "normal," "healthy," and "able-bodied," which have been sustained by narratives of "fixing" and "curing." Instilling new epistemologies also means recognizing the limits of biomedical methods because, as the sociologist Arthur Frank has noted, "The

body I experience cannot be reduced to the body someone else measures."[52] According to Eli Clare,

> *The medical-industrial complex pushes normal weight, normal walking, normal ways of thinking, feeling, and communicating as if normal were a goal to achieve and maintain... This nonsense couldn't exist without the threat of unnatural and abnormal... The pressure is intense, created and sustained by the consequences and dangers of being considered abnormal and unnatural. Inside this pressure cooker, the promise of cure is continually at work.[19]*

Moving people toward an imagined, "fixed" state assumes that they were once broken. This flawed belief denies personal agency because, Clare further contends,

> *Sometimes we can claim brokenness for ourselves... But mainly it's claimed for us. We're broken because doctors and the media, our partners and families, coworkers and case managers say so. Amidst these voices, listening to our own body-minds is almost impossible.[19]*

Instead of seeing people as being broken, the 4R model reframes the labels and classifications that have been used to devalue disabled perspectives and people. Accordingly, Michael Schillmeier has emphasized that "health is not a given and universal condition that can be objectified as normal; neither are its deviances and deficiencies from an objective norm that frame the realm of illness. Rather, health and illness are intertwined signatures of life."[53] Schillmeier's analysis points to the fact that not only are categories like health dynamic, but so are we. Accordingly, the search for "voice" to which Clare refers requires reframing notions of authority by "including the patient as an expert in the decision-making and in developing appropriate medical recommendations; acknowledging one's own knowledge gaps; [and] learning from the patient."[23] It also entails practices such as "decentered sharing," which the poet and physician Shane Neilson characterizes as the process by which one places their experience adjacent to someone else's experience to avoid imposing a greater authority and to enhance constructive options for care.[54] After all, seeing the self requires seeing the impact of our professions on others.

Disability as Culture, Disability as Diversity: Teaching Students to Embrace Liminal States of Being Through Esthetics

Each of these six domains is a testament to the fact that the body is an esthetic object. Collectively, reframing deficit-oriented patterns of thought involves two paradigm shifts: moving from a source of pathology to a site of cultural expression and transforming classifications of deviance into narratives of diversity.[55] In a similar manner, Havercamp et al. argue, "The most efficient and effective approach to disability competence would recognize disability as an aspect of population diversity akin to race or ethnicity."[26] Indeed, over the past decade, a number of medical schools have begun to address disability as a diversity issue, including the University of Colorado.[56] Yet this approach has not become widespread. Therefore, by placing the work of scholars in esthetic domains into dialogue with burgeoning trends in medical education, we can better reframe deleterious narratives that have historically been positioned at the core of the medical model of disability.

And if bodies have been medically rejected using esthetic criteria,[57] then we can also use esthetic criteria to foster greater acceptance and social justice of those same bodies by disrupting binary-based patterns and educating for tolerance of ambiguity.[37] In his study *Broken Beauty*, Straus draws a parallel between stylistic traits in modernist music/literature and disability, citing three key observations. First, works conceived in this style move disability from the periphery to the center, making disability both more visible and a prominent part of cultural discourse. Second, modernist representations of disability are more likely to approach disability sympathetically, thus eschewing forms of stigma that have been assigned to various conditions. And third, disabled characters are granted an identity that is more complex and significant than any stigmatized traits.[58] These perspectives are a reversal of the "medical and eugenic rejection of disability" that has otherwise accompanied modernist techniques.[59] Accordingly, they provide the foundation for assigning esthetic value to disability that is "itself worthy of future development."[59] Using Straus' three key observations of modernist music and literature, we suggest several techniques in Table 4.3 that are representative of the ways in which esthetics can reshape our pedagogical approaches. The focus in this case is the documentary film "In My Language" by Mel Baggs[60]—a disabled writer and artist. By applying Straus' categories as an analytic lens, the reflection questions enable students to interrogate notions of disability that have historically denied agency to disabled persons. In doing so, we center the disabled voice within the discourse to reframe the medical model of disability and facilitate a critical engagement with the relationships between social justice and disability. This example is offered as a stimulus for developing further techniques across the curriculum. If medical education is a powerful force of socialization, then each institution will need to establish ways of disrupting the hidden curriculum by teaching students to find value in disability culture and to resist the coupling of disability

to notions of pain, lower quality of life, and its marginalized status outside of the framework of health.

REVOICING THE LIVED EXPERIENCE: TRANSFORMING LEARNERS INTO ADVOCATES FOR EPISTEMIC JUSTICE

This section explores the concept of revoicing as a mode of advocacy and responding to epistemic injustice. We begin by briefly discussing epistemic injustice and its impact, framing it alongside modes of humility that respond to forms of epistemic injustice. This framework serves as the foundation for methods of revoicing within medical education that work toward a model of epistemic justice and coadvocacy.

Countering Epistemic Injustice With Humility

Countering epistemic injustice requires understanding both the modes and causes of injustices. Miranda Fricker defined two modes of epistemic injustice that are widely accepted by philosophers and other scholars: **testimonial injustice** and **hermeneutical injustice.** The former occurs when a listener devalues another's narrative or lived experience because of the listener's bias; the latter occurs when historical exclusion from the creation of knowledge (e.g., scholarship, policies) prevents an individual (or others) from understanding and communicating their lived experience.[61] While these are distinct forms of epistemic injustice, they are also mutually reinforcing, creating a cycle of injustice that is difficult to break. These two branches of epistemic injustice lead to what we term **epistemic disembodiment**, whereby the impacts of epistemic injustice are mapped onto the body. Embodiment is grounded in the idea that bodies are storytellers, which can convey an individual's lived experience, even when the individual is unable to tell their story directly.[62] When epistemic disembodiment occurs, all forms of the individual's story are invalidated, including that which the body may be telling, leading to a distancing of the physical body from the knowledge and sense of self. For instance, an individual with autism may experience testimonial injustice when a health care provider dismisses their account of flourishing and hermeneutical injustice when they cannot express their flourishing because traditional knowledge and scholarship suggest living a good life is not congruent with autism.[63] These experiences of epistemic injustice result in a paradox, whereby to be flourishing must mean the individual is not autistic, and if they are autistic, then they must be suffering because of their autism.[63] This paradox can cause epistemic disembodiment, whereby the individual disassociates the autistic body from the flourishing self.

Underscoring epistemic injustice is a lack of humility by individuals and medico-scientific and sociopolitical

TABLE 4.3 Modernist Techniques Applied to Medical Education

Theme	Critical Reflection Questions
Move disability from the periphery to the center of discourse.	1. In the first half of the film, Baggs eschews the traditional technique of a narrated voice-over. How does this esthetic decision help to center hir voice? 2. How does Baggs' engagement with the environment in the first part of the film help to reframe expectations of meaning? How does Baggs find purpose with the interactions depicted?
Approach disability sympathetically, thus eschewing forms of stigma.	1. Baggs entitled the second half of the film "A Translation." What do you think Baggs means by this? 2. How does Baggs interrogate the hegemony of spoken language throughout both parts of the film?
Grant disabled characters an identity that is more complex and significant than any stigmatized traits.	1. According to Baggs, what are common requirements for being viewed as a "real person"? How does sie invert these cultural expectations? 2. On hir webpage, Baggs writes, "In the eyes of the medical profession, I've become even more of a *ballastexistenz*[a] than I used to be, ever since I got my feeding tube last year. I had no idea that once you got a feeding tube, you crossed a line into a category of people that are seen as being 'artificially kept alive.' People who maybe shouldn't be kept alive... Make no mistake about this: *I love my feeding tube with a passion.*" Compare these statements to your analysis of the film. In your own words, describe how ableism has devalued hir lived experience. How can Baggs' testimonial help you to reframe the medical model of disability to guarantee justice to disabled persons? 3. According to Baggs, "this film is not a look-at-the-autie gawking freakshow as much as it is a statement about what gets considered thought, intelligence, personhood, language, and communication, and what does not." What elements of the film shed light on concepts of personhood that transcend hir autistic identity?

[a]Baggs describes this as a "historical term that means 'ballast existence' or 'ballast life,' which was applied to disabled people in order to make us seem like useless eaters, lives unworthy of life."
Note: Baggs uses the pronouns "sie," "hir," and "hirs." And "autie" is an informal way of referring to an autistic person.

structures that reinforce categorization of bodies and marginalize stories of minoritized populations. As medical education moves away from competency to humility, it can better address the causes of testimonial injustice and related health inequities. Competency assumes having sufficient knowledge to act and/or have authority over another; as such, it perpetuates testimonial injustice and fails to support patient-centered care. The virtue of humility requires an individual to recognize the limits and biases of their knowledge and their experiences and to be open to learning from new knowledge. True humility requires an expansive understanding of knowledge, which includes that created through lived experience. Thus, humility can serve as a panacea for epistemic injustice, particularly in the ways in which it can help to reimagine a more inclusive creation of knowledge. **Epistemic humility** looks to how external factors influence

knowledge creation and requires reflection on influences and biases in the construction of knowledge, recognition of the uncertainty of knowing, and the willingness to modify beliefs.[36,64] **Structural humility** requires reflecting on external structural forces (historical, political, medical) that perpetuate difference and oppress populations, including one's role in these structures, and learning from individuals and communities to address structural vulnerability.[65] **Cultural humility** entails community- and identity-focused reflection on how one's culture influences one's beliefs and how one can learn from and honor others' cultures without assuming the ability to know them fully in order to reduce cultural hegemony.[66] Finally, **narrative humility** necessitates reflection on the limitations of knowing another's story fully, the boundaries of narrative expression, and narrative biases that influence how one receives, processes, and values stories.[67,68] Fig. 4.5

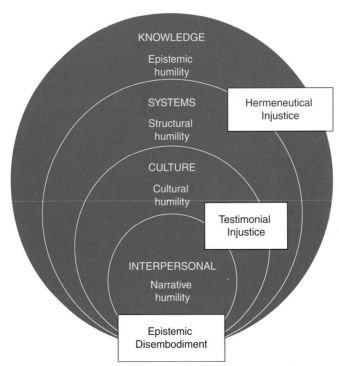

Fig. 4.5 Socioecological model of disability humility.

provides a socioecological model of disability humility as aligned with epistemic injustice.

Models of Revoicing

The process of revoicing is a means of embodying the socioecological model of humility in order to counter the manufactured silences of epistemic injustice. Revoicing is not the same as retelling, which involves narrative influence, nor is it the same as voicing, which is initial vocalized expression. Revoicing is the act of echoing a vocalized or nonvocalized expression, whereby the expression is both reflected outward and returned, creating the space for further reflection. While revoicing suggests verbalization of epistemologies, we use this term to include any models of communication. We have developed three revoicing modes: (1) verbatim revoicing, (2) precision revoicing, and (3) liberation revoicing. While each of these models counters specific modes of epistemic injustice, deployed collectively, they are a model of how to reduce epistemic injustice in all forms and ease epistemic disembodiment.

Verbatim Revoicing

Verbatim revoicing is based on the very literal communication assistance of a revoicer, which is an individual or technology that listens to and repeats the communication from an individual who has a speech impairment. Devva Kasnitz describes revoicing as an act of embodiment, explaining how the revoicer's voice and mouth function not only as stand-ins for her own but as physical entities that are hers during the act of revoicing.[69] Kasnitz argues that as a means of accessibility, a revoicer does not need to understand but to "listen, repeat, forget"; yet the very act of revoicing can lead to understanding. Within the context of medical education, revoicing is a means for learners to counter testimonial injustice by elevating the voice of an individual with a disability: in the act of conveying their communication verbatim, the medical professional's mouth speaks the voice of another, thereby dissolving the power dynamic of medical professional and disabled patient. Verbatim revoicing occurs within a framework of narrative humility, whereby the learner is led by the narrative structure used by the disabled person, which cannot be altered by their biases. Through this narrative positionality, the learner cannot devalue the disabled person's experience or means of narratively conveying that experience.

Precision Revoicing

Precision revoicing is based on the educational model used to reinforce and validate learning by repeating a learner's utterance and confirming accuracy with concluding questions like "is that right?"[70-72] This mode of revoicing has been successfully employed in a number of educational settings, including with English-language learners.[70,73] Precision revoicing involves repeating a communication in order to convey the revoicer's learning (not the original speaker) and to elevate the speaker by encouraging their correction of the revoicer's communication.

Confirming accuracy of communication makes legible the way in which meaning is received and conveyed, thereby exposing any epistemic gaps or biases. It also forces the revoicer to be accurate in how they understand and repeat a disabled person's communication. Precision revoicing is an enactment of cultural humility in that it denies the cultural hegemony associated with a dominant voice's assumption of the experience of others. Thus, a medical professional cannot tell a disabled person what their experience with disability is like (or represent this experience to others); rather, they must honor how that disabled person communicates their experience. Precision revoicing challenges testimonial injustice by preventing a health care provider from dismissing a disabled person's account and instead elevating it by communicating it accurately and by positioning the disabled person as the sole source of authority about their own experience.

Liberation Revoicing

Liberation revoicing is derived from postcolonialism and its focus on decolonization. Postcolonialism examines the ways in which colonial subjects were exploited and marginalized by colonizers. To counter colonial hegemony, postcolonial writers have retaken the dominant accounts by decentering colonizers, rejecting the notion of a monolithic and authentic postcolonial subject, and rewriting histories to include their experiences, perspectives, and values.[74,75] Political decolonization restored stolen land to Indigenous populations; however, decolonization of history, language, literature, and ultimately knowledge is an ongoing imperative.[76,77] In the context of disability, decolonization is a call to overthrow the "oppressive social structures of power that create and recreate disability out of difference in part as a system of control."[78]

Liberation revoicing is the communicative act of decolonizing medicine that is enacted through initial and echoed accounts of disability from persons with disabilities. Such revoicing actively engages with existing oppressive narratives and engages with "epistemic (de)centering."[79] Liberation revoicing disrupts epistemological dividing practices and erasure of persons with disability by centering accounts from persons with disabilities and reaffirming them in educational and clinical spaces. This involves not only including persons with disability in the creation and dissemination of knowledge about disability but also the purposeful and accurate echoing of their voices in scholarship, educational,

and clinical spaces. Liberation revoicing rebalances **evidence-based medicine** so that the patient's values, expressed through their experiences, are centered, and the health care provider's experience is decentered. Enacted through both epistemic and structural humility, it challenges health care providers and learners to both learn from those with disabilities and to reflect upon medicine's marginalization of disabled person's knowledge and power. In doing so, liberation revoicing counters hermeneutical injustice by recreating epistemologies that center experiences of persons with disabilities and by assigning meaning to these experiences that can help disabled persons communicate their experiences through this new mode of communication.

Toward a Model of Advocacy

Revoicing is a means to learn about/from persons with disabilities and to use that knowledge for advocacy. In speaking out against ableism, learners can practice revoicing in echoing the experience of disabled persons and honoring the accuracy and value of their experience. In advocating for dignity in care, learners can use liberation revoicing to counter narratives that impose medicalized values of flourishing and definitions of quality of life that are external to the individualized experience of a disabled person. In this model of advocacy, learners and health care providers are not speakers for persons with disabilities; rather, they are revoicing disabled lives and experiences as a means of coconstructing narratives that encourage ongoing reflection by learners, thus continually working toward epistemic justice.

REVISITING LINGERING ASSUMPTIONS: TOWARD AN ONGOING EFFORT OF PERSONAL AND EDUCATIONAL TRANSFORMATION

In this section, we outline the final component of the 4R model—revisiting, which functions as a metatextual evaluation of learning within the model. Foundational to this work is lifelong personal and professional reflection, which we position within both theories of professional identity formation and practices of humility.

Personal Reflection as a Path to Lifelong Professional Development

Professional identity formation (PIF) is considered foundational to medical education and professional socialization in medicine.[80,81] Monrouxe and Rees[82] distinguish PIF into two main approaches: individualist, which focuses on internal identity formation, and social-contextual, which posits that identity is shaped by external forces.

Individualist approaches rely heavily on self-reflective writing to assess PIF, whereas social-contextual interventions are group-based, whether through group activity, such as interprofessional education (IPE)[83] or patient partnerships,[84] or via group-based reflections.[85] Many implementations of PIF in medical school curricula fall within the spectrum of these approaches or even implement aspects of both.[85] Professional identity formation begins during medical school but is a lifelong process of self and professional evaluation.

Deploying the 4R model involves both developing a sense of belonging within the profession and continuing to interrogate ways in which the medical profession can cause harm to marginalized communities, such as those with disabilities, by adhering to problematic and inaccurate categorization of bodies. This intervention involves a longitudinal application of both the individualist and social-contextual approaches, whereby learners are encouraged to revisit the process of reflecting, reframing, and revoicing throughout medical school and their careers within the framework of the representative dimensions and zones (Fig. 4.3). Continued reflection beyond medical school is foundational to developing humility as a medical professional.[64-67] Within the context of revoicing, ongoing reflection is part of the echoing back what has been learned and what learning is still needed. As part of the 4R's cyclical learning process, revisiting promotes reflection within the context of new information or experiences, encouraging learners to continually engage with disability reframing and revoicing as a means of practicing humility, amplifying the lived experiences of persons with disabilities, and combatting testimonial injustice.

Revisiting can take several forms within the 4R model. Within undergraduate medical education, it can involve additional reflection after revoicing practices, whereby students revisit the reflection questions with their new knowledge from revoicing and within a disability humility framework. This practice is best employed through a reinforcing process of individual and group reflection, whereby learners first revisit reflections on their own, then share within a group, and revisit their reflections again in light of their group discussions. Group reflection focuses on the echoing process of revoicing, whereby what was learned by individuals from revoicing is expressed to others and reverberated back. Such revisiting can also occur within a learner-patient model,[84] whereby students explore the lessons of revoicing directly to the individuals who they revoiced. These same practices can be deployed within graduate medical education.

The 4R model should be situated within the context of lifelong learning, whereby learners are encouraged to revisit this dynamic model beyond the scope of formalized instruction in undergraduate and graduate medical education. Such revisiting supports efforts to enhance physician humility and encourages continued engagement of disability epistemologies in order to resist epistemic injustice.

CONCLUSION

History reminds us that words are sticky. They pick up new meanings across space and time. For example, the various meanings tied to the notion of "normal" swelled across the 19th century, transforming it from a synonym of the "standard body" to a symbol of the "ideal body." As a result, this category became an enforceable imperative by requiring citizens to meet the increasing demands of both form and function—obligations that contributed to the dehumanizing of people with disabilities.[38] Paradoxically, words can also be slippery. For instance, the descriptor "invalid" gave way to a whole new category of people during this same period: the invalid. This slippage from adjective to noun gave birth to a new constellation of labels such as feebleminded, idiot, and imbecile—all intended to disqualify people from personhood. The residue of this oppressive logic remains in many sectors of medical education today. It resides in the false assumptions of quality of life, the conflation of disability with pain and suffering, and the barriers to epistemic justice that are woven into our curricula. Also similar to the 19th century, research has shown that words have a way of constructing people.[17] People remain susceptible to becoming their diagnostic labels in the eyes of observers and, as a result, are forced to contend with undemocratic health inequities. And despite the many years that separate our current practices from those of the first dawn of eugenics, a stubborn commonality can be found in the propensity to pathologize forms of perceived deviance. Consequently, the complex term "disability" has become a repository for any condition deemed undesirable by hegemonic authorities.

For these reasons, we offer the 4R model as a method for turning back these oppressive forces and granting epistemic justice to those who have been marginalized by the pathologization of deviance. By imbricating the processes of reflecting, reframing, revoicing, and revisiting across the many sectors of medical education, we can impart the ameliorating properties of critical reflexivity and use the arts and humanities as a catalyst for justice. This methodology is offered not as an ending, but as the beginning of a process we must perpetually instill in ourselves and our students. As part of this reconceptualization of medical education, future research is needed to establish ways of assessing the way learners' beliefs and assumptions of disability are linked to professional identity formation. Developing milestones for self-reflection and personal transformation across domains can also enable learners and educators alike to develop the forms of humility needed to thrive in the epistemic space created by uncomfortable knowledge. Artificial intelligence (AI) remains both a source of potential problems and promise in this regard. Further research is needed to determine the extent to which AI-assisted analysis of students' writing is helpful in uncovering bias and evaluating empathetic experiences.[86] Furthermore, this process must coincide with addressing the lack of support that students with disabilities are commonly offered in medical schools. We believe that the 4R model can be implemented at individual, institutional, and structural levels to create new types of sociocultural expectations that value different forms of knowing and ways of being. In addition, scholars, educators, and clinicians need to work across disciplines to develop transdisciplinary methods for implementing this process within existing curricula. In this manner, the 4R model can become an integrated and transformative lens instead of an additive and reductive paradigm. Collectively, these vectors can help to unmoor traditional methodologies from long-standing barriers to inclusion and impart a more dignified and diversified notion of personhood, at the center of which lies a critical notion of self and society. Doing so can help put an end to the "un-choosing of disability"[19] that has permeated medical education and create new forms of justice for people with disabilities amid the liminal spaces of belonging.

VIGNETTE: CRIP POETRY AND MODES OF REVOICING: "POEMS WITH DISABILITIES," JIM FERRIS

Crip poetry "seeks to explore and validate the lived experience of moving through the world with a disability […and] embodies a disability consciousness; it is informed by and contributes to disability culture."[87] By centering the disabled experience, crip poetry challenges biases of narrative construction and ableist values and epistemologies. The act of reading crip poetry aloud is an act of verbatim revoicing of text and liberation revoicing by decolonizing the poetic cannon, with the potential for precision liberation through analysis and validation.

Jim Ferris's "Poems with Disabilities" challenges assumptions about sociopolitical constructions of disability and our gaze of/on disability. It serves to ground discussions of how concepts such as "differently abled" contribute to oppressive narratives that sustain epistemic injustice and epistemic disembodiment.

We use this poem to demonstrate how revoicing disability through both personal and sociopolitical engagements functions as an open space to reclaim language and power.

1. How does the incorporation of crip poetics into medical education dismantle sociopolitical and sociolinguistic narratives of oppression and disembodiment?
2. How can crip poetics encourage a revoicing of disability that is foundational to epistemic justice in medicine?

REFERENCES

1. Galasiński D, Ziółkowska J, Elwyn G. Epistemic justice is the basis of shared decision making. *Patient Educ Couns.* 2023;111:107681.
2. Pohlhaus J. Gaile Varieties of epistemic justice. In: Kidd IJ, Medina J, Pohlhaus JG, eds. *The Routledge handbook of epistemic injustice. Routledge Handbooks in Philosophy.* 1st ed. Routledge, Taylor & Francis Group; 2017:13–26.
3. Leonardi M, Bickenbach J, Ustun TB, Kostanjsek N, Chatterji S. The definition of disability: what is in a name? *Lancet.* 2006;368(9543):1219–1221.
4. Reynolds JM. Theories of Disability. In: Reynolds JM, Wieseler C, eds. *The Disability Bioethics Reader.* 1st ed. Routledge; 2022:156–169.
5. Seidel E, Crowe S. The State of Disability Awareness in American Medical Schools. *Am J Phys Med Rehabil.* 2017;96(9):673–676.
6. Core Competencies on Disability for Health Care Education 2019; 2023. https://adhce.org/Core-Competencies-on-Disability-for-Health-Care-Education..
7. Lee D, Pollack SW, Mroz T, Frogner BK, Skillman SM. Disability competency training in medical education. *Med Educ Online.* 2023;28(1):2207773.
8. Meeks L, Jain N. *Accessibility, Inclusion, and Action in Medical Education: Lived Experiences of Learners and Physicians With Disabilities.* Association of American Medical Colleges; 2018.
9. Nouri Z, Dill MJ, Conrad SS, Moreland CJ, Meeks LM. Estimated prevalence of US physicians with disabilities. *JAMA Network Open.* 2021;4(3):e211254. -e.
10. Iezzoni LI, Rao SR, Ressalam J, Bolcic-Jankovic D, Agaronnik ND, Donelan K, et al. Physicians' perceptions of people with disability and their health care. *Health Aff (Millwood).* 2021;40(2):297–306.
11. Mezirow J. Transformative learning theory. In: Illeris K, ed. *Contemporary Theories of Learning: Learning Theorists in Their Own Words.* 2nd ed. Routledge; 2018:114–128.
12. McGuire A. *War on Autism: On the Cultural Logic of Normative Violence.* Michigan Publishing, University of Michigan Press; 2016.
13. Kegan R. What 'Form' transforms: a constructive-developmental approach to transformative learning. In: Illeris K, ed. *Contemporary Theories of Learning: Learning Theorists in Their Own Words.* 2nd ed. Routledge; 2018:29–45.
14. Eisner E. *Handbook of the Arts in Qualitative Research: Perspectives, Methodologies, Examples, and Issues.* SAGE Publications, Inc; 2008. 2023/10/11.
15. Mennin S, Eoyang G, Nations M. Health, health care, and health education: problems, paradigms, and patterns.

In: Bleakley A, ed. *Routledge Handbook of the Medical Humanities*. Routledge, Taylor & Francis Group; 2020:55–71.

16. Landry LN. Chronic Illness, Well-Being, and Social Values. In: Reynolds JM, Wieseler C, eds. *The Disability v Reader*. 1st ed. London: Routledge; 2022:156–169.

17. Hacking I. Making Up People. *London Review of Books*. August 17, 2006:23–26.

18. Reynolds J. Three things clinicians should know about disability. *AMA J Ethics*. 2018;20:1181–1187.

19. Clare E. *Brilliant Imperfection: Grappling With Cure*. Duke University Press; 2017.

20. Borowsky H, Morinis L, Garg M. Disability and ableism in medicine: a curriculum for medical students. *MedEdPORTAL*. 2021;17:11073.

21. Dhanani Z, Huynh N, Tan L, Kottakota H, Lee R, Poullos P. Deconstructing ableism in health care settings through case-based learning. *MedEdPORTAL*. 2022;18:11253.

22. Campbell FK. *Contours of Ableism: The Production of Disability and Ableness*. 1st ed. Palgrave Macmillan UK; 2009. Imprint: Palgrave Macmillan; 2009.

23. Hearn SL, Hearn PJ. Working with people with disabilities: an interactive video/lecture session for first- and second-year medical students. *MedEdPORTAL*. 2020;16:10913.

24. Burke TB. In: Reynolds JM, Wieseler C, eds. *Bioethics and the Deaf Community*. 1st ed. Routledge; 2022.

25. Goodley D. *Disability Studies: An Interdisciplinary Introduction*. SAGE Publications; 2017.

26. Havercamp SM, Barnhart WR, Robinson AC, Whalen Smith CN. What should we teach about disability? National consensus on disability competencies for health care education. *Disabil Health J*. 2021;14(2):100989.

27. Jain NR. Frameworks for inclusion: toward a transformative approach. In: Meeks L, Neal-Boylan L, eds. *Disability as Diversity*. Springer; 2020:1–13.

28. Howe B. *Music and Disability Studies: An Introduction*. 2014. https://musicologynow.org/music-disability-studies-an-introduction/.

29. Albrecht GL, Devlieger PJ. The disability paradox: high quality of life against all odds. *Soc Sci Med*. 1999;48(8):977–988.

30. Bacherini A, Havercamp SM, Balboni G. A new measure of physicians' erroneous assumptions towards adults with intellectual disability: A first study. *J Intellect Disabil Res*. 2023;67(5):447–461.

31. Fellinghauer B, Reinhardt JD, Stucki G, Bickenbach J. Explaining the disability paradox: a cross-sectional analysis of the Swiss general population. *BMC Public Health*. 2012;12(1):655.

32. Wilson R. In: Reynolds JM, Wieseler C, eds. *Eugenics, Disability, and Bioethics*. 1st ed. Routledge; 2022.

33. Reynolds JM. *The Life Worth Living: Disability, Pain, and Morality*. University of Minnesota Press; 2022.

34. Segal JZ. Ageism and Rhetoric. In: Bleakley A, ed. *Routledge Handbook of the Medical Humanities*. Routledge Taylor & Francis Group; 2020:163–175.

35. Jóhannsdóttir Á, Egilson S, Haraldsdóttir F. Implications of internalised ableism for the health and wellbeing of disabled young people. *Sociol Health Illn*. 2022;44(2):360–376.

36. Medina Y. *The Epistemology of Resistance: Gender and Racial Oppression, Epistemic Injustice, and Resistant Imaginations*. Oxford University Press; 2013.

37. Bleakley A. *Medical Education, Politics and Social Justice: The Contradiction Cure*. Routledge Advances in the Medical Humanities. 1st ed. Routledge; 2020.

38. Rose SF. *No Right to be Idle: The Invention of Disability, 1840s-1930s*. University of North Carolina Press; 2017.

39. Davis LJ. *Enforcing Normalcy: Disability, Deafness, and the Body*. Verso; 1995.

40. Russell M, Rosenthal K. *Capitalism & Disability: Essays by Marta Russell*. Haymarket Books; 2019.

41. Rhode PC, Froehlich-Grobe K, Hockemeyer JR, Carlson JA, Lee J. Assessing stress in disability: developing and piloting the Disability Related Stress Scale. *Disabil Health J*. 2012;5(3):168–176.

42. Ljuslinder K, Ellis K, Vikström L. Cripping time – understanding the life course through the lens of ableism. *Scand J Disabil Res*. 2020;22(1):35–38.

43. Kafer A. *Feminist, Queer, Crip*. Indiana University Press; 2013.

44. Kuppers P. Crip Time. *Tikkun*. 2014;29(4):29–30.

45. Garland-Thomson R. *Extraordinary Bodies: Figuring Physical Disability in American Culture and Literature*. Columbia University Press; 1997.

46. Schweik SM. *The Ugly Laws: Disability in Public*. New York University Press; 2010.

47. Piemonte NM. Medical Slang: Symptom or Solution? In: Bleakley A, ed. *Routledge Handbook of the Medical Humanities*. Routledge. Taylor & Francis Group; 2020:155–162.

48. Loja E, Costa ME, Hughes B, Menezes I. Disability, embodiment and ableism: stories of resistance. *Disabil Soc*. 2013;28(2):190–203.

49. Johnson ML, Mcruer R. Cripistemologies: Introduction. *J Lit Cult Disabil Stud*. 2014;8:127–147.

50. Hamascha S. Cripistemologies of the body: knowing through disability. In: Mica A, Pawlak M, Horolets A, Kubicki P, eds. *Routledge International Handbooks*. Routledge; 2023.

51. Bleakley A. *Routledge Handbook of the Medical Humanities*. Routledge, Taylor & Francis Group; 2020.

52. Frank AW. *At the Will of the Body: Reflections on Illness*. New ed. Houghton Mifflin; 2002.

53. Schillmeier MWJ. *Eventful Bodies: The Cosmopolitics of Illness*. Ashgate; 2014.

54. Neilson S. The Practice of Metaphor. In: Bleakley A, ed. *Routledge Handbook of the Medical Humanities*. Routledge Taylor & Francis Group; 2020:144–154.

55. Andrews EE. *Disability as Diversity: Developing Cultural Competence*. 1st ed. Oxford University Press; 2020.

56. Wong A. *Disability As a Diversity Issue in Medical Education*. University of Colorado Anschutz Medical

Campus; 2020. https://medschool.cuanschutz.edu/family-medicine/about/news/disrupting-the-status-quo-blog/disrupting-the-status-quo/disability-as-a-diversity-issue-in-medical-education.

57. Snyder SL, Mitchell DT. *Cultural Locations of Disability*. University of Chicago Press Chicago; 2006.

58. Straus J. *Broken Beauty: Musical Modernism and the Representation of Disability*. Oxford University Press; 2018. 24 May 2018.

59. Siebers T. *Disability Aesthetics*. University of Michigan Press; 2010.

60. Baggs A. I*n My Language. Video*. 2007. https://www.youtube.com/watch?v=JnylM1hI2jc.

61. Fricker M. *Epistemic Injustice: Power and the Ethics of Knowing*. Oxford University Press; 2007.

62. Krieger N. Embodiment: a conceptual glossary for epidemiology. *J Epidemiol Community Health*. 2005;59(5):350–355.

63. Chapman R, Carel H. Neurodiversity, epistemic injustice, and the good human life. *J Social Phil*. 2022;53: 614–631.

64. Stone JR. Cultivating humility and diagnostic openness in clinical judgment. *AMA J Ethics*. 2017;19(10):970–977.

65. Metzl JM, Hansen H. Structural competency: theorizing a new medical engagement with stigma and inequality. *Soc Sci Med*. 2014;103:126–133.

66. Tervalon M, Murray-García J. Cultural humility versus cultural competence: a critical distinction in defining physician training outcomes in multicultural education. *J Health Care Poor Underserved*. 1998;9(2):117–125.

67. DasGupta S. Narrative humility. *Lancet*. 2008;371(9617):980–981.

68. Tsevat RK, Sinha AA, Gutierrez KJ, DasGupta S. Bringing home the health humanities: narrative humility, structural competency, and engaged pedagogy. *Acad Med*. 2015;90(11):1462–1465.

69. Kasnitz D. The politics of disability performativity. *Curr Anthropol*. 2020;61(S21):S16–S25.

70. Ferris SJ. Revoicing: a tool to engage all learners in academic conversations. *Read Teach*. 2014;67(5):353–357.

71. O'Connor MC, Michaels S. Aligning academic task and participation status through revoicing: analysis of a classroom discourse strategy. *Anthropol Educ Quart*. 1993;24:318–335.

72. O'Connor MC, Michaels S. Shifting participant frameworks: orchestrating thinking practices in group discussions. In: Hicks D, ed. *Discourse, Learning, and Schooling*. Cambridge University Press; 1996:63–103.

73. Shein P. Seeing with two eyes: a teacher's use of gestures in questioning and revoicing to engage English language learners in the repair of mathematical errors. *J Res Math Educ*. 2012;43:182–222.

74. Ashcroft B, Griffiths G, Tiffin H. *The Empire Writes Back: Theory and Practice in Post-colonial Literatures*. 2nd ed. Routledge; 1989.

75. Spivak GC. Can the Subaltern Speak?. In: Nelson C, Grossberg L, eds. *Marxism and the Interpretation of Culture*. Urbana University of Illinois Press; 1989:271–313.

76. Dreyer J. Practical theology and the call for the decolonisation of higher education in South Africa: reflections and proposals. *HTS Teologiese Studies/Theological Studies*. 2017;73

77. Heleta S. Decolonizing knowledge in South Africa: dismantling the 'pedagogy of big lies.' *Ufahamu*. 2018;40

78. Nishida A, McGee M, Erevelles N. Neoliberal academia and a critique from disability studies. In: Block P, Kasnitz D, Nishida A, Pollard N, eds. *Occupying Disability: Critical Approaches to Community, Justice, and Decolonizing Disability*. 1st ed. Springer Netherlands; 2016:145–157. 2015.

79. Boda P. On the methodological and epistemological power of epistemic (de)centering as a reflexive praxis of resistance toward disability justice. *Qual Res J*. 2022;23

80. Cruess RL, Cruess SR, Boudreau JD, Snell L, Steinert Y. A schematic representation of the professional identity formation and socialization of medical students and residents: a guide for medical educators. *Acad Med*. 2015;90(6):718–725.

81. Sarraf-Yazdi S, Teo YN, How AEH, Teo YH, Goh S, Kow CS, et al. A scoping review of professional identity formation in undergraduate medical education. *J Gen Intern Med*. 2021;36(11):3511–3521.

82. Monrouxe L, Rees C. Theoretical perspectives on identity: researching identities in hHealthcare education. In: Cleland J, Durning S, eds. *Researching Medical Education*. Wiley-Blackwell; 2015:129–140.

83. Stull CL, Blue CM. Examining the influence of professional identity formation on the attitudes of students towards interprofessional collaboration. *J Interprof Care*. 2016;30(1):90–96.

84. Barr J, Bull R, Rooney K. Developing a patient focussed professional identity: an exploratory investigation of medical students' encounters with patient partnership in learning. *Adv Health Sci Educ Theory Pract*. 2015;20(2):325–338.

85. Mount GR, Kahlke R, Melton J, Varpio L. A critical review of professional identity formation interventions in medical education. *Acad Med*. 2022;97(11s):S96–s106.

86. Hanlon CD, Frosch EM, Shochet RB, Buckingham Shum SJ, Gibson A, Goldberg HR. Recognizing reflection: computer-assisted analysis of first year medical students' reflective writing. *Med Sci Educ*. 2021;31(1):109–116.

87. Ferris J. Crip poetry, or how I love learned to love the limp. *Wordgathering*. 2007;1(1).

PART III

Case Studies: Curriculum and Pedagogy

5

Healing-Centered Pedagogy
Understanding and Addressing Minoritized and Marginalized Trauma, Stress, and Healing in Medical Education

Javeed Sukhera, Justin L. Bullock, Mytien Nguyen, and Lisa M. Meeks

OUTLINE

SUMMARY

Systemic inequities influence the mental health and well-being of both patients and learners from minoritized and marginalized groups. The effects of oppression and discrimination contribute to psychological distress and hypervigilance that result from experiencing or witnessing discrimination, mistreatment, threats, violence, and intimidation. In the context of medical education, historically rooted and culturally reinforced forms of discrimination such as structural racism, sexism, ableism, classism, and homophobia perpetuate psychological distress for health professionals and learners with minoritized and marginalized identities. For example, such individuals disproportionately experience marginalization, leading to a sense of impaired well-being which further contributes to helplessness, hopelessness, and attrition from medicine.

The human consequence of psychological trauma and stress within medical education can contribute to significant burnout as well as impaired learning and workforce challenges. Yet, medical education can also be a catalyst for transformation. In this chapter, we outline several key concepts for medical educators that can help inform a framework for cultural and structural change.

UNDERSTANDING THE RELATIONSHIP BETWEEN OPPRESSION, DISCRIMINATION, TRAUMA, AND STRESS

Oppression relates to how an unequal distribution of power across groups leads to more dominant groups leveraging their power to marginalize, discriminate against, exploit, or subject less dominant groups to derogatory stereotypes.[1]

Oppression is both a process and a state of existence. For example, the state of oppression encompasses the ongoing process of oppression which maintains asymmetries of power.[2]

Research demonstrates that the cumulative impact of oppression, victimization, and discriminatory experiences affects an individual's mental and physical well-being.[3] When individuals experience oppression through discrimination, such incidents contribute to chronic stress, thus increasing the overall risk of illness and morbidity.[4] Key concepts that highlight the relationship between oppression, discrimination, trauma, and stress include racial trauma, minority stress, and internalized ableism.

Racial Trauma

Racial trauma is generally defined as psychological distress and hypervigilance that result from experiencing or witnessing discrimination, threats of harm, violence, and intimidation.[5-8] Racial trauma does not typically result from the traumatic stress of racist experiences in isolation, but rather a combination of exposure to race-based traumatic stress and the processing of such incidents as occurring in relation to the pervasive existence of various forms of systemic racism.[5]

There are both physical and psychological sequelae of racial trauma. Exposure to racism activates the body's stress response, leading to high levels of cortisol and autonomic system activation. Cumulative impacts of chronic stress increase the risk of physical health disorders such as cardiovascular, metabolic, and autoimmune diseases.[5,9,10] Psychological symptoms of racial trauma may be akin to posttraumatic stress disorder (PTSD) and include anxiety, mood changes, sleep disturbances, and hypervigilance.[10] For example, there may be intrusive thoughts regarding experiences of discrimination, avoidance of any reminders of racially traumatizing experiences and groups associated with such discrimination, and mood changes accompanied with feelings of self-blame, guilt, or anger.[6]

There are many ways that racial trauma may be inflicted on individuals who experience discrimination. Experiences of direct racism or indirect racism such as microaggressions, stories of friends, peers, or family pulled over in traffic stops, witnessing strangers who we identify with undergoing trauma, or public narratives about racist violence can erode well-being and adversely impact academic and social functioning.[6] For example, Black and Hispanic students living in communities with high rates of police violence demonstrate the most negative impact on their grades following police killings of racially minoritized individuals.[11,12] Similarly, racially minoritized individuals also commonly experience racism in working or learning environments. For example, workplace racism includes a disproportionate sense of access to resources or a sense of agency, contributing to findings suggesting that the workplace is an especially stressful environment for racially minoritized individuals.[6]

Minority Stress Theory

Minority stress theory originated in research on prejudice and discrimination against sexual and gender minorities. Examples of minority stress may range from discriminatory everyday experiences to the impact of discriminatory policies and laws.[13] Minority stress can also arise through the gradual internalization of negative self-concept,[14,15] and those affected are more highly sensitized to feeling rejected or avoided,[16] leading to stress due to excessive self-censorship and concealment of their minoritized identity.[17] Collectively, such stressors have an adverse impact on the health and well-being of sexual and gender minorities.[13]

There are several complex ways that minority stress may contribute to physical and psychological problems. Minority stress can contribute to emotional dysregulation and have a negative impact on social and interpersonal functioning.[18] There is also research suggesting that minority stress can become amplified within romantic and sexual relationships through minority stress contagion, thus compounding the negative effects of individual minority stress among couples.[19,20]

Ableism and Internalized Ableism

Ableism is another form of oppression and is defined as "a network of beliefs, processes, and practices that produce a particular type of self and body."[21] In doing so, it positions individuals with disabilities as less capable, less valuable, and less desired. These belief systems then impact behaviors toward disabled people, either overt or covert, that may prevent disabled people from fully engaging in employment, studies, medical care, and social events. Ableism often rests on the assumption that disabled people need to be "fixed" in one form or the other.

Routine oppression and the insidious trauma of ableism on disabled people can lead to the internalized belief in this dominant discourse. The internalized version of ableism is a complex and often overlooked aspect of disability discourse that delves into the internal struggles individuals with disabilities may face because of societal biases and stigmas.

Historical harm, shame, negative dominant discourse, and lack of role models stymy any counter narrative about disability, leading people to seek the desired state of health and to disavow any relationship with disability identity—fostering internalized ableism.[22,23] This internalization may lead to the adoption of ableist language or beliefs about one's own abilities. Individuals may downplay their achievements, attribute success to luck, or engage in self-deprecating behavior, denying disability status, embracing an inability narrative, and distancing from other disabled individuals.[24] Moreover, internalized ableism may lead to a reluctance to seek accommodation or support, as individuals may perceive such assistance as a sign of weakness or failure.

At the extreme, disabled people will attempt to pass as non-disabled to keep the status quo and not disrupt the system, reinforcing the systems of power that perpetuate ableism.

DISCRIMINATION TRAUMA AND STRESS IN A MEDICAL EDUCATION CONTEXT

Given that racial trauma accumulates over generations, medical education must acknowledge that the existing system has served to perpetuate racial trauma over centuries. First, by contributing to systemic health and social inequities, medical education takes place within a health care system where structural racism persists despite a preponderance of data proving the damaging effects of structural racism on individual and community health. Medical education has a history of experimentation on slaves without consent.[25] Black physicians have also been systematically excluded from organized medicine,[26] and the Flexner report left a longstanding racist legacy that continues to influence how future physicians are educated across North America.[27,28]

Racially minoritized health workers and learners continue to experience discrimination and mistreatment. Most notably, there is a significant amount of racism from patients and colleagues toward Black doctors and trainees, which influences decisions about which career path to pursue and which settings to practice in.[29] Such experiences of discrimination are compounded when racism is minimized or repeatedly ignored,[30] contributing to a diminished sense of agency.[31,32] Racial trauma is also worsened by ongoing experiences of stereotype threat[33–35] and the ubiquitous minority tax,[36] contributing to fear of further discrimination, devaluing, and a pervasive sense of not belonging or fitting in unless one conforms.

Even though racially minoritized individuals and communities are more likely to encounter racism throughout their lives, conversations about racism are often discouraged in working or learning environments because they produce cognitive dissonance.[37] Therefore, there is a compound effect of experiencing racial trauma and simultaneously feeling that such experiences are not valid or real that erodes an individual's psychological well-being.[30] In the context of medical education, research suggests that Black trainees and faculty experience public incidents of racism and police brutality in

a vicarious manner. Even though such individuals may not be direct victims of racial violence, they may trigger memories of intergenerational racial trauma, perpetuating a sense of retraumatization. Such trauma was worsened when Black trainees and faculty realized that their white colleagues were seemingly unaware of their centuries-long experiences of historical trauma.[38]

Existing paradigms of medical education may also perpetuate the ill effects of internalized racism. When an individual experiences racism, they begin to internalize the racist ideologies perpetuated through systemic racism about themselves, contributing to a sense of disrespect for oneself and one's racial identity.[39–42] Internalized racism therefore involves internalizing such negative ideologies, thus adopting a more racist worldview and self-destructive behaviors. For example, the more an individual internalizes racism, the less they believe that racism exists.[2,43] The more individuals experience racism and internalize it, the more they rationalize and propagate racism,[2] oppress others,[44] and normalize racism for themselves and others.[45–47]

EFFECTS OF ABLEISM AND INTERNALIZED ABLEISM

Exposure to ableism for health care professionals can lead to inaccessible environments, physical barriers, and unsupportive work environments broadly and can cause considerable harm at the individual level via negative attitudes, bullying, and harassment.[48] Indeed, a study of physicians with disabilities demonstrates significantly more mistreatment and harm in that population when compared to their non-disabled peers.[49] The source of mistreatment and harm stems from both the medical community (i.e., other physicians) and patients.

Ableism does not just impact providers. Indeed, ableism is dangerous for patients as well through lack of essential screenings[50–52] and a lack of diagnosis and treatments.[53] Peña-Guzman and Reynolds[53] suggest that ableism is harmful to patients through epistemic error. These epistemic schemas are linked to specific group identities such as race, sex, gender, sexuality, and disability that are deeply rooted in bias.[53]

While the outward effects of ableism are highly detrimental to both providers and patients, the same level of harm and trauma can result from internalized ableism. Internalized ableism carries complex psychological, social, and physical consequences. The constant internal struggle to measure up to societal standards can contribute to anxiety, depression, and low self-esteem, which may hinder people from realizing their full potential. Internalized ableism may also lead to reduced help-seeking, believing that one is not disabled enough to warrant medical or psychological treatment and that those mechanisms are only reserved for the few cases that neatly fit into a pre-prescribed category of disability or for conditions that are well received by the medical establishment.

Given the consequences of existing in a highly ableist environment, it is not difficult to understand why disability identity may be tightly held. The fear of stigma and effects on well-being, career development, and opportunities are known barriers to disclosure within medical training.[54–56] The consequences of nondisclosure or inadequate support for medical trainees and providers with disabilities are far-reaching. For example, nondisclosure and subsequent lack of accommodation have a considerable impact on mental health for disabled trainees and physicians alike. Studies show that trainees and physicians with disabilities experience higher levels of depressive symptoms and burnout compared to their non-disabled peers.[57–59] This impact is exponential for those from minoritized populations.[60] Medical professionals fear that the use of accommodations signals incompetence. This belief, especially in medical practice, forces individuals to conceal their disabilities, inadvertently perpetuating a cycle of invisibility.

Combatting ableism and internalized ableism requires a multifaceted approach that dismantles dominant attitudes, challenges societal norms, and promotes positive representation. One effective approach is counter storytelling.[61,62] Education and awareness campaigns can play a crucial role in dismantling ableist stereotypes and promoting a more accurate and empowering portrayal of disability. Additionally, creating safe spaces for open dialogue within the disabled community can help individuals confront and overcome internalized and societal ableism by fostering a sense of belonging and shared experiences, ultimately fostering an inclusive and equitable future for all and reducing the trauma that accompanies this form of oppression.

TOWARD HEALING-CENTERED PEDAGOGY

Given the role that medical education has played in perpetuating historical trauma and injustice, medical education must also play a role in moving toward healing while dismantling injustice. There is increasing recognition that existing systems must move away from an exclusive focus on bio-medical symptom control, to a system that embraces diverse ways of healing. Fostering a healing-centered approach goes beyond buzzwords to encourage a holistic and intergenerational perspective on an individual's recovery from suffering or pain. From a pedagogical perspective, medical schools and teaching hospitals must move toward embedding cultural sensitivity and advocacy into all aspects of the school's mission. Ultimately, healing-centered organizations ground social justice work in restorative principles to heal from identity-based discrimination and injustice through community, collectivism, and cultural authenticity.

Radical Healing

The radical healing framework may provide specific ways that medical education can foster healing-centered pedagogy (HCP). Table 5.1 provides specific examples. In the context of rising structural and racist violence, a group of thought leaders in psychology highlighted that greater exposure to discrimination contributes to emotional distress and that individual healing must occur in tandem with collective healing. The group developed the concept of radical healing, noting that "conventional healing focuses on individual symptom reduction…radical healing incorporates strategies that address the root causes of the trauma by building on the strengths of individuals and engaging the general and culture-specific practices of their community that promote resilience and well-being."[63]

Radical healing is anchored on five principles including (1) collectivism, (2) critical consciousness, (3) radical hope, (4) strength and resistance, and (5) cultural authenticity and self-knowledge.[64] Taken together, the main concept of the radical healing framework involves both the acknowledgment of and active resistance to oppression, as well as a vision of possibilities for freedom and wellness as part of pride and hope for the future.[64]

Some authors have used radical healing as a method to create interventions for mental health concerns in racially minoritized populations. Specifically, a radical healing therapeutic approach created by Adames et al.[65] was used to treat clients experiencing racial trauma to resist self-blame, racism, and oppression and to develop and nurture healing through the five pillars of radical healing. This approach has shown promise in validating clients' experiences of the distressing reality of racial trauma, as well as support in acknowledging impacts on well-being.[65] Overall, there are many different interventions that have been grounded in a radical healing framework (i.e., storying survival[66] and the Blafemme Healing Framework[67]). However, none of these interventions has been effectively evaluated for racially minoritized learners or workers in a health care context.

Collectivism

The radical healing framework suggests that collectivism is a necessary prerequisite for healing from the trauma of racism and discrimination. Healing requires support from within a community where an individual feels they can be their authentic selves without the need to self-censor or conform to oppressive ideologies. Collectivism can foster healing through co-creating spaces where there is a sense of validation and refuge from the ongoing harms of racism.

TABLE 5.1 Integrating Radical Healing Into Healing-Centered Pedagogy in Medical Education

Component	Definition	Components in Medical Education Example
Collectivism	Cocreating spaces where individuals can validate experiences of discrimination and seek refuge while building solidarity to advance antioppressive praxis.	Addressing saviorism. Integrating racial and cultural affinity groups.
Critical consciousness	Fostering an individual's capacity to critically reflect and act upon oppression.	Fostering critical reflection and reflection in action. Developing faculty role models who embrace humility, vulnerability, and candor.
Radical hope	Foregrounding the narrative that discrimination can end and oppressive systems can be dismantled.	Strengthening health advocacy curricula. Integrating community advocates and individuals with lived/living experience as medical teachers, role models, and mentors.
Strength and resistance	Reframing narratives about individuals and communities who face discrimination away from deficit-centered and toward strength-centered portrayals.	Iteratively auditing content and case-based narratives for deficit framing and revising.
Cultural authenticity and self-knowledge	Cultivating working and learning environments where individuals can bring their authentic selves.	Identity safety. Preventing and responding to microaggressions.

Collectivism serves as an opportunity for communities to reflect, label, and engage with their racial trauma.[68] It is based on the idea of sociotherapy—using facilitated group processes (i.e., storytelling) to address mental health and well-being.[69] A group's shared understanding of the recent or distant racist incident(s) coupled with their shared racial identity can aid in the healing process.[64,69] Through community, there is an existing foundation of trust that enables honest and open discourse that acknowledges racism while fostering a sense of solidarity. Overall, embracing collectivism can help to restore self-worth, community efficacy, and connection with one's racial identity.[64]

Advancing a collectivist approach in medical education requires acknowledging the role of saviorism in community frameworks for service learning. Saviorism can be perpetuated through various forms of global mediation where learners benefit from an imbalance of power that maintains a racist and economically exploitative status quo, thus further entrenching systems of exploitation.[70]

One example of collectivism in medical education is the increasing proliferation of cultural affinity or resource groups.[71] Affinity groups facilitate sessions among individuals who share a self-identified racial identity. Such groups can facilitate community and integrate theory, self-reflection, and improved well-being.[71] Such groups have been studied in K-12 education, undergraduate education, and workplace environments and are increasingly being organized in medical education and health systems. For example, at the University of California, San Francisco, School of Medicine, the implementation of affinity groups allowed learners to explore their experiences of racism, while embracing a sense of cultural authenticity, building community, and complementing antiracist praxis.[72]

Critical Consciousness

Critical consciousness has been defined as "an individual's capacity to critically reflect and act upon their sociopolitical environment."[73] The concept of critical consciousness has roots in transformative pedagogies and was introduced as a mechanism to move medical education beyond cultural competence toward fostering critical consciousness in all areas of medical education through dialogic forms of learning.[74] Recent reviews suggest that critical consciousness may foster reflective practice, promote equity, and illuminate power structures.[75] However, there is a pervasive tension between a critical consciousness orientation and a more competency-focused approach and the existing culture of medical education.[76,77] Zaidi and colleagues[77] found that medical education faculty were able to facilitate critical consciousness by creating a sense of safety, recognizing and naming forms of oppression, building relationships, and role modeling the courage to speak up.

Radical Hope

Radical hope in the context of radical healing refers to an unwavering sense that the struggle to break free from discrimination is audacious yet possible.[64] Individuals who experience the psychological harm of oppression are often paralyzed by a sense of hopelessness and helplessness. Therefore, for medical education to foster radical hope, there must be a proliferation of stories and tangible examples of how inequities can be reduced and liberation can truly advance. For example, medical education can and should not only teach about the ways in which existing health systems have perpetuated discrimination, but also how systems of oppression have been dismantled through activism. There should also be more active and sustained implementation of health advocacy curricula and integration of community advocates and activists as teachers, role models, and mentors for medical students.

Strength and Resistance

The scholars who developed the radical healing framework conceptualized strength and resistance to reflect the importance of affirming joy, shifting away from deficit-centered narratives, and drawing from ancestral and intergenerational narratives of resilience.[64]

Cultural Authenticity and Self-Knowledge

Cultural authenticity refers to the therapeutic power of bringing one's full authentic self into a working or learning environment, while self-knowledge means knowledge about one's ancestors, communities of origin, and intergenerational histories. An example of fostering cultural authenticity and self-knowledge—as well as other components of radical healing—in medical education involves embracing decoloniality through decolonial epistemologies. Decoloniality refers to a theoretical perspective that allows medical educators and learners to interrogate how medicine may perpetuate colonialism through various sociohistorical, geopolitical, and economic contexts.[78,79] Decolonizing medical education can also advance healing by teaching learners how racial trauma and colonization affect mental well-being, as well as explicitly teaching about

how Indigenous or Afro-centric epistemologies are healing from the destructive effects of colonialism through community, relationships, and ancestral wisdom.

Protective factors that serve to buffer against the negative effects of racial trauma include family support and social connectedness. Similarly, a sense of cultural affirmation buffers against anxiety and mood symptoms in Black Americans but not European Americans.[80,81] In medical education, cultural affirmation may occur through authentic sharing of individual stories and role modeling of vulnerability among faculty preceptors.[77,82,83]

Detailed next is the emerging concept of identity safety, which is another example of how medical education may foster cultural authenticity and self-knowledge.

Identity Safety

Moving toward a healing-centered pedagogy requires educators to not only consider ways in which we can mitigate the harm we inflict upon learners in the learning environment but also to consider ways in which we can foster a state of safety. Identity safety has been proposed as an identity-conscious form of safety in which learners are able to exist as their authentic selves without a need to self-monitor how others perceive their identities.[84] Identity safety is constructed upon three pillars, the first driven by the learner themself, the second driven by direct interpersonal interactions with peers and colleagues, and the final by direct and indirect experiences in the learning community.[84]

Minority stressors such as microaggressions, discrimination, and stereotype threat are psychologically, physiologically, and cognitively impactful.[33,85-88] There is a proliferation of literature supporting interventions against these threats in the learning environment.[82,89-93] A true construct of safety likely represents more than simply intervening against harmful social interactions.[84]

Psychological safety, the dominant conceptualization of safety in medical education, emphasizes mitigating power imbalances. It recognizes that in states of high power imbalance, trainees do not feel safe to disclose errors, challenge authority, or speak openly. We articulate two main critiques of psychological safety.[94,95] First, those who most need safety (e.g., learners and patients) are dependent upon others to create safety for them. In psychological safety, those who self-perceive low social power are never seen as agentic. Second, while acknowledging the importance of diversity, psychological safety adopts a power-centered, identity-agnostic lens to safety and articulates that after individuals are psychologically safe, *then* they will bring their diverse perspectives and opinions. For many minoritized trainees, an inability to bring their diversity to the workplace inhibits them from ever feeling a sense of true safety. Our identities are not an afterthought, but rather the lens through which we see the world. In contrast, identity-safe environments are not colorblind,[96] but rather recognize and value what one's identities bring.

Identity safety, as articulated by Bullock et al., refers to a state in which a learner can exist as their authentic self. It is built upon three main pillars: agency to serve, upholding personhood, and belonging. Agency to serve refers to the ways that learners fostered their own identity safety by leveraging their identities to serve patients (i.e., speaking the same language as a patient or using their own experience as a patient to help other patients). Upholding personhood refers to supervisors' and colleagues' respectful efforts to know a learner as a human being. Participants felt that their personhood was upheld when supervisors invested in knowing them during breaks in clinical duties. Belonging describes a sense of fitting in with and feeling anchored to a larger group.

There are many unknowns about identity safety in health professions education. For instance, it is unclear whether all three needs must be met simultaneously to feel a sense of identity safety or how identity safety evolves through time. The authors propose that identity safety is necessary but insufficient to create healing-centered spaces in medicine. Educators must both foster identity safety within a team and develop teams that are able to recognize and respond to novel identity threats which inevitably arise as the team interacts with different individuals throughout the hospital.

CONCLUSION

Discrimination and prejudice adversely affect the psychological well-being of minoritized patients, learners, and health professionals. Racial trauma, minority stress, and internalized ableism are several examples of discrimination adversely influencing well-being. Medical educators can play an important role in healing from the wounds of identity-based discrimination by incorporating healing-centered pedagogy and identity safety into practice. Healing-centered pedagogy ultimately refers to embedding cultural sensitivity and advocacy into medical education through collectivism, critical consciousness, radical hope, strength-based narratives, and cultural authenticity.

TAKE-HOME POINTS

1. Structural racism, ableism, sexism, homophobia, classism, and other forms of discrimination adversely affect the psychological well-being of minoritized patients, learners, and health professionals.
2. Medical educators can play a role in healing from the trauma of oppression and discrimination by understanding

concepts from the psychology literature such as racial trauma and minority stress.
3. The medical education community can be a catalyst for transformation by supporting healing from the trauma of oppression and discrimination.

REFERENCES

1. Prilleltensky I, Gonick L. Polities change, oppression remains: on the psychology and politics of oppression. *Polit Psychol.* 1996:127–148. doi:10.2307/3791946
2. David E, Schroeder TM, Fernandez J. Internalized racism: a systematic review of the psychological literature on racism's most insidious consequence. *J Soc Issues.* 2019;75(4):1057–1086. https://doi.org/10.1111/josi.12350.
3. Kirkinis K, Pieterse AL, Martin C, Agiliga A, Brownell A. Racism, racial discrimination, and trauma: a systematic review of the social science literature. *Ethn Health.* 2021;26(3):392–412. https://doi.org/10.1080/13557858.2018.1514453.
4. Geronimus AT. The weathering hypothesis and the health of African-American women and infants: evidence and speculations. *Ethn Dis.* 1992;2(3):207–221. PMID:1467758.
5. Akerele O, McCall M, Aragam G. Healing ethno-racial trauma in black communities: cultural humility as a driver of innovation. *JAMA Psychiatry.* 2021;78(7):703–704. https://doi.org/10.1001/jamapsychiatry.2021.0537.
6. Williams MT, Osman M, Gran-Ruaz S, Lopez J. Intersection of racism and PTSD: Assessment and treatment of racial stress and trauma. *Curr Treat Options Psychiatry.* 2021;8(4):167–185. https://doi.org/10.1007/s40501-021-00250-2.
7. Carter RT, Johnson VE, Roberson K, Mazzula SL, Kirkinis K, Sant-Barket S. Race-based traumatic stress, racial identity statuses, and psychological functioning: An exploratory investigation. *Prof Psychol Res Pr.* 2017;48(1):30. https://doi.org/10.1037/pro0000116.
8. Makoff E. Racial trauma: a palliative care perspective. *J Palliat Med.* 2020;23(4):577–578. https://doi.org/10.1089/jpm.2019.0484.
9. Carter RT. Racism and psychological and emotional injury: recognizing and assessing race-based traumatic stress. *Couns Psychol.* 2007;35(1):13–105. https://doi.org/10.1177/0011000006292033.
10. Williams M, Halstead M. Racial microaggressions as barriers to treatment in clinical care. *Dir Psychiatry.* 2019;39(4):265–280.
11. Bor J, Venkataramani AS, Williams DR, Tsai AC. Police killings and their spillover effects on the mental health of black Americans: a population-based, quasi-experimental study. *Lancet.* 2018;392(10144):302–310. https://doi.org/10.1016/S0140-6736(18)31130-9.
12. Ang D. *Wider Effects of Police Killings in Minority Neighborhoods.* Crime and Criminal Justice; 2020.
13. Frost DM, Meyer IH. Minority stress theory: application, critique, and continued relevance. *Curr*

Opin Psychol. 2023;51:101579. https://doi.org/10.1016/j.copsyc.2023.101579.

14. Jaspal R, Lopes B, Rehman Z. A structural equation model for predicting depressive symptomatology in Black, Asian and Minority Ethnic gay, lesbian and bisexual people in the UK. *Psychol Sex.* 2021;12(3):217–234. https://doi.org/10.1080/19419899.2019.1690560.

15. Liang Z, Huang YT. "Strong Together": minority stress, internalized homophobia, relationship satisfaction, and depressive symptoms among taiwanese young gay men. *J Sex Res.* 2022;59(5):621–631. https://doi.org/10.1080/00224499.2021.1947954.

16. Douglass RP, Conlin SE, Duffy RD. Beyond happiness: minority stress and life meaning among LGB individuals. *J Homosex.* 2020;67(11):1587–1602. https://doi.org/10.1080/00918369.2019.1600900.

17. Pachankis JE, Mahon CP, Jackson SD, Fetzner BK, Bränström R. Sexual orientation concealment and mental health: a conceptual and meta-analytic review. *Psychol Bull.* 2020;146(10):831. https://doi.org/10.1037/bul0000271.

18. Sarno EL, Newcomb ME, Mustanski B. Rumination longitudinally mediates the association of minority stress and depression in sexual and gender minority individuals. *J Abnorm Psychol.* 2020;129(4):355. https://doi.org/10.1037/abn0000508.

19. LeBlanc AJ, Frost DM. Couple-level minority stress and mental health among people in same-sex relationships: Extending minority stress theory. *Soc Ment Health.* 2020;10(3):276–290. https://doi.org/10.1177/2156869319884472.

20. Rostosky SS, Riggle ED. Same-sex relationships and minority stress. *Curr Opin Psychol.* 2017;13:29–38. https://doi.org/10.1016/j.copsyc.2016.04.011.

21. Campbell FA. Inciting legal fictions-disability's date with ontology and the abieist body of the law. *Griffith L Rev.* 2001;10:42.

22. Campbell FAK. Exploring internalized ableism using critical race theory. *Disabil Soc.* 2008;23(2):151–162. https://doi.org/10.1080/09687590701841190.

23. Burstow B. Toward a radical understanding of trauma and trauma work. *Violence Against Women.* 2003;9(11):1293–1317. https://doi.org/10.1177/1077801203255.

24. Rosenwasser P. Tool for transformation: co-operative inquiry as a process for healing from internalized oppression. In: *Paper Presented at Adult Education Research Conference (AERC)*; June 2–4, 2000; British Columbia, Canada.

25. Washington H. *Medical Apartheid: The Dark History of Medical Experimentation on Black Americans from Colonial Times to Present.* Doubleday Broadway Publishing Group; 2006.

26. DeShazo RD. *The Racial Divide in American Medicine: Black Physicians and the Struggle for Justice in Health Care.* Univ. Press of Mississippi; 2018.

27. Flexner A. *Medical Education in the United States and Canada, A Report From the Carnegie Foundation for the Advancement of Teaching.* 1910.

28. Laws T. How should we respond to racist legacies in health professions education originating in the flexner report?

AMA J Ethics. 2021;23(3):E271–275. https://doi.org/10.1001/amajethics.2021.271.

29. Mpalirwa J, Lofters A, Nnorom O, Hanson MD. Patients, pride, and prejudice: exploring Black Ontarian physicians' experiences of racism and discrimination. *Acad Med.* 2020;95(11S):S51–S57.

30. Watson-Creed G. Gaslighting in academic medicine: where anti-Black racism lives. *CMAJ.* 2022;194(42):E1451–E1454. https://doi.org/10.1503/cmaj.212145.

31. Filut A, Alvarez M, Carnes M. Discrimination toward physicians of color: a systematic review. *J Natl Med Assoc.* 2020;112(2):117–140. https://doi.org/10.1016/j.jnma.2020.02.008.

32. Smith WA, Yosso TJ, Solórzano DG. Challenging racial battle fatigue on historically White campuses: A critical race examination of race-related stress. In: Coates RD, ed. *Covert Racism.* Brill; 2011:211–237.

33. Bullock JL, Lockspeiser T, Del Pino-Jones A, Richards R, Teherani A, Hauer KE. They don't see a lot of people my color: a mixed methods study of racial/ethnic stereotype threat among medical students on core clerkships. *Acad Med.* 2020;95:S58–S66. https://doi.org/10.1097/ACM.0000000000003628. (11S Association of American Medical Colleges Learn Serve Lead: Proceedings of the 59th Annual Research in Medical Education Presentations).

34. Teherani A, Hauer KE, Fernandez A, King TE, Lucey C. How small differences in assessed clinical performance amplify to large differences in grades and awards: a cascade with serious consequences for students underrepresented in medicine. *Acad Med.* 2018;93(9):1286–1292. https://doi.org/10.1097/ACM.0000000000002323.

35. Rojek AE, Khanna R, Yim JWL, et al. Differences in narrative language in evaluations of medical students by gender and under-represented minority status. *J Gen Intern Med.* 2019;34(5):684–691. https://doi.org/10.1007/s11606-019-04889-9.

36. Osseo-Asare A, Balasuriya L, Huot SJ, et al. Minority resident physicians' views on the role of race/ethnicity in their training experiences in the workplace. *JAMA Netw Open.* 2018;1(5):e182723. https://doi.org/10.1001/jamanetworkopen.2018.2723.

37. Wyatt TR, Taylor TR, White D, Rockich-Winston N. "When No One Sees You as Black": the effect of racial violence on Black trainees and physicians. *Acad Med.* 2021;96(11S):S17–S22. https://doi.org/10.1097/ACM.0000000000004263.

38. Sharma M, Kuper A. The elephant in the room: talking race in medical education. *Adv Health Sci Educ Theory Pract.* 2017;22(3):761–764. https://doi.org/10.1007/s10459-016-9732-3.

39. Fanon F. *A Dying Colonialism.* Grove/Atlantic, Inc; 1965.

40. Freire P. *Cultural Action for Freedom.* Harvard Educational Review; 1970.

41. Lipsky S. *Internalized Racism.* Rational Island Publishers Seattle, Wash; 1987.

42. Pyke KD. What is internalized racial oppression and why don't we study it? Acknowledging racism's hidden injuries. *Sociol Perspect.* 2010;53(4):551–572. https://doi.org/10.1525/sop.2010.53.4.551.

43. Neville HA, Coleman MN, Falconer JW, Holmes D. Color-blind racial ideology and psychological false consciousness among African Americans. *J Black Psychol*. 2005;31(1):27–45. https://doi.org/10.1177/0095798404268287.

44. Lipsky S. *Internalized Oppression*. 2nd ed. Black Re-Emergence; 1977.

45. David E, ed. *Internalized Oppression: The Psychology of Marginalized Groups*. Springer Publishing Company; 2013.

46. David EJR, Nadal KL. The colonial context of Filipino American immigrants' psychological experiences. *Cultur Divers Ethnic Minor Psychol*. 2013;19(3):298–309. https://doi.org/10.1037/a0032903.

47. David E, Okazaki S. Biculturalism. In: Jackson Y, ed. *Encyclopedia of Multicultural Psychology*. Sage Publications; 2006:67–68.

48. Lindsay S, Fuentes K, Ragunathan S, Lamaj L, Dyson J. Ableism within health care professions: a systematic review of the experiences and impact of discrimination against health care providers with disabilities. *Disabil Rehabil*. 2023;45(17):2715–2731. https://doi.org/10.1080/09638288.2022.2107086.

49. Meeks LM, Conrad SS, Nouri Z, Moreland CJ, Hu X, Dill MJ. Patient and coworker mistreatment of physicians with disabilities. *Health Aff (Millwood)*. 2022;41(10):1396–1402. https://doi.org/10.1377/hlthaff.2022.00502.

50. Iezzoni LI, Wint AJ, Smeltzer SC, Ecker JL. Physical accessibility of routine prenatal care for women with mobility disability. *J Womens Health (Larchmt)*. 2015;24(12):1006–1012. https://doi.org/10.1089/jwh.2015.5385.

51. Horner-Johnson W, Dobbertin K, Iezzoni LI. Disparities in receipt of breast and cervical cancer screening for rural women age 18 to 64 with disabilities. *Women Health Iss*. 2015;25(3):246–253. https://doi.org/10.1016/j.whi.2015.02.004.

52. Iezzoni LI, Agaronnik ND. Healthcare Disparities for Individuals with Disability: Informing the Practice. In: Meeks LM, Neal-Boylan L, eds. *Disability as Diversity: A Guidebook for Inclusion in Medicine, Nursing, and the Health Professions*. Springer International Publishing; 2020:15–31. http://doi.org/10.1007/978-3-030-46187-4_2.

53. Peña-Guzmán DM, Reynolds JM. The harm of ableism: medical error and epistemic injustice. *Kennedy Inst Ethics J*. 2019;29(3):205–242. https://doi.org/10.1353/ken.2019.0023.

54. Pereira-Lima K, Meeks LM, Ross KET, et al. Barriers to disclosure of disability and request for accommodations among first-year resident physicians in the US. *JAMA Netw Open*. 2023;6(5):e239981. https://doi.org/10.1001/jamanetworkopen.2023.9981.

55. Meeks L, Jain N. *Accessibility, Inclusion, and Action in Medical Education: Lived Experiences of Learners and Physicians with Disabilities*. Association of American Medical Colleges (AAMC); 2018.

56. Jain NR. The capability imperative: theorizing ableism in medical education. *Soc Sci Med*. 2022;315:115549. https://doi.org/10.1016/j.socscimed.2022.115549.

57. Meeks LM, Pereira-Lima K, Frank E, Stergiopoulos E, Ross KET, Sen S. Program access, depressive symptoms, and medical errors among resident physicians with disability. *JAMA Netw Open*. 2021;4(12):e2141511. https://doi.org/10.1001/jamanetworkopen.2021.41511.

58. Meeks LM, Pereira-Lima K, Plegue M, et al. Disability, program access, empathy and burnout in US medical students: a national study. *Med Educ*. 2023;57(6):523–534. https://doi.org/10.1111/medu.14995.

59. Meeks LM, Conrad SS, Nouri Z, et al. Burnout among physicians with disabilities. *JAMA Netw Open*. 2024;7(5):e2410701. https://doi.org/10.1001/jamanetworkopen.2024.10701.

60. Nguyen M, Meeks LM, Pereira-Lima K, et al. Association of race, ethnicity, and multiple disability status on medical student burnout. *JAMA Netw Open Preprint*. 2024;7(1):e2351046. https://doi.org/10.1001/jamanetworkopen.2023.51046.

61. Panzer KV, Maraki I, Cross T, Meeks LM. Podcast possibilities: asynchronous mentoring for learners with disabilities. *Med Educ*. 2020;54(5):448–449. https://doi.org/10.1111/medu.14084.

62. Parker L, Stovall DO. Actions following words: critical race theory connects to critical pedagogy. *Educ Theory*. 2004;36(2):167–182. https://doi.org/10.1111/j.1469-5812.2004.00059.x.

63. Neville HA, Adames HY, Chavez-Dueñas NY, et al. The psychology of radical healing: what can psychology tell us about healing from racial and ethnic trauma? *Psychology Today Blog: Healing through Social Justice*; 2019.

64. French BH, Lewis JA, Mosley DV, et al. Toward a psychological framework of radical healing in communities of color. *Couns Psychol*. 2020;48(1):14–46. https://doi.org/10.1177/0011000019843506.

65. Adames HY, Chavez-Dueñas NY, Lewis JA, et al. Radical healing in psychotherapy: addressing the wounds of racism-related stress and trauma. *Psychotherapy (Chic)*. 2023;60(1):39–50. https://doi.org/10.1037/pst0000435.

66. McNeil-Young VA, Mosley DV, Bellamy P, Lewis A, Hernandez C. Storying survival: an approach to radical healing for the Black community. *J Couns Psychol*. 2023;70(3):276–292. https://doi.org/10.1037/cou0000635.

67. Mosley DV. A biomythography introducing the Blafemme Healing framework. *Am Psychol*. 2023;78(5):678–694. https://doi.org/10.1037/amp0001146.

68. Tummala-Narra P. Racial trauma and dissociated worlds within psychotherapy: a discussion of "racial difference, rupture, and repair: a view from the couch and back. *Psychoanal Dialogues*. 2020;30(6):732–741. https://doi.org/10.1080/10481885.2020.1829437.

69. Chioneso NA, Hunter CD, Gobin RL, McNeil Smith S, Mendenhall R, Neville HA. Community healing and resistance through storytelling: a framework to address racial trauma in Africana Communities. *J Black Psychol*. 2020;46(2-3):95–121. https://doi.org/10.1177/0095798420929468.

70. Banerjee AT, Bandara S, Senga J, González-Domínguez N, Pai M. Are we training our students to be white saviours in

global health? *Lancet.* 2023;402(10401):520–521. https://doi.org/10.1016/S0140-6736(23)01629-X.

71. Lewis L, Cribb Fabersunne C, Iacopetti CL, et al. Racial affinity group caucusing in medical education - a key supplement to antiracism curricula. *N Engl J Med.* 2023;388(17):1542–1545. https://doi.org/10.1056/NEJMp2212866.

72. Lewis JA. Contributions of Black psychology scholars to models of racism and health: Applying intersectionality to center Black women. *Am Psychol.* 2023;78(4):576–588. https://doi.org/10.1037/amp0001141.

73. Diemer MA, Kauffman A, Koenig N, Trahan E, Hsieh CA. Challenging racism, sexism, and social injustice: support for urban adolescents' critical consciousness development. *Cultur Divers Ethnic Minor Psychol.* 2006;12(3):444–460. https://doi.org/10.1037/1099-9809.12.3.444.

74. Kumagai AK, Lypson ML. Beyond cultural competence: critical consciousness, social justice, and multicultural education. *Acad Med.* 2009;84(6):782–787. https://doi.org/10.1097/ACM.0b013e3181a42398.

75. Halman M, Baker L, Ng S. Using critical consciousness to inform health professions education : A literature review. *Perspect Med Educ.* 2017;6(1):12–20. https://doi.org/10.1007/s40037-016-0324-y.

76. Manca A, Gormley GJ, Johnston JL, Hart ND. Honoring medicine's social contract: a scoping review of critical consciousness in medical education. *Acad Med.* 2020;95(6):958–967. https://doi.org/10.1097/ACM.0000000000003059.

77. Zaidi Z, Vyas R, Verstegen D, Morahan P, Dornan T. Medical education to enhance critical consciousness: facilitators' experiences. *Acad Med.* 2017;92:S93–S99. https://doi.org/10.1097/ACM.0000000000001907. (11S Association of American Medical Colleges Learn Serve Lead: Proceedings of the 56th Annual Research in Medical Education Sessions).

78. Naidu T. Modern medicine is a colonial artifact: introducing decoloniality to medical education research. *Acad Med.* 2021;96(11S):S9–S12. https://doi.org/10.1097/ACM.0000000000004339.

79. Lokugamage AU, Ahillan T, Pathberiya SDC. Decolonising ideas of healing in medical education. *J Med Ethics.* 2020;46(4):265–272. https://doi.org/10.1136/medethics-2019-105866.

80. Williams MT, Chapman LK, Wong J, Turkheimer E. The role of ethnic identity in symptoms of anxiety and depression in African Americans. *Psychiatry Res.* 2012;199(1):31–36. https://doi.org/10.1016/j.psychres.2012.03.049.

81. Watson LB, DeBlaere C, Langrehr KJ, Zelaya DG, Flores MJ. The influence of multiple oppressions on women of color's experiences with insidious trauma. *J Couns Psychol.* 2016;63(6):656–667. https://doi.org/10.1037/cou0000165.

82. O'Brien MT, Bullock JL, Minhas PK, et al. From eggshells to action: a qualitative study of faculty experience responding to microaggressions targeting medical students. *Acad Med.* 2023;98(11S):S79–S89. https://doi.org/10.1097/ACM.0000000000005424.

83. Sukhera J, Kulkarni C, Taylor T. Structural distress: experiences of moral distress related to structural stigma during the COVID-19 pandemic. *Perspect Med Educ.* 2021;10(4):222–229. https://doi.org/10.1007/s40037-021-00663-y.

84. Bullock JL, Sukhera J, Del Pino-Jones A, et al. "Yourself in all your forms": a grounded theory exploration of identity safety in medical students. *Med Educ.* 2023 https://doi.org/10.1111/medu.15174. Published online July 30,.

85. Sue DW, Capodilupo CM, Torino GC, et al. Racial microaggressions in everyday life: implications for clinical practice. *Am Psychol.* 2007;62(4):271–286. https://doi.org/10.1037/0003-066X.62.4.271.

86. Torres L, Driscoll MW, Burrow AL. Racial microaggressions and psychological functioning among highly achieving African-Americans: a mixed-methods approach. *J Soc Clin Psychol.* 2010;29(10):1074–1099. https://doi.org/10.1521/jscp.2010.29.10.1074.

87. Zeiders KH, Landor AM, Flores M, Brown A. Microaggressions and diurnal cortisol: examining within-person associations among African-American and Latino Young Adults. *J Adolesc Health.* 2018;63(4):482–488. https://doi.org/10.1016/j.jadohealth.2018.04.018.

88. Steele CM, Spencer SJ, Aronson J. Contending with group image: the psychology of stereotype and social identity threat. *Adv Exp Soc Psychol.* 2002;34:379–440. https://doi.org/10.1016/S0065-2601(02)80009-0.

89. Diaz T, Navarro JR, Chen EH. An institutional approach to fostering inclusion and addressing racial bias: implications for diversity in academic medicine. *Teach Learn Med.* 2020;32(1):110–116. https://doi.org/10.1080/10401334.2019.1670665.

90. Thurber A, DiAngelo R. Microaggressions: intervening in three acts. *J Ethn Cult Divers Soc Work.* 2018;27(1):17–27. https://doi.org/10.1080/15313204.2017.1417941.

91. Wheeler DJ, Zapata J, Davis D, Chou C. Twelve tips for responding to microaggressions and overt discrimination: when the patient offends the learner. *Med Teach.* 2019;41(10):1112–1117. https://doi.org/10.1080/0142159X.2018.1506097.

92. Byrd CM. Microaggressions self-defense: a role-playing workshop for responding to microaggressions. *Soc Sci.* 2018;7(6). https://doi.org/10.3390/socsci7060096.

93. Bullock JL, O'Brien MT, Minhas PK, Fernandez A, Lupton KL, Hauer KE. No one size fits all: a qualitative study of clerkship medical students' perceptions of ideal supervisor responses to microaggressions. *Acad Med.* 2021;96(11S):S71–S80. https://doi.org/10.1097/ACM.0000000000004288.

94. Edmondson A. Psychological safety and learning behavior in work teams. *Adm Sci Q.* 1999;44(2):350–383. https://doi.org/10.2307/2666999.

95. Edmondson AC. *The Fearless Organization: Creating Psychological Safety in the Workplace for Learning, Innovation, and Growth.* John Wiley & Sons, Inc; 2019.

96. Steele DM, Cohn-Vargas B. *Identity Safe Classrooms: Places to Belong and Learn.* Corwin, a Sage Company; 2013.

6

Dismantling Ableism in Interprofessional Medical Education to Promote Health Equity for People With Disabilities

Deana Herrman, Amanda Sharp, Cara N. Whalen Smith, Zoie C. Sheets, Ryan McGraw, Janine Salameh, Erin Hickey, and Kristin Berg

SUMMARY

Ableism is pervasive in medical education and practice. A form of systemic oppression, ableism assigns people value based on societal ideals of normal, ability, and wellness/health to disadvantage anyone not meeting these ideals, especially disabled people. This framing, in conjunction with the predominantly medical model of disability taught in health professions education, results in focusing students primarily on curing impairments. Thus, students may overlook the social, political, and cultural aspects of disability and ignore the intersections of disability with other marginalized identities. Research demonstrates that health care providers are inadequately prepared to meet the health care needs of people with disabilities (PWD). This results in disparate access to equitable health care and consequently poorer health outcomes for PWD than for patients without disabilities. We contend that to improve care and outcomes for PWD, ableist notions and practices within health professions education must be intentionally dismantled and replaced with education which includes the **social model of disability** and the expertise of disabled people.

In this chapter, we reimagine the future of **interprofessional medical education** with an interprofessional team of disabled and nondisabled educators, clinicians, and advocates. We first discuss experiences with disability instruction from the lens of our home disciplines and personal positioning. We then present how disability competencies align with interprofessional values as a jumping-off point for instruction inclusive of disability. Next, using **critical disability studies** and an **intersectional disability justice** framework we present areas for enhancement and redress in education to prepare health professions students to address ableism.

Our imagined future of medical education breaks down silos between professional clinical knowledge and lived disability expertise, elevating disability justice across the curriculum. Our model, The Path to Anti-Ableist Transformation in Health Professions Education (PATH), guides our process and offers a path to transformation with strategies for programs to facilitate disability consciousness raising for their students. We propose actions to transform traditional interprofessional patient/provider hierarchies, thereby preparing students to collaborate with the disability community. We discuss strategies for teaching students to minimize the accompanying systemic barriers which result from ableism in the health care system. We invite readers to imagine anti-ableist interprofessional medical education and to spark ideas to initiate change in their own knowledge base and education programs around disability instruction.

POSITION STATEMENT FROM THE AUTHORS

We represent different identities and backgrounds. We are collectively disability self-advocates and allies to the disability community. We are disabled. We are nondisabled. Some of us are parents to disabled children, and others of us learn from our disabled siblings, friends, colleagues, patients, and educators. We are health care providers, educators, and recipients of care. We have been on the receiving end of ableist comments about functioning, movement, abilities, and needs; we have inevitably perpetuated ableism. We have upheld norms and barriers to care as we worked in health systems that do not allow flexibility, nuance, or a method for complete full care. We have experienced frustration in getting our own or a family member's social and health care needs met. We are not limited to our disability identities and understand the limits of our own experiences. These positions influence how we understand disability positioning and medical education approaches to disability.

INTRO VIGNETTE

In an hour-long session entitled "Interprofessional Experience with Disability," students from the schools of medicine, physical therapy, public health, and social work at Harmony University hear about the medical experiences and needs of the disabled community directly from a panel of disabled patients. The aim of this session is to help students from a myriad of educational backgrounds learn how to work together toward improving access to health care for people with disabilities. Topics raised by the panelists do not carry into other classes or discussions. Educators feel that while it is not the most ideal, the panel is better than nothing.

Harmony University is an unfortunate example of the missed opportunities that exist in medical education. With little to no direct content about disability and minimal

time dedicated to training with disabled communities, health care providers who graduate from Harmony lack the context, perspective, and foundational skills needed to maximize outcomes across all populations. As this chapter unfolds, we offer solutions to Harmony University's approach and close with an updated vignette designed to inspire institutions to aim higher regarding disability-inclusive education.

BACKGROUND

People with disabilities (PWD) are the largest historically underserved and marginalized population in the United States. Despite an estimated 26% of American adults having a disability, this group often has unaddressed health needs and has been recognized as a health disparities population.[1-5] The reasons for these disparities and inequities are often multifactorial, spanning from a lack of accessible equipment to perform necessary screening exams and treatments[6-12] and ineffective communication accommodations[13-15] to the unfounded assumption that disabled lives do not warrant the same level of protection as others.[7,16,17] Negative health outcomes experienced by PWD as the result of inaccessible health care practices are worsened by additional systemic obstacles and decreased resource availability in their everyday lives and in their communities (i.e., inadequate insurance coverage, lower quality housing, or neighborhood amenities). Compared to people without disabilities, PWD are more likely to be unemployed or underemployed, have inadequate housing, have lower household income, have less education, and have inadequate transportation.[18-20] Structural racism (i.e., how society fosters racial discrimination)[21] is also a factor in health inequities for people with disabilities. Accordingly, disabled people of color show higher rates of poor health outcomes, less self-reporting of good overall health, and higher mortality rates.[15,18,22-24] Economic concerns, isolation, and historic trauma from structural racism added to the stress and trauma experienced by disabled people during the COVID-19 pandemic.[25,26]

Doctors report being unprepared to address the health needs of people with disabilities, partially due to ableism in medical education and practice.[27] Ableism, a form of systemic oppression, assigns people value based on societal ideals of normal, ability, and wellness/health to disadvantage anyone not meeting these ideals, especially disabled people.[28-30] These thoughts and actions prioritize certain types of bodies and minds over others, creating a hierarchy of ability over assumedly inferior disability.[28] Ableism positions disability outside a predetermined societal "norm," and as such, has social, political, economic, and physical implications. Ableism further assumes monolithic experiences for disabled people, ignoring the fluid, fluctuating nature of disability. Ableism shapes the "normative construct" whereby any deviation requires interventions and rehabilitation to attain the norm.[30] Through an ableist lens, PWD are seen as burdens, with certain support and care needs devalued. Interdependence—a reliance on one another to achieve daily activities and goals—is viewed as being needy or overly dependent, despite the reality that interdependence is needed by most people to navigate modern society. Ableism further frames disability as an individual and isolated experience, often thinking of disability as an individual's problem to be corrected.[28-30] This framing ignores the ways in which additional social prejudices such as racism and sexism and systems of oppression including capitalism reinforce the negative framing of disability. Within these systems that prioritize particular ways of working, looking, and achieving, those at the intersections of identities outside of these ways of being are at higher risk of discrimination and harm. Disabled people of color, as an example, may experience the confounding impact of medical racism and ableism, leaving them to be disbelieved, ignored, or viewed as "challenging" patients.[24,31-33]

Ableism, so inherent in medical education, may be rooted in the medical model of disability, the prevailing disability model in medical practice. The medical model[34] posits disability itself as the problem, rather than the inaccessibility of our society or prevailing harmful beliefs. With disability as a "problem," the key solution is cure or medical intervention. Further, the medical model positions the provider as the keeper of the cure and serves to emphasize power dynamics in medicine. The social model of disability[34] directly responds to the medical model to position disability as a social construct faced by disabled people living with minds and bodies that fall outside of the prescribed "norm" and occurs because of physical, attitudinal, and institutional barriers. Physical barriers may include inaccessible building entrances or a lack of accessible medical examination equipment,[10,11] while attitudinal barriers are often based on broad assumptions and biases, including an assumption that people with disabilities experience poorer quality of life.[27] Institutional barriers may include a lack of employee training about disability culture or strict policies that do not allow the reality of living in an inaccessible world to be considered (i.e., inflexible policies regarding appointment arrival times combined with unrealistic health care provider productivity expectations resulting in unhappy patients and providers). The influence of the medical model and an ableist ideology entitles nondisabled people to avoid learning about disability as a sociopolitical experience, as this type of understanding is not necessary for medical intervention. Indeed, medical students are not required to take courses that focus on the social model of disability (in which ableism and inaccessibility are the problem) or to understand the impact of ableism on health outcomes. This leads to a medical education system that upholds ableist notions of disability, sending providers into the world unprepared to properly meet the needs of PWD and at risk of perpetuating harm.

Research documents significant gaps in the knowledge, attitudes, and skills that physicians and other health care professionals need to competently care for people with disabilities.[12,35] Iezzoni et al. found that among 714 practicing physicians in the United States, 82.4% believed incorrectly that PWD have worse quality of life than people without disabilities.[27] That same study reported that only 40.7% of physicians were "very confident" in their ability to provide the same quality of care to PWD as they do for patients without disabilities.[27] Most physicians were unaware of the ableism and biases experienced by PWD within the health care system, with only 18.1% strongly agreeing that the health care system often treats PWD unfairly.[27] Furthermore, in anonymous focus groups with physicians, Lagu et al. found that participants revealed negative attitudes toward PWD and readily used ableist language.[36] These physicians acknowledged a lack of sufficient knowledge, experience, and skills to care for PWD, reported little or no training around the Americans with Disabilities Act (ADA)[37] and its implication for clinical practice, and described instances of denying care for PWD or attempting to discharge PWD from their clinic without clear justification.[36] Indeed, PWD report negative health outcomes and difficulties getting care arising from negative interactions with health care providers.[38,39] The impact of ableist assumptions was particularly notable during the emergence of the COVID-19 pandemic as unlike other high-risk groups, specific public health guidelines for PWD were not available, and unsurprisingly, poor outcomes resulted.[22,40]

These studies suggest that providers are unprepared, uncomfortable, and unwilling to care for PWD. The reasons behind this are likely complex, rooted in the ableist pervasiveness of the medical model in medical education and the widespread ableism in our general society. Currently, a minimal number of undergraduate and graduate medical education programs offer any disability-related training, despite the National Council on Disability's 2022 Health Equity Framework including comprehensive training as a top priority.[17,27,38] A 2017 study examining disability awareness programs in US medical schools revealed that only 39 out of 75 responding institutions (50%) implemented "disability awareness" programs.[41] These programs were defined as providing education not solely focused on the medical/biological aspects but extending to encompass psychosocial aspects of living with a disability.[41] Similarly, in a survey of practicing internal medicine and family medicine residents, only 34.6% of residents reported receiving any disability-specific education in medical school.[42] When curricula have been developed and changes in both confidence and attitudes studied, teaching disability-related competencies to medical students has led to a clear improvement in these areas.[43–46] Unfortunately, these shortcomings persist despite demands from PWD, medical trainees, faculty, and allies for updated medical and health care provider curricula and despite demands for representation of PWD in all medical and health care education programs.[47,48]

One root of health disparities for PWD is the very biases that disability awareness programs attempt to address: it is often not that physicians lack medical knowledge about the population but that they do not apply their knowledge to PWD in the same way.[5] For example, PWD require the same preventive services as the general population under the United States Preventive Services Task Force (USPSTF); however, females with disabilities are less likely than those without disabilities to be up to date on pap smears and mammograms.[8–11,49,50] Females with disabilities diagnosed with breast cancer are less likely to undergo standard therapy after breast-conserving surgery and are more likely to experience inequities in their care for breast cancer than females without disabilities.[10,11] Despite training that most USPSTF recommendations apply to all patients, providers are often not applying this standard to PWD, resulting in a stark inequity for both rates of screening and intervention. This unequal application of medical knowledge as a provider starts in medical training due to absent disability-specific training and inadequate disability awareness programming.

To improve care and outcomes for PWD, ableist notions and practices within health professions education must be intentionally dismantled and replaced by disability-inclusive education with approaches like the social model of disability, critical disability studies, and disability justice to intentionally critique and analyze the way ableism influences policies and health equity. Our knowledge of these complex, intersecting barriers that impact health disparities of PWD makes clear that not only do physicians need adequate training on disability from a social and clinical standpoint, but the entire health care team must be equipped to dismantle these barriers using a collaborative approach. Educators must focus on the ableist biases in thinking and processes that lead providers to conclude that PWD do not require or are not deserving of the same level of care as people without disabilities.

Informed by our interprofessional team of disabled and nondisabled educators, clinicians, and advocates, we share

our own positioning in society and related to disability, as well as our discipline-specific roles and understanding of disability. We then build a transformational model of disability-inclusive/anti-ableist education for health professions and present tangible takeaways for readers.

PERSPECTIVES ABOUT DISABILITY AND HEALTH PROFESSIONALS' EDUCATION FROM AN INTERPROFESSIONAL COLLECTIVE

We learn, teach, practice, and engage with health professions education in an interprofessional education (IPE) framework. IPE is most simply collaborative learning between two or more professions with the goal of fostering a patient-centered practice.[51] Domains of IPE organize education and pedagogy to help us create a climate of shared respect and to enhance a student's eagerness to learn and develop active listening skills.[51] Additionally, in IPE we value the diversity of experiences of all learners and work collectively to impact health outcomes by improving effectiveness and equity of care.[51] We share our experiences to educate our health care providers, peers, and students in our home disciplines to better understand the complex disability phenomena, to understand the impact of upholding ableism, and to encourage the inclusion of disability in ongoing diversity work. The perspectives that follow reflect our shared positions and help frame our understanding of spaces we believe will enable us all to move beyond the ableist notions that currently exist across medical education programs.

Self-Advocates

We experience disability as an identity and as a culture. Disability is not something to be fixed by medicine. As advocates for our own needs, we expect medical care centered around our own goals. We must guide treatment and decisions in collaboration with medical professionals. Health care providers need excellent training around disability culture and identity, as well as training to develop clinical skills to deliver our care. Increasing the number of disabled clinicians and the number of clinicians who understand how to discuss disability in a respectful, informed, and anti-ableist way is critical. These changes are needed because the medical system can be very complicated for a person with a disability. These types of anti-ableist practices both set an example for colleagues and increase patient-provider trust and concordance. People with disabilities who themselves have experience navigating the medical system are more equipped to listen to and mentor based on their first-hand experiences. Having shared experiences enhances capacity for empathy and understanding and may offer this support needed for the patient with a disability to have the confidence to become their own self-advocates.

Social Work

Although the field of social work has made progress in recent decades, an individual, medical model of disability continues to persist both in education and clinical practice. Social work clinical approaches are often centered on supporting individuals (i.e., changing individual behaviors or collecting supportive resources) to help manage their medical condition, as opposed to addressing the socioeconomic and political conditions that undergird social and health inequities experienced by PWD. Classroom and clinical discussions about social work with marginalized and oppressed populations, including strategies to address implicit bias in practice, often fail to include PWD. Additionally, PWD are underrepresented in both the faculty body as well as the social work curriculum (i.e., readings, authorship), further marginalizing the voices and perspectives of the disability community from social work education and practice. Disabled students in social work are consequently subject to micro and overt aggressions as the language about disability can be pathologizing, resulting in implicit if not overt exclusion. A move toward greater representation of PWD in social work education and practice, as well as the promotion of disability cultural competencies with updated curricula and a strength-based model of interventions, could shift social work education and practice toward greater inclusion and empowerment of PWD.

Physical Therapy

Disability is still largely in the medical model and in an ableist perspective, framed as something that needs to be fixed with walking as the gold standard of mobility. This framing contradicts our position as movement experts who should embrace and promote multiple forms of mobility for society, including disabled students who seek to matriculate through our programs. In the absence of diversity, we miss celebrating the impacts from disability representation across the profession. This leads to a lack of creativity in our intervention approaches but also minimizes opportunities for change as we move past outdated curricula and competencies, update standards for matriculation, embrace technology advances, and ultimately improve language and systems of exclusion around disability.

Medicine

Disability in both medical education and practice is focused on the medical model; we are taught that disability is to be prevented or cured. The goal of medicine is often framed as identifying the pathology, then eliminating it. When not possible, we alleviate its impact. While promoting quality of life and reestablishing a functional baseline are important goals, using this type of model without a nuanced understanding of disability as a sociopolitical identity can lead to an assumption that the desired goal is the elimination of disability. Beyond the elimination of disability in an individual, medicine often seeks to avoid the reproduction of disability in others. History has proven the dangers of this model, with disabled people subjected to forced sterilization and inadequate life-saving interventions. Many medical schools have lectures about specific disabilities such as Down syndrome but focus more on the medical implications of the diagnosis rather than the lived experience of the person. A disability justice lens must be incorporated to better address not only the social experience of disability but also the responsibility of a provider to promote inclusion and access for all patients. Additionally, when a disability justice lens is incorporated, there must not be a disconnect between understanding disability justice principles and applying them to clinical care. For example, one principle of disability justice reminds us to "recognize wholeness," understanding that disabled people are indeed full people, with goals, strengths, weaknesses, relationships, and all the nuance of being human. This calls for providers to take a full social history for disabled patients, taking care not to skip critical sections due to an assumption that these patients may not have jobs, sexual relationships, or specific goals for their lives and futures. Recent movements have called for both an increase in disability education and increased representation of disabled physicians.[52-54]

Public Health

Public health still teaches about disability as an isolated population that has unique issues that need to be addressed rather than addressing the removal of barriers in society that disproportionately affect PWD and that would be beneficial to all populations, not just those with disabilities. Much of the focus in public health is on children with disabilities. There is less focus on transition age from youth to becoming an adult with a disability, community living, post-secondary education opportunities, and the many other areas intersecting with disability. Education promotes an emphasis on preventing death and disability without addressing the nuance in disability prevention. For example, preventing disability that results from gun violence makes sense, but endorsing genetic screening or genetic manipulation to prevent Down syndrome impacts how society views and acts toward people with Down syndrome. Universally validating Down syndrome as a disability to avoid applies a negative context, normalizes inferior feelings toward disabled people, and has the potential to lead down a path of eugenics. There is an opportunity for public health to provide guidance through the lens of the social model of disability, especially as we think about the barriers that impact societal health.

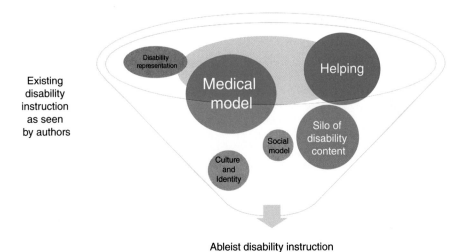

Existing disability instruction as seen by authors

Fig. 6.1 Elements that produce ableist disability instruction.

Our shared perspective is that disability is complex and not fully addressed in any of our professions' educational approaches or interventions. Fig. 6.1 shows how the elements we identify in current educational practices funnel together to produce the ableist disability instruction we see in our programs. The larger blue circles represent what was common across our perspectives and which currently have an outsize influence in education. Gray circles are the smaller elements that are less integrated throughout instruction.

But, while deficits are present, our perspectives highlight opportunities for change across our stories. Fig. 6.2 shows the interactions described in our perspectives, that if present will allow us to engage with the full spectrum of experiences that encompass disability, decrease responsibility on advocates to bring these elements to the forefront in interactions with health care providers, and ensure that instruction is without ableist perspectives.

INTERPROFESSIONAL EDUCATION FRAMEWORK FOR COMBATING ABLEISM IN HEALTH PROFESSIONS EDUCATION

We believe that utilizing an IPE framework in health professions education is one step toward combating ableism. The collaborative IPE approach and collective work to promote health lead students toward the social model of disability recognizing the responsibility of everyone to remove barriers to health for PWD. The IPE focus of centering of patients, including in this case patients with disabilities, along with the climate of respect and valuing of diverse experiences directly parallels the disability mantra "nothing about us

without us," and creates a disability-inclusive space for learning. The IPE framework offers a unique opportunity to add a disability curriculum and to address this topic with students from across all specialties. As all providers will likely work with patients with disabilities at some point in their education and careers, disability as a content area is relevant to all. The Alliance for Disability in Health Care Education (ADHCE) Core Competencies on Disability for Healthcare Education are a set of interprofessional disability-specific competencies developed with PWD and designed for all health care professionals across disability types that can be adopted and embedded in health care professions education.[35,55] The competencies act as a starting point for programs to help students shift away from the medical model thinking of disability and instead focus on treating PWD with respect and to recognize and guard against the bias of incorrect assumptions and low expectations when caring for patients with disabilities.[55] The competencies expect students to learn their legal obligations and responsibilities related to PWD in addition to developing clinical skills to meet the health needs of PWD. Finally, these competencies engage with topics of health equity and factors which impact the health of PWD including health promotion interventions.[55] Table 6.1 shows how the ADHCE and IPE competencies connect in relation to disability health equity.

We build upon these intersections to amplify efforts to dismantle barriers related to ableism that require self-examination and a broader review of structures or policies that uphold barriers. Competencies may address lack of skills and cultural awareness of disability, but assessing true impacts from changed attitudes may be harder to ascertain, particularly as the concept of disability identity as a

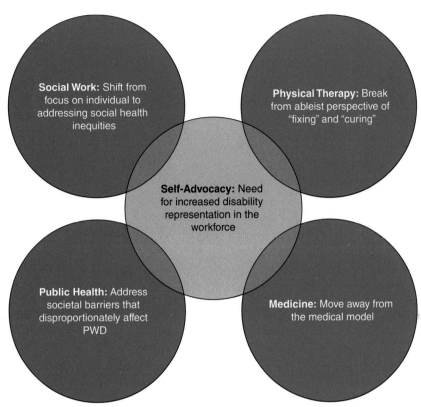

Fig. 6.2: Opportunities and necessary actions to highlight disability in education. *PWD*, People with disabilities.

TABLE 6.1.   Alliance for Disability in Health Care Education (ADHCE) and Interprofessional Education Competencies Related to Disability-Inclusive Education

Shared value	Core Competencies on Disability for Health Care Education (ADHCE)	Core Competencies for Interprofessional Collaborative Practice	Disability-Inclusive Education Emphasis
Collaboration	Competency 2: Professionalism and Patient-Centered Care Competency 4: Teams and Systems-Based Practice Competency 6: Clinical Care over the Lifespan and during Transitions	Competency 1: Values/Ethics for Interprofessional Practice Competency 2: Roles/Responsibilities Competency 3: Interprofessional Communication Competency 4: Teams and Teamwork	Health equity and health promotion for PWD; address social determinants of health for PWD
Person-Centered Care	Competency 2: Professionalism and Patient-Centered Care Competency 4: Teams and Systems-Based Practice Competency 5: Clinical Assessment Competency 6: Clinical Care over the Lifespan and during Transitions	Competency 1: Values/Ethics for Interprofessional Practice	Clinical Skills to deliver quality teams-based care to PWD

(Continued)

TABLE 6.1.   Alliance for Disability in Health Care Education (ADHCE) and Interprofessional Education Competencies Related to Disability-Inclusive Education—cont'd

Respect	Competency 2: Professionalism and Patient-Centered Care Competency 3: Legal Obligations and Responsibilities for Caring for Patients with Disabilities	Competency 1: Values/Ethics for Interprofessional Practice Competency 3: Interprofessional Communication	Recognize legal responsibilities; accommodations
Active Listening	Competency 2: Professionalism and Patient-Centered Care Competency 5: Clinical Assessment	Competency 3: Interprofessional Communication	Clinical Skills to deliver quality teams-based care to PWD; recognize disability culture and identity
Valuing Diversity	Competency 1: Contextual and Conceptual Frameworks on Disability Competency 2: Professionalism and Patient-Centered Care Competency 5: Clinical Assessment Competency 6: Clinical Care over the Lifespan and during Transitions	Competency 1: Values/Ethics for Interprofessional Practice Competency 2: Roles/Responsibilities Competency 3: Interprofessional Communication	Shift from medical model, incorporate social model and biopsychosocial model; recognize disability culture and identity
Collective Work to Impact Health Equity	Competency 1: Contextual and Conceptual Frameworks on Disability Competency 4: Teams and Systems-Based Practice Competency 5: Clinical Assessment Competency 6: Clinical Care over the Lifespan and during Transitions	Competency 1: Values/Ethics for Interprofessional Practice Competency 2: Roles/Responsibilities Competency 4: Teams and Teamwork	Health equity and health promotion for PWD; address social determinants of health for PWD

PWD, People with disabilities.

form of diversity has not been integrated into all medical education training.[47,48,56] As such, we consider these necessary to weave within and integrate across IPE education. Competencies can guide education, yet intentional guidance is necessary to truly be transformative and to dismantle the harms of ableism. Foundational work grounded in the perspectives of disabled people, like those found in critical disability studies and across the disability justice movement, is covered in the next section.

CRITICAL DISABILITY STUDIES AND DISABILITY JUSTICE

Critical disability studies (CDSs) recognize how ableism influences structures, policies, and approaches to equity.[57–60] CDS analyzes disability as a cultural, historical, social, and political phenomenon, centering the experiences and expertise of PWD. CDS positions disability as diversity—a complex social construct, culture, and identity to transform systems.[57–60] Contextualizing disability challenges the objectivity of standards and the idea that disability is not an avenue for social change, questioning the positioning of disability in systems of privilege and oppression.[57–60] CDS rejects the idea of disability as less than, but rather notes that, like all social identities, it is an experience that is shaped entirely by its surroundings. While this approach allows us to identify areas for change and collaboration, CDS has historically been centered on the experience of white disabled people, failing to recognize the critical implications of intersectionality. A movement, #DisabilityTooWhite, has called for CDS to center those who are most impacted by ableism, those living at the intersection of multiple marginalized identities.[61]

The disability justice movement was born out of a recognition that the disability rights movement also centered on only a relatively few members of the disability community. Formally named in 2005—although active long before—the disability justice movement was founded by queer, disabled, people of color, including Patricia Berne, Mia Mingus, and Leroy Moore.[62] The disability justice movement acknowledges gains made by disabled people while recognizing that progress for multiple marginalized disabled people has not been realized, with solutions unable to combat the root causes of ableism that keep disabled people isolated, in poverty, and targets for surveillance.[62,63] Disability justice focuses on queer, trans, Black, Indigenous, person/people of color (QTBIPOC) and what they need to live and thrive and how they organize to work together with movements and communities working to transform justice (i.e., antiracist, reproductive justice).[62,64] Intentionally intersectional, the disability justice movement works to celebrate and elevate the stories, needs, and contributions of historically marginalized disabled people with multiple identities.[62,64] Using 10 guiding principles,[62] it calls for the movement to not only be intersectional and focused on cross-disability solidarity but to hold firm against capitalism and the prioritization of productivity and money over the well-being of people. The intersectional nature of race and disability highlights the markers of identity alongside social class and gender to reveal knowledge and uncover embedded racism and ableism in medical education and health care systems to show how positioning of multiple identities (i.e., Black and disabled) experience inequality.[65] This approach moves us toward a more whole and complete understanding of experiences aligning with multiple disability justice principles, moving students to see disability as a societal responsibility to be considered with collective action from multiple people, not solely reliant on individual interventions.

It is through an understanding and integration of critical disability studies, disability justice, and the social model of disability that both physical and social accessibility in medicine will occur, and disability consciousness will be raised. Relying on the wisdom of these frameworks will promote the dismantling of barriers and structures that promote negative and incomplete views of disability. Not only can this improve outcomes for disabled patients, but it can also increase the inclusion of disabled learners across the health professions. The frameworks promote inclusion of cultural elements of disability and models of disability as relevant underpinnings of how students are taught to implement interventions,[56] and thus shift teaching strategies to include additional expertise from PWD and encourage new teaching approaches. The intersection of disability across populations will be highlighted as students learn that disability does not exist in a silo but is relevant to and the responsibility of all.

We envision a transformation informed by elements of cultural competence, humility, and consciousness centering disability.[48,66-68] The Path to Anti-Ableist Transformation in Health Professions Education (PATH), depicted in Fig. 6.3, moves from existing ableism to a disability awareness, to competence, and finally a disability consciousness recognized as an ongoing evolving process symbolized by the ongoing arrow direction.

THE PATH TO DISMANTLING ABLEISM AND REIMAGINING EDUCATION

Dismantling ableism in medical education is possible and, in the process, creates opportunities for productive changes that will ultimately impact health equity for PWD. In addition to following IPE values and meeting competencies

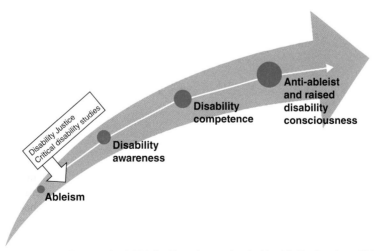

Fig. 6.3: Model: the Path to Anti-Ableist Transformation in Health Professions Education.

around disability, integrating CDS and disability justice throughout the curriculum broadens a student's knowledge base to increase disability cultural humility and disability consciousness. The **PATH** to transformation begins as programs move away from ableism to help students develop an awareness of the social context of disability and an awareness of one's own bias and knowledge base of disability. Next programs promote disability competence as disability content and competencies are threaded across curricula. Educators prepare to teach students content, and IPE experiences with PWD are considered core experiences. Disability consciousness is without a firm endpoint but rather an ongoing process for students. As programs evolve over time and continue to refine instruction, they will graduate disability-conscious providers. Fig. 6.4 details additional strategies for programs to employ within our PATH, as we imagine the outcomes from this transformation in this section, concluding with the transformation of Harmony University as they embrace our model.

A disability justice and critical disability studies lens as foundational and integrated across IPE education will push the understanding of these competencies to raise disability consciousness[48] through the PATH. Health professions education programs will dedicate resources and time to train educators around disability and health equity. Retention strategies will be implemented to keep and support educators, disabled students, and PWD who are sharing expertise. With the PATH as the guide, experiential learning opportunities are integrated across curricula with a minimum set number of courses in an IPE setting related to disability (e.g., accessibility of the health care environment, psychosocial aspects of health and disability, disability lab practicum, evidence-based practice, health promotion of PWD, disability in US society). Interprofessional clinics that focus on best practices for PWD are commonplace. Simulations where students "pretend" to have a disability, activities known to be harmful to the disabled community,[69-71] are discarded as an educational practice. Instead, students engage with the disability experience from the lens of a peer, collaborator, friend, and ally to integrate social, political, and cultural elements into their own understanding of disability. This translates into how students collaborate with patients and recognize interdependence. Student teams will work collaboratively with patients until their needs are sufficiently met. Student assessment measures expand to include metrics of care and support given, efforts to address barriers to health

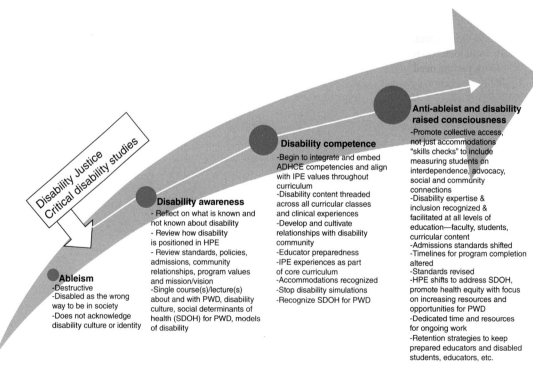

Fig. 6.4: Path to Anti-Ableist Transformation in Health Professions Education with strategies to move toward anti-ableism and disability consciousness.

care, and collaboration skills. Additional skills that are valued in this new model include reflection, evidence of growth in learning, and efforts to decrease bias.

A "new" generalist option for future health care providers is created across health professions education. Students continue to learn didactically relevant material, but clinical experiences change to reflect student preference for practice and their abilities, as well as community needs. Care is reconceptualized in terms of communities rather than just strictly providers and patients.[48] Accessibility audits of spaces, policies, and communities become a standard part of coursework to fully engage with community needs. Students will work in interprofessional teams to remove health care access barriers and community resource-related barriers. One can imagine a health professions education program specifically set in a community without adequate access to health care services (i.e., rural areas, under-resourced, health professional shortage areas). This program will train providers to specifically serve the needs of the community while training them in the community. For example, physicians will be geared toward primary care to serve a void while physical therapist students hone their primary care skills in addition to focusing on musculoskeletal impairments. Social workers, public health, and nursing professionals will work with community members to create resources, spaces for community collaboration, and peer health worker programs to involve the community in a more collective and communal approach. Students across all professions will focus on mobile and home health, delivering care where people need it.

Additionally, programs will make efforts to review who is entering programs as students and how they are supported. Students admitted to health professions education programs will come from humanities and nonmedical undergraduate majors. Programs will make time and space in the curricula for these students to learn the hard sciences and expand the length of time allowed to complete health professions education programs. Accessible, functional technical standards, universal design learning strategies, and a commitment to the success of disabled students in programs will be a core part of programs following the PATH. Creative approaches that pair students with and without disabilities become common in individual health profession curricula and across programs. Importantly, students learn that their success is dependent on the success of their peers and communities, and they work toward a collaborative shared goal.

CONCLUDING VIGNETTE

Harmony University now promotes inclusion, diversity, health equity, and justice in its mission and vision statements.

They meet these aims with a comprehensive, thoughtful, and interprofessional approach to medical education based on the PATH, one that threads intersectionality, disability expertise, and disability justice throughout. Unlike in previous years, people with disabilities are now represented both as faculty and as students. They regularly self-assess and adapt to avoid exclusion and to ensure graduates have the contemporary knowledge to meet the needs of all patients. Beyond just preparing graduates to effectively oversee a visit to a doctor, the school embeds learning activities to promote critical reflection on factors which influence health. Because of the intentional scaffolding of curricular components and the consistent way in which content is delivered, students are prepared to address barriers and facilitators of health in ways that best meet societal needs.

Students first gain disability awareness and become fluent in social, cultural, and political domains of disability and engage collaboratively with a broad group of interprofessional students. Trainees meet the Core Competencies on Disability for Health Care Education[55] to raise disability competence. Students are educated on ableism, the disability rights movement, and on existing barriers that impede access to society. During coursework, students work with standardized patients who have physical, mobility, intellectual, developmental, emotional, and mental health disabilities. Students participate in interprofessional roundtable sessions and discuss decisions impacting patients.

Responsibility for maintaining this level of preparedness and transformation is not just left to a few educator champions. All administrators and faculty are expected to serve and contribute across the program. Harmony University includes a focus on scholars, clinical preceptors, and faculty who have embraced change and on hiring disabled experts across all levels, documenting and reporting these hiring metrics on annual reports. Harmony has also prioritized community involvement in education. This is achieved over a period of years, where administrators, educators, and clinical faculty listen to the needs of communities and by participating in community-based social and cultural events. Learning circles of interprofessional teams are developed to foster shared accountability for care. Teams engage in community-based experiences embedded longitudinally across program curricula. As a result of these program shifts, student assessment expands. Reflective activities and engagement with communities are recognized and assessed as essential components of learning. Now, students have opportunities to integrate technical knowledge in a manner that is acceptable for diverse communities. Additionally, students meet "growth checkpoints" where students are asked to demonstrate their growth and aptitude to the language of development, impairments, and illness from normal and abnormal to a way that respects the dignity, autonomy, and rights of PWD.

The school is an exemplar and administrators are working with accreditation bodies to change required program and curricular elements to include measures found on the PATH. At the winter gala, the school's dean (a proudly disabled doctor of color herself), celebrated successes of the school. She delivered a rousing call to action imploring the students, faculty, and staff to continue raising their own disability consciousness and encouraging others to do the same.

CONCLUSION

Ableism present in health professions education impacts health outcomes for PWD. To transform health professions education and move toward a disability consciousness, programs need to understand and integrate critical disability studies, disability justice, and the social model of disability. Our proposed PATH model gives tangible strategies to offer opportunities for students to include voices and expertise of disabled people, value interdependence, and work toward collective access. As readers move along the PATH to integrate disability justice and strategies into their own programs, questions to consider are the following:

How is disability expertise integrated across curricula and into clinical or experiential learning experiences at your institution?

How will you dismantle ableism in your health profession education program?

REFERENCES

1. Varadaraj V, Deal JA, Campanile J, Reed N, Swenor BK. National prevalence of disability and disability types among adults in the US, 2019. *JAMA Netw Open.* 2021;4(10):e2130358. https://doi.org/10.1001/jamanetworkopen.2021.30358.
2. National Institutes of Health. *NIH Designated People With Disabilities as a Population for Health Disparities Research.* 2023https://www.nih.gov/news-events/news-releases/nih-designates-people-disabilities-population-health-disparities
3. Videlefsky A, Reznik JM, Nodvin J, Heiman HJ. Addressing health disparities in adults with developmental disabilities. *Ethn Dis.* 2019;29(Supp2):355–358. https://doi.org/10.18865/ed.29.s2.355.
4. Mahmoudi E, Meade MA. Disparities in access to health care among adults with physical disabilities: analysis of a representative national sample for a ten-year period. *Disabil Health J.* 2015;8(2):182–190. https://doi.org/10.1016/j.dhjo.2014.08.007.
5. Krahn GL, Walker DK, Correa-De-Araujo R. Persons with disabilities as an unrecognized health disparity population. *Am J Public Health.* 2015;105(Suppl 2):S198–S206. https://doi.org/10.2105/AJPH.2014.302182.
6. National Council on Disability. *Enforceable Accessible Medical Equipment Standard.* 2021https://ncd.gov/publications/2021/enforceable-accessible-medical-equipment-standards. Page no longer available.
7. Matin BK, Williamson HJ, Karyani AK, Rezaei S, Soofi M, Soltani S. Barriers in access to healthcare for women with disabilities: a systematic review in qualitative studies. *BMC Women's Health.* 2021;21(1). https://doi.org/10.1186/s12905-021-01189-5.
8. Baruch L, Bilitzky-Kopit A, Rosen K, Adler L. Cervical cancer screening among patients with physical disability. *J Womens Health (Larchmt).* 2022;31(8):1173–1178. https://doi.org/10.1089/jwh.2021.0447.
9. Kilic A, Tastan S, Guvenc G, Akyuz A. Breast and cervical cancer screening for women with physical disabilities: a qualitative study of experiences and barriers. *J Adv Nurs.* 2019;75(9):1976–1986. https://doi.org/10.1111/jan.14048.
10. Agaronnik N, El-Jawahri A, Iezzoni LI. Implications of physical access barriers for breast cancer diagnosis and treatment in women with mobility disability. *J Disabil Policy Stud.* 2021;33(1):46–54. https://doi.org/10.1177/10442073211010124.
11. Agaronnik N, El-Jawahri A, Kirschner KL, Iezzoni LI. Exploring cancer treatment experiences for patients with preexisting mobility disability. *Am J Phys Med Rehabil.* 2020;100(2):113–119. https://doi.org/10.1097/phm.0000000000001622.
12. World Health Organization. Global Report on Health Equity for Persons With Disabilities. 2022. https://www.who.int/publications/i/item/9789240063600.
13. Agaronnik N, Campbell EG, Ressalam J, Iezzoni LI. Communicating with patients with disability: Perspectives of practicing physicians. *J Gen Intern Med.* 2019;34(7):1139–1145. https://doi.org/10.1007/s11606-019-04911-0.
14. Sharby N, Martire K, Iversen MD. Decreasing health disparities for people with disabilities through improved communication strategies and awareness. *Int J Environ Res Public Health.* 2015;12(3):3301–3316. https://doi.org/10.3390/ijerph120303301.
15. Yee S, Breslin M, Goode T, Havercamp S, Horner-Johnson W, Iezzoni L, Krahn G. *Compound Disparities: Health Equity at the Intersection of Disability, Race, and Ethnicity.* National Academics; 2017. https://dredf.org/wp-content/uploads/2018/01/Compounded-Disparities-Intersection-of-Disabilities-Race-and-Ethnicity.pdf.
16. Stainton T. Disability, vulnerability and assisted death: commentary on Tuffrey-Wijne, Curfs, Finlay and Hollins. *BMC Med Ethics.* 2019;20(1). https://doi.org/10.1186/s12910-019-0426-2.
17. National Council on Disability. *The Current State of Health Care for People With Disabilities.* NCD; 2009. https://files.eric.ed.gov/fulltext/ED507726.pdf.
18. Courtney-Long EA, Romano S, Carroll DD, Fox MH. Socioeconomic factors at the intersection of race and ethnicity influencing health risks for people with disabilities. *J Racial Ethn Health Disparities.* 2016;4(2):213–222. https://doi.org/10.1007/s40615-016-0220-5.

19. Erickson W, Lee C, von Schrader S. *Disability Status Report: United States.* Cornell University Yang-Tan Institute on Employment and Disability; 2017.
20. Bureau of Labor Statistics. *Labor Force Statistics From the Current Population Survey: Supplemental Data Measuring the Effects of the Coronavirus (COVID-19) Pandemic on the Labor Market.* https://www.bls.gov/cps/effects-of-the-coronavirus-COVID-19-pandemic.htm#highlights%20Oct%202020.
21. American Medical Association. *What Is Structural Racism.* https://www.ama-assn.org/delivering-care/health-equity/what-structural-racism.
22. Verduzco-Gutierrez M, Lara AM, Annaswamy TM. When disparities and disabilities collide: inequities during the COVID-19 pandemic. *PM&R.* 2021;13(4):412–414. https://doi.org/10.1002/pmrj.12551.
23. Velasco-Mondragón E, Angela J, Palladino-Davis AG, Davis D, Escamilla-Cejudo JA. Hispanic health in the USA: a scoping review of the literature. *Public Health Rev.* 2016;37(1). https://doi.org/10.1186/s40985-016-0043-2.
24. Dorsey Holliman B, Stransky M, Dieujuste N, Morris M. Disability doesn't discriminate: health inequities at the intersection of race and disability. *Front Rehabil Sci.* 2023;4:1075775. https://doi.org/10.3389/fresc.2023.1075775. Published 2023 Jul 6.
25. Lund EM, Forber-Pratt AJ, Wilson C, Mona LR. The COVID-19 pandemic, stress, and trauma in the disability community: a call to action. *Rehabil Psychol.* 2020;65(4):313–322. https://doi.org/10.1037/rep0000368.
26. Jashinsky TL, King CL, Kwiat NM, Henry BL, Lockett-Glover A. Disability and COVID-19: impact on workers, intersectionality with race, and inclusion strategies. *Career Dev Q.* 2021;69(4):313–325. https://doi.org/10.1002/cdq.12276.
27. Iezzoni LI, Rao SR, Ressalam J, et al. Physicians' perceptions of people with disability and their health care. *Health Aff (Millwood).* 2021;40(2):297–306. https://doi.org/10.1377/hlthaff.2020.01452.
28. Campbell FK. Inciting legal fictions: disability's date with ontology and the ableist body of the law. *Griffith Law Rev.* 2001;10:42–62.
29. Lewis TA. *Working Definition of Ableism.* 2019. https://www.talilalewis.com/blog/january-2021-working-definition-of-ableism.
30. Nario-Redmond MR. *Ableism: The Causes and Consequences of Disability Prejudice.* John Wiley & Sons; 2019.
31. Hall WJ, Chapman MV, Lee KM, et al. Implicit racial/ethnic bias among health care professionals and its influence on health care outcomes: a systematic review. *Am J Public Health.* 2015;105(12):e60–e76. https://doi.org/10.2105/ajph.2015.302903.
32. Hoffman KM, Trawalter S, Axt JR, Oliver MN. Racial bias in pain assessment and treatment recommendations, and false beliefs about biological differences between blacks and whites. *Proc Natl Acad Sci U S A.* 2016;113(16):4296–4301. https://doi.org/10.1073/pnas.1516047113.
33. Brown C, Marshall A, Snyder CR, et al. Perspectives about racism and patient-clinician communication among Black adults with serious illness. *JAMA Network Open.* 2023;6(7):e2321746. https://doi.org/10.1001/jamanetworkopen.2023.21746.
34. Oliver M. *The Politics of Disablement: A Sociological Approach.* St. Martin's Press; 1990.
35. Havercamp SM, Barnhart WR, Robinson AC, Whalen Smith CN. What should we teach about disability? National consensus on disability competencies for health care education. *Disabil Health J.* 2021;14(2):100989. https://doi.org/10.1016/j.dhjo.2020.100989.
36. Lagu T, Haywood C, Reimold K, DeJong C, Sterling RW, Iezzoni LI. 'I Am Not The Doctor For You': physicians' attitudes about caring for people with disabilities. *Health Aff (Millwood).* 2022;41(10):1387–1395. https://doi.org/10.1377/hlthaff.2022.00475.
37. Americans with Disabilities Act of 1990, Pub L No. 101-336, 104 Stat 327. 1990.
38. National Council on Disability. *Health Equity Framework for People With Disabilities.* 2022. https://ncd.gov/sites/default/files/NCD_Health_Equity_Framework.pdf. No longer available.
39. Herrman D, Papadimitriou C, Green B, LeFlore A, Magasi S. Relationships at Work: Integrating the perspectives of disability partners to enhance a peer navigation intervention. *Front Rehab Sci.* 2022;3 https://doi.org/10.3389/fresc.2022.876636.
40. Desroches ML, Ailey SH, Fisher K, Stych J. Impact of COVID-19: nursing challenges to meeting the care needs of people with developmental disabilities. *Disabil Health J.* 2021;14(1):101015. https://doi.org/10.1016/j.dhjo.2020.101015.
41. Seidel E, Crowe S. The state of disability awareness in American Medical Schools. *Am J Phys Med Rehabil.* 2017;96(9):673–676. https://doi.org/10.1097/PHM.0000000000000719.
42. Stillman MD, Ankam N, Mallow M, Capron M, Williams S. A survey of internal and family medicine residents: assessment of disability-specific education and knowledge. *Disabil Health J.* 2021;14(2):101011. https://doi.org/10.1016/j.dhjo.2020.101011.
43. Symons AB, Morley CP, McGuigan D, Akl EA. A curriculum on care for people with disabilities: effects on medical student self-reported attitudes and comfort level. *Disabil Health J.* 2014;7(1):88–95. https://doi.org/10.1016/j.dhjo.2013.08.006.
44. Borowsky H, Morinis L, Garg M. Disability and ableism in medicine: a curriculum for medical students. *MedEdPORTAL.* 2021;17:11073. https://doi.org/10.15766/mep_2374-8265.11073. Published 2021 Jan 25.
45. Sarmiento CM, Miller SR, Chang E, Zazove P, Kumagai AK. From impairment to empowerment. *Acad Med.* 2016;91(7):954–957. https://doi.org/10.1097/acm.0000000000000935.
46. Ali R, Amin I. Adding disability lectures to medical school curriculums. *Med Educ.* 2023;57(5):466. https://doi.org/10.1111/medu.15055.
47. Feldner HA, Evans HD, Chamblin K, et al. Infusing disability equity within rehabilitation education and practice: a

qualitative study of lived experiences of ableism, allyship, and healthcare partnership. *Front Rehabil Sci.* 2022;3:947592. https://doi.org/10.3389/fresc.2022.947592. Published 2022 Aug 2.

48. Doebrich A, Quirici M, Lunsford C. COVID-19 and the need for disability conscious medical education, training, and practice. *J Pediatr Rehabil Med.* 2020;13(3):393–404. https://doi.org/10.3233/PRM-200763.

49. Xu X, Mann JR, Hardin JW, Gustafson E, McDermott SW, Deroche CB. Adherence to US Preventive Services Task Force recommendations for breast and cervical cancer screening for women who have a spinal cord injury. *J Spinal Cord Med.* 2017;40(1):76–84. https://doi.org/10.1080/10790268.2016.1153293.

50. Xu X, McDermott SW, Mann JR, et al. A longitudinal assessment of adherence to breast and cervical cancer screening recommendations among women with and without intellectual disability. *Prev Med.* 2017;100:167–172. https://doi.org/10.1016/j.ypmed.2017.04.034.

51. Interprofessional Education Collaborative. *Core Competencies for Interprofessional Collaborative Practice: 2023 Update.* ipecollaborative.org.

52. Meeks LM, Herzer K, Jain NR. Removing barriers and facilitating access: increasing the number of physicians with disabilities. *Acad Med.* 2018;93(4):540–543. https://doi.org/10.1097/ACM.0000000000002112.

53. Schwarz CM, Zetkulic M. You belong in the room: addressing the underrepresentation of physicians with physical disabilities. *Acad Med.* 2019;94(1):17–19. https://doi.org/10.1097/ACM.0000000000002435.

54. Singh S, Meeks LM. Disability inclusion in medical education towards a quality improvement approach. *Med Educ.* 2022;57(1):102–107. https://doi.org/10.1111/medu.14878.

55. Alliance for Disability in Health Care Education. *Core Competencies on Disability for Health Care Education.* 2019. https://www.adhce.org/Core-Competencies-on-Disability-for-Health-Care-Education.

56. Kaundinya T, Schroth S. Dismantle ableism, accept disability: making the case for Anti-Ableism in medical education. *J Med Educ Curric Dev.* 2022;9 https://doi.org/10.1177/23821205221076660. 238212052210766.

57. Gibson B. *Rehabilitation: A Post-Critical Approach.* CRC Press; 2016.

58. Schalk S. Critical disability studies as methodology. *Lateral: Journal of the Cultural Studies Association.* https://csalateral.org/issue/6-1/forum-alt-humanities-critical-disability-studies-methodology-schalk/.

59. Schalk S. *Black Disability Politics.* Duke University Press; 2022. https://www.dukeupress.edu/black-disability-politics.

60. Kafer A. *Feminist, Queer, Crip.* Indiana University Press; 2013. https://iupress.org/9780253009340/feminist-queer-crip/.

61. Thompson V. *#DisabilityTooWhite, Twitter.* https://twitter.com/search?q=disabilitytoowhite&src=recent_search_click..

62. Sins Invalid. *10 Principles of Disability Justice.* 2015. https://www.sinsinvalid.org/blog/10-principles-of-disability-justice.

63. Mingus M. *Changing the Framework: Disability Justice.* Leaving Evidence; 2011. https://leavingevidence.wordpress.com/2011/02/12/changing-the-framework-disability-justice/.

64. Piepzna-Samarasinha L. *The Future Is Disabled.* Arsenal Pulp Press. https://arsenalpulp.com/Books/T/The-Future-Is-Disabled.

65. Annamma SA, Connor D, Ferri B. Dis/ability critical race studies (DisCrit): theorizing at the intersections of race and dis/ability. *Race Ethn Educ.* 2013;16(1):1–31.

66. Schwab SM, Silva PL. Intellectual humility: how recognizing the fallibility of our beliefs and owning our limits may create a better relationship between the physical therapy profession and disability. *Phys Ther.* 2023;103(8). https://doi.org/10.1093/ptj/pzad056.

67. Grandpierre V, Milloy V, Sikora L, Fitzpatrick E, Thomas R, Potter BK. Barriers and facilitators to cultural competence in rehabilitation services: a scoping review. *BMC Health Serv Res.* 2018;18(1). https://doi.org/10.1186/s12913-017-2811-1.

68. Center for Culturally Proficient Education. *What Is Cultural Proficiency?* 2020. https://ccpep.org/home/what-is-cultural-proficiency/the-continuum/.

69. Caston S, Sharp A. Cultivating disability humility: opportunities for course correction in healthcare. *J Allied Health.* 2024;55(3):227-230.

70. Nario-Redmond MR, Gospodinov D, Cobb A. Crip for a day: the unintended negative consequences of disability simulations. *Rehabil Psychol.* 2017;62(3):324–333. https://doi.org/10.1037/rep0000127.

71. Hicks EC, Traci MA, Korb K. "Sympathy" vs."Empathy": comparing experiences of I2Audits and disability simulations. *Front Rehabil Sci.* 2022;3 https://doi.org/10.3389/fresc.2022.876099.

7

The "Add-A-Slide" Approach
A Practical Solution for Integrating LGBTQ+ Health Topics into Undergraduate Medical Education

Kelly E. Bowen, Jeffrey Shu, Anthony Tizzano, Maeve K. Hopkins, and Jason V. Lambrese

SUMMARY

LGBTQ+ populations experience significant health inequities and have unique health needs, and medical students must be trained to address these in an affirming and competent manner. However, current medical school curricula have very little time dedicated to teaching medical students about LGBTQ+ health care. In this chapter, we outline our approach to increasing coverage of LGBTQ+ health care in our institution's preclinical curriculum. We discuss our methodologies for identifying what content to add and how to integrate it into the existing curriculum, highlighting our "Add-A-Slide" approach. Further, we review our process for iteratively reviewing our progress and adapting to address challenges or gaps in curricular coverage.

INTRODUCTION

Lesbian, gay, bisexual, transgender, and queer plus (LGBTQ+) populations experience health inequities, unequal access to care, and special health needs.[1,2] These inequities in care are due to an array of sociopolitical factors including systemic discrimination and high rates of minority stress.[2,3] In 2023 the political climate included a surge of state legislation restricting rights for LGBTQ+ populations, with over 520 bills introduced and 70 laws enacted. These bills and laws particularly affect transgender and gender-diverse youth, ranging from limiting health education in schools to banning gender-affirming health care.[4]

The LGBTQ+ population is estimated to comprise over 4% of the US population (over 20 million people), which is likely an underrepresentation given the difficulty in accurately measuring this population due to the reliance on self-reporting a minoritized identity.[3] However, LGBTQ+ patients face disproportionate barriers to accessing care, including prior experiences or fears of discrimination in the medical space, often leading sexual and gender minority (SGM) patients to present later in the course of disease, with missed opportunities for preventive care and early intervention. It is imperative that medical students are comfortable with and capable of addressing the unique health needs of the LGBTQ+ population.

While public support for same-sex marriage in the United States is at an all-time high and public discourse around LGBTQ+ identities has become more mainstream, medical education has lagged behind in adopting LGBTQ+ health topics.[2,5,6] Previous studies estimate a median of five hours is dedicated to education about sexual and gender minorities in undergraduate medical education[5] and limited discussion of SGM care in graduate medical education, with the amount of time spent differing by specialty. Notably, 67% of emergency medicine programs and 59%–80% of obstetrics and gynecology programs report no teaching on LGBTQ+ health.[6]

Previous studies have shown that increasing exposure to LGBTQ+ health topics in medical education increases student and physician skills and comfort when working with LGBTQ+ patients.[7] While elective courses and curricular add-ons have been successfully implemented in many medical schools to address this gap in education, these electives tend to self-select for students who are already interested in LGBTQ+ health, limiting the reach of these curricular interventions.[6,8] In clinical practice, every physician will inevitably treat LGBTQ+ patients during their careers. Consequently, all future physicians must have the core skills and knowledge to provide affirming and effective care, regardless of their clinical specialty.[2]

In this chapter, we present a cohesive initiative in which LGBTQ+ topics are not an elective course or standalone lecture in a "Doctoring" course, but integrated into standard, preexisting basic science seminars and discussions on clinical diagnosis and management. We describe how integration and dispersion of these learning objectives organically throughout the medical curriculum provides sufficient education in core competencies for caring for LGBTQ+ patients, regardless of specialty interest or practice area.

This "Add-A-Slide" model is a process for integrating LGBTQ+ health topics into undergraduate medical education. We developed and implemented this model at a small, research-focused medical school with a goal of continued and sustained exposure to LGBTQ+ learning objectives in the preclinical curriculum.[9] This model for curricular integration is broadly applicable to medical education and can be utilized for a variety of educational topics, particularly those that address the needs of underserved and minoritized patients (Fig. 7.1).

FORMING THE ACTION GROUP

The Cleveland Clinic Lerner College of Medicine (CCLCM) of Case Western Reserve University is a five-year medical

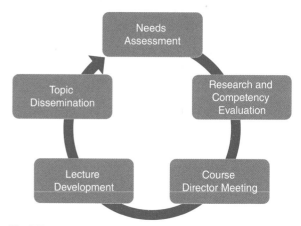

Fig. 7.1 Iterative process of the "Add-A-Slide" model for LGBTQ+ health topic integration.

school that offers a unique research-focused curriculum to a small class of 32 medical students per year. Students are encouraged to play an active role in feedback; this includes course evaluations and participation in diversity, equity, and inclusion (DEI) initiatives. The preclinical curriculum is divided into organ system blocks, with most organ systems covered in both the first ("normal physiology") and second ("abnormal pathology") years.

In Fall 2020 the CCLCM DEI Steering Committee issued a call to action in response to national events, emphasizing structural racism as a public health crisis and advocating for more inclusive and concrete steps toward positive change. As a response, the LGBTQ+ Curricular Change Action Group was started as a collaboration between students and faculty to address a gap in the observed curriculum, specific to LGBTQ+ health inequities.[10]

The goal of the action group was to incorporate LGBTQ+ health topics into the preclinical curriculum to promote greater exposure to LGBTQ+ populations and needs, with a long-term goal of preparing students for caring for a diverse patient population in their future careers.

Identifying Involved Parties

A key starting point for developing our action plan was to identify parties who would be affected by our curricular changes and the potential impacts of our project on each group. The ideal curricular intervention would need to be accepted, implemented, and sustained by each of the groups impacted by these changes. We identified the following as key parties for our program:

1. Current students undergoing preclinical medical education: One group most impacted by our curricular change project was the first- and second-year medical students who were progressing through the preclinical curriculum

during the time of the intervention. While implementing these adjustments over the course of the academic year can enhance students' education on LGBTQ+ patient care, making sweeping modifications to seminars, clinical cases, and activity scheduling would have been disruptive to the learning process. We identified strategies to alter the curriculum in a way that would minimally interfere with the planned curriculum and schedule but maximize the exposure to key health needs of LGBTQ+ patients.

2. Future students undergoing preclinical medical education: Similarly, we considered the needs of future students, as our curricular changes became a part of the standard curriculum and would be carried forward each year. We designed them to be sustainable and adaptable with future iterations of the preclinical curriculum. We highlighted key educational topics and competencies in learning objectives communicated to both students and faculty that would be maintained throughout curricular revisions.

3. Course directors: At CCLCM, course directors are responsible for (1) establishing and communicating learning objectives for each organ-system block in the preclinical curriculum, (2) coordinating seminars and educational materials for each organ block, (3) coordinating seminar leaders and seminar content, and (4) acting as liaisons between students and seminar leaders. Our curricular changes required the support of course directors to integrate LGBTQ+ specific learning objectives into their courses. Additionally, our changes balanced the breadth and depth of LGBTQ+ curricular topics to allow for adequate coverage of other key learning objectives in the course. In order to be successful, our intervention avoided asking for substantial additional curricular time in an already condensed preclinical curriculum. Instead we found creative ways to integrate LGBTQ+ health topics into pre-existing seminars and patient cases.

4. Seminar leaders: Within each course, basic science and clinical experts on a topic are recruited to give 1- to 2-hour seminars pertaining to each organ system. Options we considered for curricular changes included: (1) additions or modifications to the existing seminars or (2) new seminars dedicated to LGBTQ+ topics within each course, typically requiring new seminar leaders comfortable with the topic. Nevertheless, any changes required flexibility and adaptability with the teaching styles and content knowledge of a variety of faculty members and needed to have minimal barriers to implementation.

5. Office of Diversity, Equity, and Inclusion (DEI): On a larger scale, the Office of DEI has roadmaps for changing the climate of the hospital and medical school to be more inclusive and equitable. Our LGBTQ+ learning objectives were in accordance with the Office of DEI's roadmap and vision for climate change. The LGBTQ+ integration points suggested by our group successfully aligned with educational efforts for other marginalized groups and supplement ongoing DEI projects.

6. LGBTQ+ patients: Most importantly, we created our intervention to improve the knowledge, attitudes, and beliefs of medical students about the SGM community. The "Add-A-Slide" approach improves the quality of care for LGBTQ+ patients by training future physicians to be more knowledgeable about LGBTQ+ health care and to be more comfortable addressing a wide range of pertinent health topics.

Garnering Institutional Buy-In

With a small group of dedicated students and faculty, many of whom self-identify as members of the LGBTQ+ community, the action group released a "call to action" to recruit additional interested faculty members across the college. This "call to action" was essential for identifying students, faculty, and administrators who were supportive of these efforts. Action group members consisted of students from all years in the medical school, physicians practicing in various departments and specialties, preclinical course directors, retired emeritus physicians involved in medical education, and administrative staff. Each group member offered diverse strengths to the group—from clinical expertise treating LGBTQ+ populations, experience navigating medical education and curriculum design, existing relationships with educators in the medical school, or time to dedicate to action group tasks.

After solidifying the members of the action group, the team worked with the DEI office to formally designate the group as a committee of the Diversity, Equity, and Inclusion Task Force.[10] In addition to recruiting members to assist in activities of the action group, the formal establishment as part of the task force helped formalize its legitimacy and presence on the campus; in addition, educators with ideas for LGBTQ+ integration now had a designated contact to discuss ideas for engaging with LGBTQ+ topics in the curriculum. Collaboration with the larger DEI office enabled synergy with ongoing DEI efforts on anti-racism, microaggression training, and community outreach, and LGBTQ+ health became an endorsed curricular focus for the medical school.

CURRICULAR INTEGRATION

Needs Assessment

The Association of American Medical Colleges (AAMC) Advisory Committee on Sexual Orientation, Gender Identity, and Sex Development introduced 30 core competencies for physicians to best treat SGM populations.[11] Among these core competencies are recommended skills and tools for improving LGBTQ+ patient care in the domains of knowledge for practice, practice-based learning, interpersonal and communication skills, professionalism, systems-based practice, interprofessional collaboration, and personal/professional development. The 30 core competencies recommended by the AAMC provided a foundation from which we could build the specific learning points we sought to include in the preclinical curriculum.[12]

As first- and second-year medical students in our action group progressed through the preclinical courses in the 2020–21 academic year, they documented areas within each organ block course where integration of LGBTQ+ health topics easily fit. Students then mapped the suggested areas of integration onto and in line with the core competencies recommended by the AAMC with the goal that all CCLCM students would meet each AAMC core competency by participating in the standard curriculum. Students then conducted a comprehensive literature review of PubMed, using the keywords: "LGBTQ health," "queer," and each organ system ("cardiovascular," "renal," "infectious diseases," etc.). Students then identified health equity and disparities outcomes that had special concern for LGBTQ+ populations, with related and appropriate health care interventions. We consulted faculty content experts on the clinical relevance of these interventions and the identified educational gaps.

Alongside the literature review, the action group also conducted a survey of first- and second-year medical students to assess their knowledge and comfort with caring for LGBTQ+ patients. The survey provided a baseline for student knowledge and comfort in SGM health care at our medical school and assessed the current exposure to LGBTQ+ patients that students were receiving. Results from the survey provided guidance on specific integration points and which resources would best benefit students and educators; the survey results indicated that a majority of students were interested in receiving more LGBTQ+ education.[9]

Implementation

Following the systematic process of needs assessment and review of the literature to identify gaps in the curricula, the team mapped 59 new learning points to each of the 30 core competencies recommended by AAMC.

Applying the "Add-A-Slide" Approach

While identifying learning needs was a critical and humbling learning activity for the entire program, this information was useless unless we had an effective strategy for meaningfully integrating the 59 learning points into the curriculum. We recognized that the proposed integration approach would need to be accepted by all affected parties identified—students, course directors, seminar leaders, etc.

Additionally, the integration approach would need to be sustainable and have the ability to withstand changes to the curriculum from year to year.

In recognition of the 59 learning points and 30 core competencies, our group decided on a minimally disruptive integration approach that would achieve breadth and depth of LGBTQ+ medical education throughout the curriculum.

Rather than requesting additional LGBTQ-specific seminars, the deceptively simple "Add-A-Slide" approach was developed as a method of adding one or two PowerPoint-type slides to pre-existing basic science seminars during which a relevant LGBTQ+ learning point would pertain to the seminar topic. This approach is broadly applicable regardless of topic, learning objective, or seminar length. An additional benefit of the "Add-A-Slide" approach is that it creates a longitudinal and well-integrated exposure to LGBTQ+ health topics throughout the basic science curriculum. Rather than sequestering LGBTQ+ topics in a standalone "Doctoring" seminar or workshop, these health topics are incorporated into various organ systems and general medicine seminars. Lastly, the "Add-A-Slide" approach decreases the burden placed on educators, as they would need to create only one slide rather than restructure their existing presentations or cases or find time to create new dedicated seminars.

Student-Led Meetings With Course Directors and Lecturers

As part of the "Add-A-Slide" approach, students met with course directors and seminar leaders to discuss potential suggestions for integrating LGBTQ+ learning points into each organ system–based course. A table including the specific learning point, relevant seminar topic, references/learning materials, and corresponding AAMC core competency was provided to guide discussion (Table 7.1).

Seminar leaders were given the option to (1) receive references and learning materials on the LGBTQ+ learning points suggested for their topic and create the slide themselves or (2) receive a slide drafted by the action group to incorporate into their presentations (Fig. 7.2). Our curricular change efforts were met with overwhelming support from both course directors and seminar leaders. Most seminar leaders opted to create their own slides after being provided literature discussing LGBTQ+ health inequities. This collaboration between students, educators, and course organizers resulted in a synergistic relationship that fostered a supportive and inclusive climate at the institution.

Diversifying Clinical Cases Used in Small-Group Problem–Based Learning

In addition to seminars, our action group targeted clinical cases in problem-based learning (PBL) sessions present in the curriculum. During these educational sessions,

TABLE 7.1 Examples of Suggested LGBTQ+ Learning Points Provided to Course Directors

Type	Learning Point	Source	Integration Location	Association of American Medical Colleges Objective
Seminar	Puberty blockers: use in transitioning adolescents.	Rew L, Young CC, Monge M, Bogucka R. Review: Puberty blockers for transgender and gender diverse youth-a critical review of the literature. *Child Adolesc Ment Health.* 2021;26(1):3–14.	Cover in Precocious Puberty seminar	KFP 5, PC 3, SBP 6, PBL 1
Seminar	Transgender women are still at risk for prostate cancer (estrogen not as protective as previously thought) and should undergo screening.	Deebel NA, Morin JP, Autorino R, Vince R, Grob B, Hampton LJ. Prostate cancer in transgender women: incidence, etiopathogenesis, and management challenges. *Urology.* 2017;110:166–171.	Cover in PSA and Prostate Cancer seminar	KFP 4, PC 3,PC 6
Seminar	HPV susceptibility in transgender men is comparable to rates in cisgender women. There are inequities in cervical cancer screening in transgender men compared to cisgender women.	Dhillon N, Oliffe JL, Kelly MT, Krist J. Bridging barriers to cervical cancer screening in transgender men: a scoping review. *Am J Mens Health.* 2020;14(3):1557988320925691. doi:10.1177/1557988320925691.	Cover in Cervical Pathology seminar	KFP 5, PC 3, PC 6
Seminar	Breast cancer screening in transfeminine individuals occurs at lower rates. Moreover, exam is thought to be gender affirming.	Oladeru OT, Ma SJ, Miccio J, et al. Breast and cervical cancer screening disparities among transgender patients. *JCO.* 2020;38(15_suppl):7024–7024.	Cover in Breast Cancer and Pathology seminar	KFP 4, PC 6, IPCS 2
PBL	Sperm and oocyte banking options exist for transgender individuals prior to transitioning.	T'Sjoen G, Van Caenegem E, Wierckx K. Transgenderism and reproduction. *Curr Opin Endocrinol Diabetes Obes.* 2013;20(6):575–579.	Could be a learning objective or mentioned in the case for group discussion	KFP 4
PBL	Fertility options for same-sex couples.	Greenfeld DA, Seli E. Same-sex reproduction: medical treatment options and psychosocial considerations. *Curr Opin Obstet Gynecol.* 2016;28(3):202–205.	Could be a learning objective or mentioned in the case for group discussion	KFP 4

This is a subset of points integrated into the Endocrinology and Reproductive Biology block for second-year medical students. *PBL,* Problem-based learning sessions.

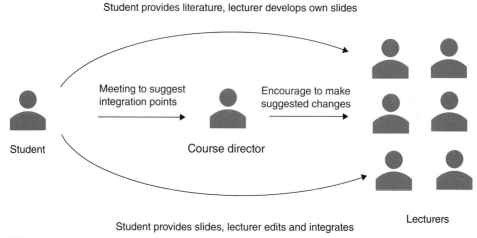

Student provides literature, lecturer develops own slides

Meeting to suggest integration points

Encourage to make suggested changes

Student

Course director

Lecturers

Student provides slides, lecturer edits and integrates

Fig. 7.2 Options for integration of LGBTQ+ educational slide(s) into existing lectures and seminars.

students would learn about the clinical presentation and management of certain pathologies through simulated clinical scenarios, following a single patient over the course of one week. In line with the efforts of the DEI office, we aimed to diversify the patient population present in these cases to expose students to intersectional identities and increase their comfort in working with a diverse patient population.

When appropriate, our group suggested an LGBTQ+ identity for some of the patients in the PBL cases. For example, we worked with case writers to change pronouns of sexual partners or alter the patient's gender expression. A key consideration during this effort was to diversify cases in a way that would not pigeonhole patients into certain diagnoses based on their sexuality or gender identity and to not introduce biases or reinforce stereotypes that are present in popular opinion. Many of our case diversification efforts were aimed at exposing students to appropriate language for discussing LGBTQ+ patients, increasing comfort with pronouns and honorifics, and spurring discussion around cognitive and diagnostic biases when presented with demographic information.

ITERATIVE EVALUATION OF THE CURRICULUM

Throughout our first academic year of curricular integration (2021–22), we established systems for continuously reviewing our progress. As first- and second-year students on our team moved through the preclinical curriculum, they took note of which integration points had been successfully incorporated and which curricular gaps persisted. We discussed our ongoing progress during our monthly

team meetings and kept running documents with tallies on integrated points and additional details on where and how they were covered. Each academic year has culminated in a comprehensive review where we determine how many of the integration points had been covered. This process has also allowed us to identify gaps in coverage, which helps guide our future focus areas and potential modifications for the next year's curriculum. At the end of our first year of implementation, we tallied that 68.8% (22/32) of points selected for the first-year curriculum and 44.4% (12/27) of points for the second-year curriculum were included. These numbers increased to 70.7% (29/41) and 76.9% (20/26), respectively, in our second year of implementation.

Faculty and student feedback has also been invaluable in our ongoing review process. Each year, we meet with course directors and other faculty members to solicit their feedback and discuss our program. In these meetings, we have also tried to identify any barriers or reasons why certain points might not have been integrated. Because course directors are the ones most familiar with the upcoming curriculum for each organ block, they have provided us with suggestions on where certain topics might fit best. This has been especially essential given the recent shortening of our program's preclinical curriculum. Some of the seminars that were initially included in our plans were removed, so course directors notified us of this and worked with us to find new potential places for the content. As part of our review process, we also consistently express our appreciation to all of the faculty who have helped us and thanked them for any of our content that they included in their seminars or courses.

At CCLCM, students regularly provide feedback on all seminars and PBL cases. This has been one avenue for students to comment on LGBTQ+ topics that have been well covered or point out areas that need improvement. Students from our team then present much of this feedback during our monthly meetings, and we incorporate this into our plans for the following year. Because students are the ones regularly interacting with the curriculum, their feedback has provided us with a lot of insight into how effectively our material resonates.

While we want as much of our content to be covered as possible, we also want to ensure that it is (1) effectively reaching students and (2) ultimately helping students provide better patient care for LGBTQ+ patients. To facilitate this goal, we designed a survey assessing medical students' knowledge and beliefs related to LGBTQ+ health care. After obtaining Cleveland Clinic institutional review board approval, the survey was sent to students at the beginning of the academic years 2021–22 and 2022–23, and we are continuing this process annually. This provides us with some additional qualitative and quantitative data on our program's effectiveness.

Overall, the process of iteratively reviewing the curriculum and our progress has helped make the program sustainable and adaptable. It has allowed us to update our content annually to reflect new educational/clinical guidelines and to address emerging needs.

DISCUSSION

In this chapter, we present our methodology for systematically improving medical school curricular coverage of topics relevant to LGBTQ+ health care.

Strengths of the Program

The overall results from our program thus far have been promising, with a wide array of LGBTQ+ health topics now covered in the preclinical years. We believe that the following elements have been strengths of our program, which may be good practices for implementation at other institutions:

1. Comprehensive needs assessment with an evidence-based foundation: Our initial needs assessment was generated using a combination of the AAMC's Core Competencies, existing peer-reviewed literature, and a thorough review of our current preclinical curriculum. This process helped us identify teaching points that aligned with both AAMC recommendations and the most current medical evidence. Additionally, we could personalize the recommended teaching points to integrate well into established seminars without needing to change any major aspects of the curriculum.

2. A collaborative team approach: The inclusion of both students and faculty on the team allowed us to review the curriculum in real time via students' observations and to generate ideas based on both learner and teacher perspectives. In meetings with course directors, for example, students led the discussions, while faculty were present to help navigate and provide insight. We also partnered with multiple offices and individuals that facilitated curricular change, including the Office of Student Affairs; the Office of Diversity, Equity, and Inclusion; and the Office of Curricular Affairs.

3. The "Add-A-Slide" approach: During our needs assessment, we realized that we needed to find creative ways to disseminate our teaching points within a curriculum that was already established and complete. Because seminars (often using PowerPoint-type presentations) are a common feature in the curriculum, the "Add-A-Slide" approach seemed like a reasonable option for covering our teaching points without requiring major curricular changes. Overall, this approach was feasible and was generally well-received by faculty, with high levels of uptake. It allowed us to integrate the desired information into lectures without placing additional burden on the faculty to research the content and edit their presentations. A single slide can also be quickly covered, which is particularly helpful given the trend toward shortening preclinical curricula. Importantly, our approach also allows for seamless integration of LGBTQ+ content into relevant organ systems-based lectures (or other clinical content), rather than separating it completely into isolated lectures on LGBTQ+ health or "Doctoring" topics.

4. Iterative review process: Our continuous improvement approach includes organizational systems that allow us to easily review our progress on an ongoing basis. We also established avenues to follow qualitative and quantitative metrics of our programs' success, including tracking the number of integration points, obtaining feedback from both students and faculty, and using a survey to measure effectiveness.

5. Increased student/faculty awareness and engagement: During our efforts, we have been fortunate to meet with faculty who are enthusiastic about integrating more LGBTQ+-related health content into their courses. As a result, we have had opportunities to add some full hour-long seminars into various places in the curriculum for topics that deserve dedicated teaching time in their own standalone seminar. In the second-year Endocrinology and Reproductive Biology course, the school added a didactic seminar on best practices for clinical care of transgender and nonbinary (TGNB) people, including information on common medications used in gender-affirming health care, discussions on fertility preservation for TGNB patients, and tips for creating affirming health care spaces for LGBTQ+-identifying patients.

Our Art and Practice of Medicine (APM) curriculum added a session on health systems-based approaches to LGBTQ+ health care, which incorporated discussions on the roles of physicians and trainees in advocacy and local/national resources for LGBTQ+-identifying patients. The inclusion of LGBTQ+ content at multiple levels, including single slides, PBL learning objectives, and even full seminars, has provided numerous opportunities to increase both student and faculty awareness.

6. Fostering a "person-first" approach: By integrating LGBTQ+ health topics into preexisting, organ system–based seminars, we relied less on standalone "LGBTQ+ 101" lectures, which can further "other" this already vulnerable group by separating out their health care needs from those of the general population. Thus, students learn to consider sexual orientation and gender identity in an integrated way, as a part of the patient's complete health history; they see the patient as a person, with their sexual orientation and gender identity as only one core facet of their identity. Not only does our approach teach core content and meet all AAMC Core Competencies, but it does so in a way that prioritizes the needs of the patient while also requiring little extra time or effort from busy seminar leaders.

7. Shifting culture toward increased belonging for LGBTQ+ students and faculty: Although our effort was initially undertaken with educational change as a key priority, a secondary benefit was more subtle yet equally as important. Through the work of our group, we have observed and experienced a shift in the culture of the school where LGBTQ+ topics and concerns are increasingly recognized, and where students and faculty feel a heightened sense of belonging. The faculty/student partnerships within our group have been mutually beneficial and have allowed all to flourish despite the time commitment of this work and the emotional toll of medical school. Incoming medical students are entering a curriculum, and a space, that is outwardly and inwardly sensitive to the needs of LGBTQ+ patients, students, and faculty. We hope that this sense of belonging is experienced by all in our school community.

Limitations

At the same time, we have faced some barriers to implementation and recognize that this process might need to be modified for optimal integration in other medical school programs or for other curricular topics. The following are some potential limitations of our approach:

1. Unique experiences with the CCLCM curriculum and student body: We created and streamlined our process based on circumstances at CCLCM, which included relatively small class sizes and required attendance

at seminars. Each medical school program will have a unique structure, and medical school curricula are always changing, so our approach may need to be modified for others. Seminars were an effective way to disseminate many of the LGBTQ+ teaching points in our program, but this may be less ideal for programs without required seminars. We also recognize that our small class sizes may have facilitated faster curriculum changes. However, we believe that the general structure of our approach (see Fig. 7.1) is adaptable and scalable for the majority of medical programs.

2. Faculty uptake: The program is largely dependent on faculty involvement, so it could be harder to implement if there is insufficient faculty engagement. Furthermore, it can be challenging for faculty to incorporate any additional content into the curriculum. This is understandable given the amount of other medical knowledge that needs to be covered and the limited time available to do so. Generally, we have found that the "Add-A-Slide" approach has largely removed this barrier. In addition to incorporation of slides into seminars, we have looked for other areas for topic integration, such as recommending inclusion of an article or notes covering the topic in the seminar syllabus. This approach can be helpful when limited lecture time is the major barrier. However, students may be less likely to learn the content if presented as an optional reading, rather than as a component of a required seminar.

3. Resource and time constraints: The initial process of establishing a group and completing a thorough review of the curriculum can be time intensive. We found that dedicating this initial time had substantial payoffs in the long term. Not as much time is required to continue the program once established, but it does still rely on having faculty involvement and recruiting students in each new class (since first- and second-year students will always be needed to prospectively monitor the curriculum).

4. Metrics of success: Identifying ways to measure long-term success of curricular change can be challenging. In our initial stages, we have used an optional survey assessing students' knowledge, attitudes, and beliefs around LGBTQ+ health care at the beginning of each academic year to compare these metrics pre- and post-curriculum. However, surveys can be limited by bias, including response bias or self-selection bias. Some of our surveys have also had suboptimal response rates, so we have tried to find methods for addressing this (e.g., a prize raffle).

5. Emotional tolls and boundaries: A significant proportion of individuals involved in our action group identify as part of the LGBTQ+ community. This has been a strength in many ways, such as adding perspectives of

lived experience. At the same time, it brings up the question of the dynamic of relying on marginalized groups themselves to undertake the responsibility of educating others, which has the potential to be emotionally taxing. While we have been fortunate to have broader institutional support and many allies in the organization, this may present a challenge if groups do not have this established support. We are grateful for the continued engagement of key stakeholders, including the oversight of the DEI Task Force and the partnerships with the Offices of Student Affairs and Curricular Affairs.

Additional Lessons Learned and Recommendations for Implementation

Central to our approach was the initial creation of a team of passionate students and faculty members who were motivated to improve coverage of important LGBTQ+ content, with the shared goal of preparing medical students to provide better care to LGBTQ+ patients. The enthusiasm and support we received from academic deans and other faculty was also fundamental in implementation. Finding project champions and supportive collaborators throughout the organization ultimately made the process much smoother and more efficient. Particularly, working with curricular deans and the Office of DEI helped us gain broader institutional support. In addition, using the AAMC Core Competencies as our foundation provided evidence-based, national guidelines to rely on when advocating for curricular change.

An initial needs assessment and complete curricular review can be time intensive as discussed, but it can simplify and streamline later implementation. At the same time, any successes, large or small, incorporating content that can improve LGBTQ+ health care should be celebrated. The addition of a few slides in a seminar somewhere in the curriculum is an important start to moving toward larger curricular and institutional change. Each year, we have continued to integrate more teaching points, and we have seen a wider institutional shift to now include dedicated LGBTQ+ topic seminars and the beginnings of adding more LGBTQ+-focused content within the clinical years.

"Add-A-Slide" confers additional novelty to our approach. It is a simple, expeditious way to incorporate LGBTQ+ health content that otherwise might have been sequestered into a single lecture or not covered at all. Our approach institutionalized this important content longitudinally, over the course of the preclinical years, in required in-person organ-system seminars and problem-based learning patient cases, without undue burden on faculty or students. Importantly, this approach can also be used to improve curricular coverage of other essential topics for medical students, including racial and ethnic health inequities. Incorporating this content

throughout the curriculum (rather than solely separated out into "Doctoring" and health systems-type seminars) can promote a larger institutional cultural change toward effectively recognizing and addressing the health inequities and needs of marginalized groups.

CONCLUSION

In summary, we present our process for increasing coverage of important topics relevant to LGBTQ+ health within our medical school's preclinical curriculum. Our methods included conducting curricular needs assessments, using the "Add-A-Slide" approach to integrate content throughout the curriculum, and creating a system to continually review our process. We believe that our core framework can be implemented at other medical schools looking to increase their students' knowledge of LGBTQ+ health. Ultimately, we hope that this will prepare current and upcoming generations of medical students to provide better care and help address the health inequities affecting LGBTQ+ populations.

TAKE-HOME POINTS

1. A combination of the Association of American Medical Colleges core competencies, the existing preclinical curriculum, and current evidence-based literature serves as a good map for an initial needs assessment.
2. Formation of an action group including students, faculty, and other key collaborators (e.g., curricular deans) is an essential component.
3. The "Add-A-Slide" approach offers one option for easily integrating LGBTQ+ teaching points into an existing curriculum without substantial time or resource requirements.
4. Early establishment of a process for iteratively reviewing the action group's progress can help ensure the program remains sustainable and adaptable.

QUESTIONS FOR FURTHER THOUGHT

1. What strategies might be helpful for integrating additional content from the Association of American Medical Colleges LGBTQ+ core competencies into the clinical years of the curriculum?
2. What are the roles of both medical students and medical schools in responding to recent upsurges in anti-LGBTQ+ legislation and LGBTQ+ health inequities? How can schools effectively promote student advocacy?
3. How can schools or action groups anticipate and respond to resistance or reluctance from faculty or others during the process of LGBTQ+ curriculum integration?

4. In addition to integration points, feedback, and survey metrics, what other methods might be used to track the success and effectiveness of curricular change? What types of long-term metrics could be used to gauge the impact of curricular change on patient care?

REFERENCES

1. Kelly T, Rodriguez SB. Expanding underrepresented in medicine to include lesbian, gay, bisexual, transgender, and queer individuals. *Acad Med.* 2022;97(11):1605–1609. https://doi.org/10.1097/ACM.0000000000004720.
2. Streed CGJ, Lunn MR, Siegel J, Obedin-Maliver J. Meeting the patient care, education, and research missions: academic medical centers must comprehensively address sexual and gender minority health. *Acad Med.* 2021;96(6):822. https://doi.org/10.1097/ACM.0000000000003703.
3. Gonzales G, Przedworski J, Henning-Smith C. Comparison of health and health risk factors between lesbian, gay, and bisexual adults and heterosexual adults in the united states: results from the national health interview survey. *JAMA Intern Med.* 2016;176(9):1344–1351. https://doi.org/10.1001/jamainternmed.2016.3432.
4. Peele C. *Roundup of Anti-LGBTQ+ Legislation Advancing In States Across the Country. Human Rights Campaign.* 2023. https://www.hrc.org/press-releases/roundup-of-anti-lgbtq-legislation-advancing-in-states-across-the-country.
5. Obedin-Maliver J, Goldsmith ES, Stewart L, et al. Lesbian, gay, bisexual, and transgender–related content in undergraduate medical education. *JAMA.* 2011;306(9):971–977. https://doi.org/10.1001/jama.2011.1255.
6. Pregnall AM, Churchwell AL, Ehrenfeld JM. A call for LGBTQ content in graduate medical education program requirements. *Acad Med.* 2021;96(6):828. https://doi.org/10.1097/ACM.0000000000003581.
7. White W, Brenman S, Paradis E, et al. Lesbian, gay, bisexual, and transgender patient care: medical students' preparedness and comfort. *Teach Learn Med.* 2015;27(3):254–263. https://doi.org/10.1080/10401334.2015.1044656.
8. Stumbar SE, Brown DR, Lupi CS. Developing and implementing curricular objectives for sexual health in undergraduate medical education: a practical approach. *Acad Med.* 2020;95(1):77. https://doi.org/10.1097/ACM.0000000000002891.
9. Greene B, Shu J, Bowen K, Hopkins M, Lambrese J. The "One Slide Approach": an adaptable model to enhance medical student pre-clinical LGBTQ+ education. *SGIM Forum.* 2022;45(10): 11,13,16.
10. Yepes-Rios M, Lad S, Dore S, Thapliyal M, Baffoe-Bonnie H, Isaacson JH. Diversity, equity, and inclusion: one model to move from commitment to action in medical education. *SN Soc Sci.* 2023;3(3):61. https://doi.org/10.1007/s43545-023-00650-6.
11. Hollenback A, Eckstrand K, Dreger A. *Implementing Curricular and Institutional Climate Changes to Improve Health Care for Individuals Who Are LGBT, Gender Nonconforming, or Born with DSD: A Resource for Medical Educators.* Association of American Medical Colleges; 2014. https://offers.aamc.org/lgbt-dsd-health
12. Zumwalt AC, Carter EE, Gell-Levey IM, Mulkey N, Streed CG, Siegel J. A novel curriculum assessment tool, based on AAMC competencies, to improve medical education about sexual and gender minority populations. *Acad Med.* 2022;97(4):524–528. https://doi.org/10.1097/ACM.0000000000004203.

8

Engaging Pediatric Providers in Racial Equity Education
Process, Reflections, and Next Steps

Avanté J. Smack and Nikita P. Rodrigues

SUMMARY

Historically, academic-focused antiracism efforts have emphasized multicultural competence, often focusing on micro-level processes in the clinical interaction. While meaningful, focusing only on micro-level processes ignores other outside factors that influence clinical interactions. Structural competency is the understanding of how history, social and economic determinants, institutional and systemic racism, and health inequities all shape health and health outcomes. We believe including structural competency in antiracism curricula is a necessary next step to help increase health care providers' effectiveness while also minimizing patient harm. We review a 10-week training curriculum created for faculty members and trainees in an academic medical center that could serve as an onboarding orientation for trainees and/or faculty. We include information about the course covering the overall structure, example content, and experiential activities. We include considerations for facilitating discussions and ideas for challenging participants to deeply engage with the material. Finally, we uphold that medical providers need to be trained to attend to the culturally relevant interpersonal
factors that happen in their patient interactions. We aim for this curriculum to support the foundation they must also learn to recognize that the systems and structures outside of the patient room impacted by identity factors hold equal importance in determining health care access and outcomes.

INTRODUCTION

Mio et al.[1] define **multicultural competence** as developing an awareness of one's own cultural values and biases, learning to value others' worldviews, and developing a set of culturally appropriate interpersonal skills. Multicultural competence has often focused on micro-level processes in clinical interactions and strayed from acknowledging a need to understand the macro-level processes that impact patients outside of the treatment room. **Structural competency**, the understanding of how history, social and economic determinants, institutional and systemic racism, and health inequities all shape health, is needed to further health care providers' effectiveness and reduce harm.

The chapter outlines a 10-week racial equity training program that can serve as an onboarding orientation for trainees or faculty of all levels. This training is grounded in the idea that providing culturally humble care[2] is only possible through understanding the systems and structures that impact patient well-being and acknowledging that racism is present in the design of those systems and structures. This program focuses on the experiences of Black/African Americans with the hope that trainees learn specifically about structural racism and its impact on the health and well-being for Black/African Americans, but also broaden their thinking to understand the importance of considering structural factors for all patients of varying identities and contexts. We assert that the power structures that uphold supremacy and oppression for Black/African Americans in our country serve as a foundation of knowledge to understand other identities that are oppressed and lay the foundation for understanding how intersectionality can impact patient interactions, treatments, and outcomes. Our trainings are co-led by two faculty members (authors of this chapter). Typically, 10 to 12 trainees participate at a time. This training could be easily adapted to larger cohorts of trainees, but we have found that group discussions need to be capped at 10 to 12 people in order to elicit meaningful engagement from all participants. Thus, if deploying this training with a larger cohort, more discussion leaders would be needed.

GROUP LEADER CONSIDERATIONS

We have faculty leaders for this program because we believe it's important that our faculty demonstrates top-down engagement in this work. Though this chapter is focused on trainee education, we would be remiss if we did not acknowledge that diversity-related training cannot be relegated to specific courses or seminars. We encourage trainees to bring material that they learn through the course to their supervisors and attendings to learn how to apply that knowledge more directly to their clinical care. With that expectation, we have to acknowledge that our faculty needs to be trained to support that learning. Thus, we have also implemented the training course outlined in this chapter with the majority of our faculty, and we include faculty supervisors and attendings in training-related communication so they can support application of course material beyond the "classroom."

Our faculty leaders strategically use self-disclosure and vulnerability to demonstrate that working toward being antiracist is an ever-developing skill with no endpoint and missteps happening along the way. For example, faculty leaders will share instances where they have navigated cultural ruptures with patients or personally navigated the tension between the desire to be antiracist in practice and the realities of working in systems where that may not be

possible. At different points in the program, we have faculty leaders chosen based on specific facets of racial identity, which is discussed in the section on small-group discussion considerations.

Our training course is led by faculty internal to our hospital, and there are pros and cons to this approach. On the positive end, the goal of this program is that trainees take structural knowledge and apply it to the clinical settings in which they work. Having faculty leaders who are familiar with the local demographics, the patient populations in various clinics, and the challenges of equitable access both within the hospital and the larger community helps in aiding trainees in applying program material to their work. Additionally, program leaders have worked to ensure that trainee supervisors are aware of training program content, in the hope that they continue to aid trainees in applying this learning to their ongoing clinical work.

On the negative side, we have at times had trainees participate in the training program who are directly supervised by program leaders. We try as much as possible to remove an evaluative component to participating in this program and discussions, but it is hard to remove that element when a supervisory relationship is introduced to the space. Additionally, an important part of leading this program and facilitating discussions is being able to challenge participants who may be intentionally or unintentionally harmful in their discussion on program content. Doing this in a way that promotes safety for all participants (both those harming and those who may be directly harmed) is challenging and requires skill that develops with time and practice. Challenging trainees who you have working relationships with can bring an added level of sensitivity to the process that could be eased by having program leaders who are external to the program.

BEGINNING TRAINING

To begin the training, all participants are invited to a 1-hour orientation. Program leaders initiate conversation by explaining that this training program will utilize discussion groups to facilitate critical thinking and understanding of presented material. The goal is for participants to always feel safe in these discussions, with facilitators present to intervene, as necessary. However, leaders define that safety, which does not guarantee comfort, noting that the goal is for conversations to challenge participants to move past their comfort zones and think about their place in systems of oppression. Specifically, trainees will be encouraged to reflect on their own histories being impacted by, perpetuating, or being a bystander of these systems. Leaders highlight that often the greatest growth in identity awareness happens when we are uncomfortable. Through many iterations of this challenge, group leaders have recognized patterns in the trainee approach to discussion that often attempt to prioritize comfort. Leaders have noticed that higher education students are comfortable with discussing curriculum content from an intellectualized approach that allows distancing from the material. For example, participants may lead with statements such as, "well, we know the literature supports. . ." or, "unfortunately, the data we base our practices on are conducted with primarily White patients . . ." While this information is useful, we want participants to personally connect with the material, so we may challenge them by asking, "Can you think of a clinical setting where you've unintentionally upheld White standards of health for non-White patients?" or "We know race is often taught to children that way. If you had to change the way you teach kids about race, either for your own children or for your patients, how would you do it?" We believe questioning like this pushes trainees out of their comfort zones and into the harder places where change can happen. However, we want to always balance that discomfort with as much provision of safety as we can.

To promote safety in discussion, group leaders outline assumptions group members should hold about each other as they enter discussion spaces:
- We are all here to learn and grow.
- We all have good intentions and acknowledge that intent and impact are not the same.
- We only speak for ourselves and our own personal lived experiences.

SAFETY CONSIDERATIONS

We recognize that all trainees approach the program with differing levels of exposure to thinking and discussing racially sensitive topics. This may be due to differences in the training program curriculum that learners receive prior to training at our institution and the trainee's personal racial identity. It may also be exacerbated by societal norms that suggest racialized talk is taboo. We find that many trainees have difficulty articulating their thoughts because they are concerned that they may say the wrong thing, say something that is not coherent, or say something that is offensive to others in the group. Group facilitators often reiterate that practice is the best way to get more comfortable talking about uncomfortable topics and highlight benefits of doing so with other people who are similarly trying to learn and grow together during the training program.

We also find that some individuals enter the program with a wealth of knowledge about the history of racism in the United States and understand structural competence and may be offended or harmed by statements made by other group members who have less knowledge of the content areas. In this instance, group leaders may approach

the trainee, provide information to the trainee, and allow them to decide whether they want to participate in the program or opt out. Additionally, we have had moments where we perceived a trainee's personal safety to be harmed. For example, in one training we had a White trainee directly address the trainees of color and apologize for the harm he was learning about for the first time in the course material. This was a great example of a mismatch between intent and impact and our trainees of color were forced into a role of representing something bigger than themselves. When moments like these happen, faculty leaders attempt to address them in the moment. We also create space in our racial identity discussion groups to process these harms that can happen in mixed-race antiracist training spaces and have even scheduled additional check-ins with trainees who may have been harmed to ensure they are supported.

Program leaders then briefly outline racial inequities in access to health care and health care providers' roles in addressing these inequities. The literature highlighting structural barriers to accessing care is well defined. This training focuses on the challenges patients face even once they connect to care, noting that racial discrimination, profiling, microaggressions, and racism exist within health service largely due to the lack of training providers receive on racial issues and inequities. It is this acknowledgment that warrants a commitment to antiracist care, meaning participants must contend that action toward social justice is needed, otherwise providers will continue to perpetuate a racist system.

Leaders then present a paper published by Jude-Mary Cenat[3] that defines four facets of providing antiracist mental health care. These facets include an awareness of racial issues, skills in assessing real needs, a treatment approach that addresses the real needs and issues related to racism, and a humanistic approach to medication. In each facet, specific skills are defined, ranging from understanding social determinants of health to having skills in conducting culturally competent assessments of symptomology. In review of this list, leaders posit that training programs have often focused on trainees developing culturally sensitive skills to use in the individual interpersonal relationships between providers and patients. However, as posited by Metzl and Hansel,[4] as clinicians enter the clinical spaces outside of the classroom, they often are faced with the reality that many of the forces that influence health outcomes are beyond the level of individual interactions. Thus, to truly embody culturally humble care, providers must not only have culturally informed interpersonal skills. They must also have structural competency or the understanding of how social structures impact social groups and individuals.

Finally, leaders explain that to address health outcomes, providers need to understand the factors underlying

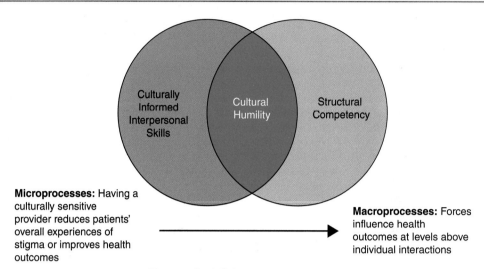

Fig. 8.1 Redefining cultural humility.

symptomology that we often do not attend to in the traditional medical model. These factors include racism, oppression, inequality, poverty, mass incarceration, sexism, transphobia, etc. Trainees are encouraged to think about how facets of identity like race, class, and gender shape interactions between the provider and patient in the exam room, but these interactions are also largely shaped by the larger structural contexts in which these interactions do or do not take place (Fig. 8.1). While we aim to treat patients as individuals, we also need to recognize how social determinants, economic determinants, biases, inequities, and blind spots shape health and should be considered in medical care.[4] Many examples of this approach are integrated and provided throughout the course. For example, trainees are encouraged to reflect on patient populations in the various clinics in which they rotate. They are asked to question why patients with public insurance are well connected to our primary care services but are less represented in our specialty care clinics which are less accessible by public transportation and have stricter no-show policies. They are asked to reflect on which cultural communities are not presenting in their clinics and whether harm committed by our health care field or cultural stigma may be contributing to those discrepancies. They are asked to look at the evidence-based practices that they implement in their clinical care and question whether the samples with which those practices were validated represent the patients they are seeing. And if they don't, they're asked to question whether there are different social or economic realities for their patients that might impact their ability to engage in treatment or their response to that treatment.

As trainees embark on the 10-week training program, they are reminded that this work can be incredibly challenging, but it is necessary. Even small steps can be meaningful. Additionally, trainees are reminded that they are well positioned to bring social justice and activism into the work they are already doing. At the end of the initial kickoff meeting, program leaders divide the group into smaller groups to discuss racial socialization. As Neblett et al.[5] defined, racial socialization refers to the process by which race-related messages about the meaning of race and racism are transmitted by parents intergenerationally. Group leaders start by disclosing their own journeys of racial socialization, starting with the ways their families taught them about race, responded to racism they have experienced or witnessed in their communities, and how their ideas of race have stayed the same or shifted as they navigated higher education and their current clinical careers. Group leaders model experiencing growth in their understanding of identity and areas where they are still growing to further acknowledge that there is no endpoint to antiracist identity formation. Group members are then invited to share their own journeys of racial socialization for 3 to 5 minutes each.

The training program is designed to be a hybrid of asynchronous learning and active learning through weekly discussions. Trainees are sent their assignments via email three times per week to complete asynchronously. Assignments are selected so that, across the three days, participants will spend no more than 1 hour completing them. Participants receive various types of assignments including empirical articles, articles from other popular media sources (e.g., *New York Times, Vice, Atlantic*), videos, podcasts, and experiential activities. Assignments are grouped together by content area throughout the program.

ASSIGNMENT SELECTION CONSIDERATIONS

This course is flexibly designed, so program leaders have the option of utilizing various types of media that pertain to each content area covered. This particular training program heavily relies on popular education (pop-ed) sources as opposed to empirical articles. This creates a program that can easily be adapted to fit the needs of various participants, regardless of training level (e.g., research assistants, postdoctoral fellows). It also allows participants the ability to share materials with other individuals who may or may not be in the medical field. Using pop-ed sources also creates opportunities to easily link content areas to real-world examples that are happening in real time. Group leaders wanted curriculum that would be engaging and easy to consume. We also wanted to move away from creating a program that would mimic traditional graduate-level coursework.

Group leaders are highly encouraged to consider the specific needs of their trainees when making decisions about selected content. For example, individuals working primarily with medical residents or nursing students may choose to customize week 7 content to focus on specific issues that may be more relevant to the specific discipline. Additional customizations might include pulling specific articles that highlight incidents of racial bias occurring in their local region or choosing to highlight specific social determinants of health that are particularly relevant to the patient population being served (e.g., focusing more on neighborhood violence for adult populations as opposed to focusing on education for pediatric populations).

To enhance learning and promote additional reflection of material, trainees participate in weekly discussions about the content with which they are interacting. Leaders share general prompts to promote reflection, as well as questions that encourage reflection about specific assignments in the program. Trainees are actively encouraged to see themselves as co-moderators within the discussion group. Trainees alternate each week between completing a paired-partner discussion or a small-group discussion. For partnered discussions, trainees have the option to select a partner or be randomly assigned to another participant in the group. They retain the same partner throughout the duration of the program. During the first partnered discussion, trainees are asked to establish rules for confidentiality and to share aspects of their identities using Pamela Hays[6] Addressing Framework. This is an effort to help partners explore and reflect on their own identities and gain comfort

in bringing their own lived experiences into the room to connect with the source material. During the remaining partner discussions, trainees are given prompts to help encourage reflection. Example questions include "Was there anything that you were exposed to in the content this past week that was surprising?" and "How did the material this week contribute to your understanding of your role in the larger system of bias, prejudice, and racism?"

On the alternating weeks, trainees are divided into smaller groups with other participants. Group assignment may be based on trainee status (e.g., interns are grouped together) depending on the composition of the overall group. Trainees also participate in at least one discussion group that is divided by self-reported racial/ethnic identity (i.e., Black, Indigenous, People of Color [BIPOC], and White). Example questions utilized in the small-group discussion include "How can we make shifts in our clinical work to validate the lived experiences of our patients?" and "We learned a lot about biases that lead to poor outcomes for Black youth and about the differential stress Black people in America may face due to systemic inequities. What is our role in recognizing these forces in our patient's lives as health professionals?" The training program concludes with a full-group discussion that has a special emphasis on goal setting (see Vignette 2 for more information).

CONSIDERATIONS FOR PARTNERED AND SMALL-GROUP DISCUSSIONS

Over the many iterations of running this course, program leaders have considered various factors in determining small-group make-up, with consideration of feedback from trainees who completed the training program.

In partner pairings, we opt to let trainees select a partner or request a random pairing. We have found some trainees find value in having a space to explore program content with a person with whom they already have a safe and trusted relationship. The potential con of this pairing is that participants may be less challenged outside of their comfort zone with someone they have chosen who may be more likely to think like them and share certain proclivities. Partners who have been randomly paired have shared positive feedback in deepening perspectives, especially when paired with someone who they wouldn't normally interact with as much. However, we have also faced challenges when trainees have been randomly placed together and are at different places on their journey toward becoming antiracist clinicians. Specifically, we have found that trainees of color report benefit from being with other trainees of color and find greater safety in those pairings. Conversely, White trainees have often requested to be paired with trainees of color in hopes of deepening their understanding of the presented material. In sum, we have landed on letting trainees choose to be paired randomly or specifically. When pairing randomly, we try to pair trainees of color together, and based on initial share of racial socialization, we try to pair trainees who we believe may be in similar areas of antiracist identity development.

In small-group discussions, we at times have groups randomly selected to just allow for more time for each group member to participate in discussion. At other times, we have found benefit in splitting trainee groups by their training status (e.g., interns or fellows). This has been helpful both in allowing trainees to participate in discussion with a group that they likely know better and eases some of the inherent power differential between trainees in various stages of training. Additionally, we have found benefit in separating trainees at different levels as they also have a different breadth of experience working clinically with patients and may have different capacity to apply the material to their clinical experiences. Small-group discussions are self-moderated, in that we provide discussion questions and ask each trainee to take one question and lead and moderate discussion for that question. We believe having some discussion spaces without program leaders allows for fewer demand characteristics and hopefully greater vulnerability in sharing.

We also have one small-group discussion during each training program that is separated by racial identity. Specifically, we have a group for BIPOC-identifying trainees and White-identifying trainees. If we have a big enough group or broad enough representation, we may further separate Black-identifying trainees, non-Black people of color-identifying trainees, White trainees with largely privileged identities, and White trainees who have a salient non-racial identity that holds less power (e.g., disability status, ethnicity, sexual identity). We believe that the use of racial affinity groups better allows for identity growth, safety in self-reflection, and more specific scaffolding of identity understanding. BIPOC affinity space group leaders, who are BIPOC-identifying themselves, are tasked with leading trainees in a conversation on how to balance self-preservation and meaningful engagement when engaging in antiracist education. They also discuss the risks and benefits of engaging in challenging conversations in mixed-race spaces. White affinity space group leaders, who are White-identifying, are tasked with leading trainees in a conversation on how to actively engage in antiracist work without centering themselves, in how to move away from performative engagement to active involvement, and how to move past White guilt, externalization, and hopelessness to a place of self-reflection and action. When we have had groups for White trainees with secondary non-racial oppressed identities, we have found group leaders with

similar identities and have asked them to lead a space with the goal of acknowledging that having other oppressed/marginalized identities can help with empathy and understanding of race-based oppression. Additionally, we want members of this group to also acknowledge that advocacy work of marginalized groups who haven't considered the intersection of race have often harmed groups who have less privilege. We consistently get positive feedback on the use of racial affinity groups. BIPOC-identifying trainees find benefit in a safer space to explore the emotional toll of engaging in this work. White trainees often at first express hesitancy about a White-only affinity space, but then acknowledge the benefit of creating safety for challenges specific to White engagement in antiracist work. Having skilled group leaders is critical for the effective deployment of these spaces.

AFTER THE INITIAL GROUP DISCUSSION

Following the initial whole-group discussion, participants receive seven weeks of content divided into the following topic areas; History of Racism in the US, Role of Bias in Black American Life, Social Determinants of Health, and Racism and Antiracism Efforts in Academic Medicine. During the first three weeks, trainees focus on understanding the history of racism in the US with a particular emphasis on the construct of race, the role of White supremacy and how it has historically shown up, and how White supremacy is engrained in current organizational culture. Weeks four and five are spent learning about bias in systems that often intersect with health, including the criminal justice system, education system, and housing practices. During weeks five and six, trainees focus on the impact of specific social determinants of health (e.g., school to prison pipeline, housing, education, poverty) on health. The final week of the curriculum focuses on ways that White supremacy exists in the field of psychology/academic medicine and reviews current efforts within the field to dismantle it. For examples of content see Table 8.1. Each week participants receive three to five assignments that will take an hour total to complete. Participants are typically sent short assignments by email on Monday, Wednesday, and Friday to space engagement through the week. They are expected to have completed the previous week's assignments when they present for the discussion group the following week.

VIGNETTE 1

During week five of the program, participants are asked to complete an experiential activity (SPENT playspent.org) that simulates decision-making while experiencing poverty. Throughout the game, players make a series of

TABLE 8.1.   Racial Equity Program Selected Curriculum Outline

History of Racism in the United States (Weeks 1–3)

Week 1	Kendi IX. Denial is the heartbeat of America. *The Atlantic.* January 27, 2021. Donald Glover. This is America [Video]. YouTube. Published May 6, 2018.
Week 2	Harvard Law School. Bryan Stevenson '85. "We can't recover from this history until we deal with it" [Video]. YouTube. Published January 30, 2019.
Week 3	Sotto, SM. 42 ways to advance racial equity in academic medicine. Indiana University School of Medicine Bioethics. October 13, 2020.

The Role of Bias in Black American Life

Week 4	Kamin, D. Home appraised with a Black owner: $472,000. With a White owner: $750,000. *The New York Times.* August 18, 2022.

The Role of Bias in Black American Life/Social Determinants of Health

Week 5	Chakara, M. From preschool to prison: The criminalization of Black girls. *American Progress.* December 8, 2017.

Social Determinants of Health

Week 6	Vallas, R., & Valenti, J. Asset limits are a barrier to economic security and mobility. *American Progress.* September 10, 2014.

Antiracism Efforts in Psychology and Academic Medicine

Week 7	Buchanan NT, Perez M, Prinstein MJ, & Thurston, IB. Upending racism in psychological science: Strategies to change how our science is conducted, reported, reviewed & disseminated. *American Psychologist.* 2021;76(7):1097–1112.

decisions that impact the balance in their checking account. For example, participants choose an entry-level job and insurance plan, often leaving their weekly pay below a few hundred dollars a week. They can choose a cheaper insurance plan but may pay for that later in the month if they have to make an urgent care visit. They then may choose to live farther from work to pay cheaper rent, but then see gas costs go up. Each decision is connected to a different dilemma and problem that is tied to health, level of education, and providing the basic needs for the player's family members. The game ends when players either run out of money before the end of the month or make it through until the next paycheck.

Participants are emailed: "*For today's assignment we would like for you to complete this activity that simulates what a month in poverty may be like. This activity takes approximately 15 to 20 minutes to complete.*"

During discussion groups the following questions about the game are asked:

1. *What was your experience playing the Spent game? What did you take away from it?*
2. *Do you think you have a good understanding of the challenges that families living in poverty face?*
3. *How important is this insight in providing appropriate mental health care to some of the families that you serve?*

Trainees are encouraged to connect their experience with the Spent game back to their patient care. *How often do they make treatment recommendations for their patients that will incur monthly expenses (e.g., travel back to clinic, travel to a pharmacy, education supplies for their child), and do they consider the family's socioeconomic status in those decisions? How do we ensure equitable care when patients are coming to us from wildly inequitable places outside of our medical clinics?*

This program concludes with a final whole-group discussion facilitated by the program leaders. The primary goal of the final discussion is to review material that was not covered during prior discussion groups and to reflect on all content presented throughout the program. Trainees are prompted to consider how they might apply information learned during the program to change/modify their own clinical practice. To promote additional engagement with curriculum beyond the program, trainees are asked to engage in brief reflection to identify goals that they are willing to commit to for the next six months.

VIGNETTE 2

In our final group discussion, participants are given time to set individual, interpersonal, and systemic-level goals that will promote antiracist health care. A group leader models goal setting for the group before breaking off for individual goal setting. Finally, participants are encouraged to share a goal with the group and consider finding accountability partners to continue this work moving forward.

Example goals shared by program leader:

Individual: *I want to learn more about housing policies in my area. I know these policies impact my patients greatly, and I don't really understand how the current systems work.*

Interpersonal: *I want to challenge myself to speak up in settings where I have the power to do so (e.g., faculty meetings, team meetings, clinic meetings). If I miss the opportunity to address racism I witness or perpetrate, I will try to re-engage in the conversation when I'm ready (attempt a cultural repair).*

Institutional: *I will sign up to participate in a community collaborative to help raise patient voices in decision-making spaces; I will raise an issue I observed in our current hospital system that perpetuates disparities in promotion potential.*

Example goals trainees have set at the end of the training program:

Individual: *I would like to identify oppressive structures I benefit from and consider ways that I can challenge those systems.*

Interpersonal: *Incorporate more intake questions to more broadly assess patients' backgrounds; stop allowing my fear of saying something wrong leading to not saying anything at all.*

Institutional: *Speak up when seeing leadership panels/positions of all White people.*

We end with discussion on how we will remain committed to this work when the training course is over and discuss systems of accountability we may need in our personal lives and with each other to ensure sustained commitment to antiracist efforts. We acknowledge the tide is pulling all of us toward perpetuating health inequity and that real change will need significant culture shifts. When enough of us turn against the tide, we can really make a difference.

We argue that while there is immense value in training focused on the interpersonal cultural skills needed to provide culturally humble care, that alone cannot lead to antiracist health care. Specifically, a focus on structural competency challenges providers to see the whole picture, to understand that we treat individual people, but to do so, we must be cognizant of the contexts in which they live. Additionally, our patients with oppressed identities deserve providers who understand and acknowledge that racism and other isms impact the contexts that shape their health outcomes.

At the end of our training programs, participants can often be left with some feelings of hopelessness as they have faced the overwhelming history and current reality of inequity in our country. Racism and structural inequities have persisted for so long, and it can feel daunting to think about the large systemic changes that are needed to truly improve patient health outcomes. We have learned that this hard and necessary work must be paired with reminders that small changes can have big impacts, and medical providers are particularly well-suited to organize and advocate for change. Ending the training with goal setting at various levels aims to remind trainees not to get stuck in hopelessness, but to instead look for places where activism can be brought into the spaces they already inhabit. Additionally, throughout the training, as we utilize identity-based reflection spaces, we emphasize the importance of acknowledging where we are on the continuum of being oppressed to benefiting from oppression. This self-reflection is vital for all of us to do if we aim to move toward antiracism. In the words of American activist, Brittany Packnett, "the more you benefit from supremacy, the more responsible you have to be to dismantle it." We hope that having this training as part of trainee onboarding sets the foundation for acknowledging advocacy and antiracism as integral parts of medical provider roles. We encourage trainees to bring the information learned during this training program into their supervisory spaces so they can learn how to apply their new knowledge and theoretical foundation to their clinical work. We also acknowledge that trainees are often in spaces where they have less power to raise concerns and issues, but we challenge them to constantly reflect on their power and what sacrifices they are willing to make. We challenge them to continue that reflection as they move through the training hierarchy and eventually become independent practitioners and leaders in their respective careers.

ADDITIONAL CONSIDERATIONS

We recognize that learners' schedules are often packed with several required educational components in addition to direct patient care. As such, obtaining support at the supervisor and/or institutional level via the division-level training directors has been helpful in sustaining this program over time at our current institution. The biggest areas where departmental/institutional support was helpful were in protecting group leaders' time to create content and facilitate the program and assistance with protecting time for trainees to engage in the various discussion formats. This program was initially created and run by group leaders in addition to their full clinical caseloads. Over time, we have secured a small portion of time coverage from the psychology division chief that helps cover part of the time and effort that ongoing program administration requires. In earlier iterations of the program, group leaders handled scheduling discussion groups throughout the duration of the program. This was a substantial time burden for the group leaders as people's availability could change prior to the groups being scheduled.

Over time, we have modified recruitment to facilitate a smoother, streamlined process. The learning opportunity is advertised during orientation at the beginning of the year to trainees and supervisors, and the total time commitment is included in the description of the program. Trainees are asked to consider whether they can commit to the synchronous and asynchronous components of the program. Trainees indicate interest in participating in the program given time commitments and verify whether the supervisor has committed to protecting the time for the trainee to participate. For some of our rounds of training we have been able to work with the training directors of the department to identify pockets of protected time to have this experience built into the trainees' annual training curriculum. We have also explored having trainees' participation be mandatory but have decided against that, so the program is completed by those who are able and willing to dedicate the time needed.

CONCLUSION

We have implemented this training with over 30 faculty members and over 50 trainees of various levels of training at a top academic hospital in the United States. After many rounds of training implementation, we strongly believe that targeted educational initiatives can support trainee growth in antiracist clinical alignment and that such initiatives should be incorporated into routine trainee onboarding. This training has been well received by faculty and trainees, and anecdotally we hear often about the shifts in clinical care participants have made following the training. In a system that is hard to change, it's inspiring to see shifts in the mentality of our trainees and hope that programs like this can contribute to the larger cultural shifts that are needed to dismantle the inequitable systems within which we practice.

REFERENCES

1. Mio JS, Barker-Hackett L, Tumambing J. *Multicultural Psychology: Understanding Our Diverse Communities.* 3rd ed. Oxford University Press; 2012.
2. Tervalon M, Murray-Garcia J. Cultural humility versus cultural competence: a critical distinction in defining physician training outcomes in multicultural education. *J Health Care Poor Underserved.* 1998;9(2):117–125.
3. Cénat JM. How to provide anti-racist mental health care. *Lancet Psychiatry.* 2020;7(11):929–931.
4. Metzl JM, Hansen H. Structural competency and psychiatry. *JAMA Psychiatry.* 2018;75(2):115–116.
5. Neblett Jr EW, Terzian M, Harriott V. From racial discrimination to substance use: the buffering effects of racial socialization. *Child Dev Perspec.* 2010;42(2):131–137.
6. Hays PA. *Addressing Cultural Complexities in Practice: A Framework for Clinicians and Counselors.* American Psychological Association; 2001.

9

Training the 21st-Century Physician
Health Equity, Cutting-Edge Technology and Pedagogy, and a Global Perspective

Daniel Z. Hodson, Amarachi I. Erondu, Akshara Malla, and Esther H. Kang

OUTLINE

SUMMARY

The turn of the 21st century has been marked by exponential growth in the volume of medical knowledge available to clinicians, increasingly sophisticated technologies to aid in clinical decision-making, greater acknowledgment of the medical community's past and continued complicity in elements of structural inequity, and increased globalization of the medical community. These changes present an incredible opportunity for the next generation of clinicians to meet the challenges of an increasingly changing world with the knowledge and skill set needed to improve outcomes for our patients. However, the current system of medical education and training must make drastic changes to meet the current moment. In this chapter, we illustrate the changing medical climate and suggest changes needed to train a fully competent physician for the 21st century.

VIGNETTE 1: A 20TH-CENTURY PATIENT ENCOUNTER

Imagine the following clinical encounter: A 57-year-old female presents for a 30-minute pre-operative visit prior to a laparoscopic partial colectomy for Stage IIB colorectal cancer detected on recent colonoscopy. Her colorectal cancer screening had been delayed. She moved to the area two years ago and initially had difficulty scheduling an appointment with a new doctor, then was not aware that she had to call to schedule the colonoscopy as well. She does not speak English. The pathology was indeterminate on the first colonoscopy, so a repeat colonoscopy and biopsy were performed. Her past medical history includes obesity, diabetes, hypertension, hyperlipidemia, as well as multiple prior surgeries including two previous cesarean sections and a cholecystectomy. The medical assistant was too busy to complete a medication reconciliation, but the electronic health record (EHR) listed eight daily medications. As the physician, you arrive at the patient's room five minutes late and call a phone interpreter while you log onto the computer. There are several EHR alerts that you close immediately without fully reading.

Before you can begin, the patient has several questions: she has seen advertisements for semaglutide on TV and wants to know if she should take it; her blood pressure has been high, but she forgot to bring or send her home blood pressure log; she reports concern about swelling in her legs because her sister was recently diagnosed with a "blood clot in her chest"; she is tearful, explaining her younger cousin recently died from a heart attack and asks if she should undergo stress testing before surgery. You review her medications, then quickly listen to her heart and lungs, palpate her abdomen, and palpate her calves. You increase one of her antihypertensives based on her office blood pressure reading, order an ultrasound of her lower extremities, and refer her to a cardiologist. You tell her you will fax the needed documentation to her surgeon tonight. With your hand on the doorknob, you end the call with the interpreter, but she asks about results from her recent blood work. You quickly sit back down and, speaking her language as best you can, review these results with her. Low-density lipoprotein level and hemoglobin A1c remain above goal. She expresses frustration as she has attempted many lifestyle changes. You encourage her to schedule a follow-up to discuss more. Later that evening, you spend another 20 minutes completing your documentation. You calculate her Revised Cardiac Risk Index and Gupta Perioperative Risk for Myocardial Infarction scores. You realize the surgeon requested an electrocardiogram, which you did not order, but remember that the cardiologist will surely obtain one. You message your office staff to fax over your note and lab results to the surgeon. Finally, you complete the necessary billing information and close the visit in the EHR.

Thought questions
1. What thoughts or emotions did you experience reading this encounter?
2. What aspects of this encounter can be improved?

INTRODUCTION: CHALLENGES FACING MEDICAL EDUCATION

A system will achieve the outcome it is designed to achieve. Innumerable times during medical school and residency, we have questioned whether faculty intend to teach how to care for the patient or how to care for the chart. What are we being trained to do and become? Are we being trained as physicians of the 21st century or even as doctors at all?

The ideals of medicine aspire to promote health and to alleviate suffering and disease. We believe health and access to health care to be an innate human right. There are several challenges and opportunities facing medicine in the 21st century. Acknowledging our biases as resident physicians in the combined specialty of Internal Medicine—Pediatrics, we discuss these challenges and propose several adaptations to ensure that trainees will emerge as healers and leaders for the 21st century. In Section 1, we describe how the roots of medical institutions in the United States are intertwined with deep running, established roots of elitism, sexism, racism, and colonialism. In part due to these roots, advances in medical science have been paralleled by failures in equitable health care delivery. In Section 2, we define and illustrate technologies currently transforming our understanding of health and disease. In Section 3, we discuss how these technologies augment and transform the history, physical, and clinical assessment. In Section 4, we argue health and disease in the 21st century are inherently global. Therefore, geographic specificity of training exists at odds with the international milieu in which physicians of our generation will live and practice. In Section 5, we advocate for adaptations to pedagogy and question current assumptions in medical education. Vignettes 1 and 2 offer an example of a preoperative visit with a middle-aged female in two contexts: the status quo and our vision for the 21st-century physician.

SECTION 1. MEDICINE AND STRUCTURAL VIOLENCE

"The assumption is that a Black [football] player started at a lower cognitive baseline."[1]

Training in medicine in the United States means that we learn and work in health care institutions *designed* to deliver inequitable care, and the institutions at which we train allow and even promote these health care disparities.[2] To dismantle violent structures that create and maintain preferential outcomes for some groups over others, medical education needs to be framed within a context that is geographically broad, historically deep, and firmly committed to establishing health care as a fundamental human right. We must acknowledge the full range of the human condition and avoid pathologizing qualities that do not meet white, cisgender (often male), heteronormative standards. To address these issues, medical education must remove race-based medicine from its curricula (explicit and implicit), invest in local partnerships, make conscious decisions to use technology to eliminate inequities rather than exacerbate them, and move beyond recognition of inequities toward practical, daily action.

Race-based medicine needs to be permanently excised from medical education. Clinical algorithms that use race are poignant examples of racism influencing the daily practice of medicine.[3,4] Some of the more egregious examples include assessment of cognitive function,[1] pulmonary function testing,[5,6] estimation of glomerular filtration rate,[7,8] risk associated with vaginal delivery following previous cesarean section,[9–11] risk of complications following cardiac surgery,[12] risk of breast cancer,[13] risk of atherosclerotic cardiovascular disease,[14] and treatment for hypertension.[15,16] As we have argued previously, these algorithms incorrectly and dangerously teach students that "race, instead of racism, is an independent risk factor for disease," thus "there is something inherently wrong with racialized minorities rather than with the systems that have harmed them."[17] In recent years, the Department of Health and Human Services recognized the harm of this practice and issued a rule to prevent discrimination "through the use of clinical algorithms."[18–20] Thus, trainees require adequate instruction in how to identify and avoid race-based medicine still present today.

Medical schools must demonstrate a commitment to health equity in both their formal and hidden curricula. While the formal curriculum "can be measured by the number of hours students receive training related to racial inequities and bias, structured service-learning, minority health activities, cultural awareness programming, and the completion of an [implicit association test]," the hidden curriculum remains "unofficial and often more powerful, consisting of faculty role modeling, institutional priorities around the interracial climate, and experiences of microaggressions."[17]

Regarding formal health equity curricula, the CHANGES study demonstrated that structured training focused on caring for LGBTQIA+ patients and racialized minorities was associated with a reduction in students' implicit biases toward these populations.[21,22] However, other studies that attempt to show the impact of these curricula are limited by a lack of a control group or in their restriction to classroom or web-based learning.[17] Because so much of medical education and medical practice are driven by evidence, institutions must commit to evaluating health equity interventions for efficacy and to disseminating these findings.

Discussion of health care inequities should be a longitudinal thread integrated into each block. Educational materials should present cases and images from diverse patient populations. For example, dermatology textbooks have historically provided illustrations of findings on lighter skin. Recent efforts to incorporate more images of skin of color were shown to increase trainees' comfort with identifying skin conditions in people of color.[23] In addition, organizing health equity rounds to discuss cases affected by structural barriers to health care delivery can normalize these conversations and model critical appraisal of health care encounters with a health equity lens.[24]

Regarding the hidden curricula, institutions can take several steps. First, academic training institutions should themselves strive to deliver care to underserved populations, for example by recruiting publicly insured and uninsured patients. Federal funds support trainee salaries; therefore, training institutions have an obligation to serve their catchment area. These opportunities also ensure that the next generation of physicians will have the cultural competence to care for an increasingly diverse patient population.[21,22] Importantly, patients with private and public insurance should be assigned to resident panels/teaching services and direct care/private teams in the same proportions.

Second, institutions should foster and support initiatives that promote increased diversity in their institutions by investing in equity, diversity, and inclusion (EDI) initiatives and pipeline programs that recruit students, trainees, and faculty who are underrepresented in medicine.[25] Often, these efforts fall to trainees, so institutions must provide both direct financial support and protected time for faculty to engage in this work as well.

Clinical dashboards within the EHR can provide feedback to trainees on their own health care delivery efforts. Trainees should review the outcomes of their patients with results stratified by key demographics to identify biases and inequities within their own practice. As an example, dashboards highlighted that residents have overestimated the complexity of their patient panels.[26] This demonstrates that a regular review of these data may help trainees better understand their patient panels and potential biases.

In summary, medicine cannot escape its roots, but the future need not be defined by the past. To achieve this, medical education must excise race-based medicine, address discrimination in formal and hidden curricula, invest in EDI initiatives at all levels, and facilitate care for underserved populations. We begin with these issues as they must inform all discussion that follows.

SECTION 2. TRANSFORMATIVE TECHNOLOGIES

"AI systems will generally make people more efficient at what they are already doing, whether that is good or bad."[27]

From ancient surgical tools to the stethoscope to portable MRIs, the practice of medicine is inexorably linked to technology.[28] Clinicians from any era are well acquainted with the need to integrate various sources of data. These data include knowledge of population epidemiology, elements of the history, physical exam findings, laboratory results, and clinical images. The EHR now contains all these data, and the quantity quickly becomes "far beyond human cognitive and decision-making capabilities."[27] "Big data" thus refers to massive amounts of highly variable data that grow and change rapidly.[29] In this section, we define and discuss how machine learning, artificial intelligence, and precision medicine make use of big data to revolutionize patient care.

Big data "cannot be analyzed, searched, interpreted, or stored using traditional data-processing methods."[30] Using traditional regressions, for example, the investigator must choose which variables to test in the model. Increasing complexity of the data requires increasingly complex models to explore these data, thus **machine learning** "is a natural extension to traditional statistical approaches."[31] Machine learning uses algorithms to identify optimal combinations of variables from patient-level observations to reliably predict outcomes.[32] This is, of course, the same process of inductive reasoning that clinicians employ over their careers of encountering thousands of patients, but machine learning can perform this reasoning at a previously impossible scale.

A prominent example of machine learning in medicine is the development of clinical prediction models. Examples include predicting outcomes following epilepsy surgery,[33] hospital visits among pediatric asthma patients,[34] presence/absence of angiography-confirmed coronary artery disease,[35,36] transfer to the pediatric intensive care unit,[37] hospital readmission,[38] and mortality.[39] These prediction models allow for interventions to improve clinical and financial outcomes. For example, identifying inpatients at risk for readmission can then help reduce readmission rates,[40] and identifying patients who may benefit from a rapid response intervention can reduce mortality.[41]

Cognitive computing and **artificial intelligence (AI)** naturally emerge from these technologies. Cognitive computing refers to "self-learning systems using machine learning, pattern recognition, and natural language processing to mimic the operation of human thought processes...to create automated computerized models that can solve problems without human assistance."[30] AI can be defined generally as "a branch of computer science that attempts to both understand and build" computerized intelligent entities capable of performing tasks previously reserved for humans.[42] The American Medical Association (AMA) and National Academy of Medicine refer to "augmented" rather than "artificial" intelligence to emphasize the "assistive role" to "enhance human intelligence rather than replace it" and reflect that "humans and machines can excel in distinct ways that the other cannot, meaning that the two combined can accomplish what neither could do alone."[27,43,44] To simplify our language, we refer to these concepts simply as "AI" throughout the rest of this chapter. Automation in machine learning and AI exists on a spectrum,[31] and Yo and colleagues quip that today's AI breakthrough becomes tomorrow's prosaic daily technology.[42] Examples of AI in daily life from industries outside

of medicine are prolific,[27] yet few of us would consider Google search or translate to be examples of AI today.[45] Application of AI to clinical settings lags behind other sectors due to difficulty training algorithms on complex, qualitative, poorly accessible, clinical data across vastly incongruent EHR.[46–48]

There are many applications of AI in medicine. These include identifying care gaps for patient panels and populations, assisting with triage, device interrogation, health coaching, chart review, note writing, automated response to in-basket questions, automated patient rooming and history taking, monitoring wearable and home devices, "just-in-time adaptive interventions" that automatically contact patients, image interpretation, population disease surveillance, monitoring and integration of environmental variables, assistance for elderly patients and patients with disabilities, clinical decision aids, molecular autopsies, and fully robotic surgery.[27,42,43,49] AI-controlled robot surgery remains in its nascent stages. As one example, an AI robot successfully completed end-to-end intestinal anastomosis in pigs.[50]

A prominent example of AI in medicine is image interpretation, and image-based diagnosis may be considered the "most successful" medical application of AI to date.[42] AI can identify diabetic retinopathy in fundus photographs,[51,52] pulmonary tuberculosis on chest radiographs,[53,54] left ventricular ejection fraction and wall motion abnormalities on cardiac MRIs,[55,56] malignant skin lesions from pictures,[57] prostate cancer on histopathologic images,[58] and breast cancer in biopsied lymph nodes.[58,59] AI can provide similar breast cancer detection rates and decrease radiologist workload as part of large-scale breast cancer screening.[60] Augmenting human capacity, AI has improved radiologists' ability to detect lung nodules[61] and breast cancer.[62] AI can also be applied to imaging obtained during procedures; for example, AI can augment gastroenterologists' polyp detection during colonoscopy.[63]

There are several limitations and points of caution. Concerns include issues of privacy, risk of bias and discrimination, initiating/perpetuating false information, difficulty in regulation, disintegration of the patient-physician relationship, difficulty understanding and explaining the logic of "black box" models, vulnerability to hackers and malware, elimination of health care job opportunities, physician "skill-rot" due to "over-reliance on computer-based systems," difficulty transferring successful models from one setting to another, difficulty defining normal variance in data drawn from homogeneous populations, and unequal delivery of new technologies that exacerbate health inequities.[27,42,43,49]

The limitations of AI also extend to its application to imaging. First, limitations in generalizability may raise concerns about wide-scale acceptance.[64] Second, previous research has shown that radiologists are less likely to detect findings when a computer misses these findings,[65] raising the concern that physicians may come to rely on AI and suffer regression of their skills. This would be especially unfortunate given that, third, a combined AI-human workflow may provide greater accuracy than either alone.[53] Fourth, nonmedical applications of AI to image recognition and generation have shown discrimination and bias,[66,67] so we must proactively seek to avoid these pitfalls within medicine.

AI technologies must be evaluated like any other medical intervention using the "traditional medical hierarchy of evidence to support adoption and continued use."[27] This places "pilot data as the lowest level of evidence, followed by observational, risk-adjusted assessments … and results of clinical trials at the top of the classification scheme."[27] Physicians will need to be trained to interpret a new literature of evaluating AI interventions. Despite this necessity, complex AI systems exist as "black boxes"[68] and provide output without insight into the inner workings of the model logic, and this makes evaluation of these models difficult.

The above technologies allow for the emergence of **precision medicine**. While other terms have been used, such as "personalized" or "individualized," we follow the semantic choice of the White House, National Institutes of Health, National Academy of Sciences, and others in using the term "precision."[69-71] The close of the 20th century touted evidence-based medicine as best practice. Unfortunately, most of the patients we see and for whom we attempt to apply the results of evidence-based medicine do *not* benefit. If the number needed to treat in a given trial is five, which is a quite low and advantageous number, 80% will *not* benefit from the intervention. Most simply then, precision medicine aims to "tailor medical treatment to the individual characteristics of each patient"[69] using **"pano*ro*mic" data** from every level of a person's existence, including zip code and environmental exposures (so-called exposome), social connections, real-time physiologic data (included in one's physiome), anatomy, metabolism profile (metabolome), microbiome, patterns of protein expression (proteome), RNA profile (transcriptome), genetic code as written in an individual's DNA (genome), and the dynamic interaction of the genome with the environment (epigenome).[49] In 2015, President Obama announced a precision medicine initiative (now the *All of Us* Research Program) "to give all of us access to the personalized information we need to keep ourselves and our families healthier."[71] Many countries have also initiated precision medicine programs.[72]

The association with oncology remains the most salient clinical application of precision medicine techniques.[73] However, precision medicine methodologies should be applied across the lifespan, including preconception counseling; understanding an individual's risk for chronic diseases; rapid and targeted diagnosis and treatment of illness from infectious disease to cancers; and "molecular autopsy" capable of providing life-saving and health-promoting information to surviving family members.[49] For example, people respond differently to the same diet, and precision nutrition counseling can reduce postprandial blood glucose levels and alter the microbiome.[74] At the genomic level, gene-editing therapies have become a reality, and in the final days of preparation of this chapter, a CRISPR (clustered regularly interspaced palindromic repeats)–based[75] gene-editing treatment for sickle cell disease and transfusion-dependent beta-thalassemia was approved in the United Kingdom.[76,77]

In summary, technology will continue to transform health care, and the 21st century will see AI incorporated into daily medical practice. Evidence-based medicine will evolve into precision medicine, and we need clinical trials to assess the impact of AI-based interventions. As issues of health equity remain paramount, we must employ 21st-century technologies to transcend, rather than amplify, humanity's biases and to eliminate, rather than expand, inequities in health care delivery.

SECTION 3. TECHNOLOGIES AND THE CLINICAL EVALUATION

"Listen to your patient, they are telling you the diagnosis."[78]

Some may assume that technological advancements will make the patient–physician encounter obsolete. On the contrary, optimal functioning of the AI–physician dyad will entrust the patient-facing tasks to the expert in human interactions—the physician. In a warped reality, even if we are relegated to serve as "data entry clerks, feeding data-hungry machines,"[27] the responsibility still falls to the physician to elicit the correct information from the patient. In this section, we illustrate how 21st-century technologies and perspectives can be applied to the clinical evaluation, including the history, physical, and point-of-care assessment.

Entire texts have been devoted to the topic of gathering medical histories,[79] and the importance of the history cannot be overemphasized. Furthermore, physicians must understand how the patient understands their own "illness narrative," as this affects the way they approach and interact with the health care system.[80] Kleinman's eight questions can help unlock this understanding and include the following: how the patient names the problem; the patient's understanding of possible etiology and tempo; the patient's expectations for treatment; the effect of the symptoms/disease on their life; and their most pressing concerns or fears about their presentation.[81] As an example, consider the varied arguments and misinformation patients may hold when declining vaccines.[82] Unfortunately, bias continuously threatens the history taking when we interpret patient complaints (e.g., chest pain) differently based on their identity.[83] Machine learning methodologies based on real health system data can help debunk assumptions of how we expect patients to describe their presenting complaint (e.g., chest pain).[84,85]

As medicine continues to push the limits of what is diagnosable, curable, and survivable, the history must include discussion of goals of care at an early stage. The physician will have to make difficult decisions about *when* advanced and expensive interventions should *not* be employed. In synchrony with training in state-of-the-art diagnostics and treatments, trainees should be introduced to principles of goals of care from the beginning of their training to be ethical stewards of medical technologies. AI can help identify patients for inpatient consults to the palliative care service to facilitate such discussions,[86] previous documentation of goals-of-care discussions in the EHR,[87] and "potential palliative care beneficiaries" using administrative data.[88]

Expert clinicians initially passed down pearls and pitfalls of the physical exams via poetic descriptions, such as the examination in acute abdominal pain[89] or congenital heart disease.[90] Next, innumerable individual studies have used traditional statistical methods to examine how well aspects of the physical exam performed against more "objective" findings. Attempts to define the test characteristics of exam maneuvers led to the emphasis on a "rational"[91] or "evidence-based"[92] physical exam. An increasing number of clinical calculators help aggregate key history, exam, and lab findings to guide the physician on the next steps in diagnostic workup and management (e.g., MDCalc, Calculate by QxMD). Still, the evidence for these exam maneuvers and calculators has been derived from limited studies in relatively homogeneous populations, so they may not well apply to every patient. Employing 21st-century methodologies, AI analysis of "panoromic" data can define which physical exam findings are relevant to a diagnosis, phenotype, or outcome for your patient.

Numerous systems exist for point-of-care testing/tests (POCT). The ever-expanding list of currently available POCT includes, but is not limited to, urine pregnancy, cell counts and differential, lymphocyte enumeration, metabolic panels and electrolytes, blood gases, blood glucose and hemoglobin A1c, lipid panel, urinalysis, urine toxicology, cardiac markers, coagulation markers, and testing for many infectious diseases. While many providers question the accuracy of POCT, their accuracy continues to improve.[93–95] Professional organizations have released guidelines on the implementation and management of POCT.[96–98] Given its widespread application and the rapid introduction and evolution of new tests, 21st-century providers will need to be comfortable with the indications, implementation, and limitations of POCT. It has also been argued that POCT should be part of the curriculum in public health training.[99] To allow these POCT results to be part of the patient's "panoroma" of data, these results should sync directly into the patient's EHR.

POCT can be effectively employed in the hospital, clinic, and community. In the inpatient setting, several POCT, such as glucose and blood gases, have been widely adopted as standard of care. In the clinic setting, patients on oral anticoagulation with warfarin traditionally were required to present to the clinic or lab for regular monitoring of the International Normalized Ratio (INR). POCT devices allow the patient to monitor their INR themselves and make adjustments following a pre-specified protocol or discuss their home test results with the clinic. Reviews of home-based INR monitoring have found this strategy reduced thromboembolic events and mortality.[100,101] POCT of INR also reflects general themes that POCT can be less accurate at extreme values (e.g., INR > 3.5) and among certain populations (e.g., congenital factor deficiency, lupus anticoagulant, chronic liver disease).[102] At the community level, POCT for human immunodeficiency virus (HIV) viral load and CD4 counts will revolutionize HIV health care delivery.[103–105] Looking ahead, HIV antibodies can even be detected using a smartphone accessory, which holds the potential of further increasing access to testing.[106]

Focused point-of-care bedside ultrasound (POCUS) has exploded in popularity. Pocket ultrasound systems (e.g., Lumify, SonoMe, Clarius, Butterfly) allow the physician to perform whole-body ultrasound immediately at the bedside. POCUS allows the physician to answer specific clinical questions.[107] Initially employed in emergency medicine, there is broad applicability.[108,109] In addition to a myriad of assessments for individual findings in specific organs (e.g., kidneys for hydronephrosis, soft-tissue structures for injury, or the biliary system for evidence of stones), many protocols exist to help guide rapid assessment. As some fundamental examples, protocols exist for the assessment of bleeding in trauma,[110,111] cardiopulmonary disease,[112–115] hypotension,[116,117] infectious disease,[118–121] and deep vein thrombosis.[122–124] Similar to trends in radiology-performed ultrasound, AI is now being used in POCUS to aid in image interpretation and diagnosis,[125] as well as to guide probe placement during image acquisition.[126] Incorporating AI into POCUS can help extend delivery into rural and underserved settings where physicians or other health care providers with significant POCUS experience may not be present.

POCUS can also be employed in the hospital, clinic, and community. In the intensive care unit, POCUS helps assess decompensating patients.[127] In clinic, one-time screening for abdominal aortic aneurysm with ultrasonography is recommended for males aged 65 to 75 years who have ever smoked,[128] and this scan could be performed by the primary care physician during the annual exam.[129,130] In rural areas, POCUS can help identify extrapulmonary tuberculosis in patients with HIV.[131]

Consumer products, such as wearable smart watches (e.g., Apple Watch, Samsung Galaxy Watch, FitBit) and pocket ECG devices (e.g., Kardia, EMAY, Omron, Wellue, Eko) are readily available. A wearable ultrasound device was also recently developed.[132] These devices provide real-time physiologic data that can be analyzed as part of an individual's "physiome" and overall "panoromic" profile. The ability of wearable and pocket devices to detect atrial fibrillation (Afib) has received considerable attention and provides an example of the potential impact and pitfalls of these technologies. Early identification of Afib using wearable devices may provide the opportunity for stroke prevention. When compared to 12-lead ECG, an early review found high sensitivity and specificity among several handheld products.[133] Two years later, however, the Apple Heart Study raised several important questions about the accuracy, implementation, and ramifications of smartwatch-based detection of irregular peripheral pulses.[134-137] Further, a more recent review found that consumer devices were more often used in younger and healthier people, who were therefore at lower risk for Afib, and an association with lower risk of stroke had not yet been established.[138] Thus, the potential to reduce both morbidity and inequities depends on the accuracy of these devices and their delivery to populations most likely to benefit. Given concerns of inappropriate use of these devices among populations for which they were not intended and overuse of health resources based on device alerts,[139] 21st-century providers will need to be fluent in the technical details, promises, and pitfalls of these devices.

Applying a 21st-century lens, AI is well suited to analyze data from mobile and wearable devices and has proven its ability to exhume novel interpretations from such data. Using the example of a 12-lead ECG, AI can identify preclinical left ventricular systolic dysfunction[140,141] and intensive care unit patients with life-threatening findings.[142] AI can also provide "just-in-time adaptive interventions"[27]; thus we could imagine AI detecting a rhythm change on a wearable device, instructing the patient to perform a multi-lead ECG at home, then alerting the physician or instructing the patient to implement a preestablished plan. In addition, AI on mobile devices can help interpret clinical images; for example, AI models used to identify malignant skin lesions can be used on mobile devices.[57]

In summary, clinical assessment changes as technologies evolve, but fundamental principles remain the same

whether we listen to the heart with our head against the patient's chest, auscultate with our stethoscope, or perform cardiac POCUS. The physician will remain the expert in accurately eliciting the patient's complaints, framing these complaints within the context of the patient's values and overall illness narrative, and performing targeted and meaningful exam maneuvers for the clinical context. POCT, POCUS, and home devices augment the clinical encounter, and AI allows the physician to integrate data from the patient's entire "panoroma" into the clinical assessment. Rather than ruminate over the physical exam as it *has been*, we must actively engage in enduring, iterative adaptation to reimagine and create the clinical assessment *as it will be*.

SECTION 4. AN INTERCONNECTED WORLD

"[R]esearchers can justify a study or publication on the basis of a gap in the literature, as if the literature could be considered the sum of all available knowledge..."[143]

Medicine in the 21st century requires a global perspective for several reasons. First, repeated examples (e.g., influenza, COVID-19, ebola, mpox) emphasize infectious diseases do not respect international borders.[144-146] Second, noncommunicable diseases (NCD) remain among the leading causes of morbidity and mortality worldwide,[147] and low- or middle-income countries (LMIC) will face the dual burden of both communicable and noncommunicable diseases due to the growing prevalence of NCD.[148] Third, climate change is a driving force behind environmental risk and dramatically alters the state of health and disease for entire populations.[149,150] Fourth, Western medicine remains a small drop in the sea of global medical knowledge and experience.[143] In each of these four areas, 21st-century technology can help us address these issues in both high-income countries (HIC) and LMIC, and in some cases, early adoption of these technologies may allow LMIC to make a technologic leap ahead of HIC.

As both communicable and noncommunicable diseases equilibrate across the globe, American physicians have considerable experience to share and even more to learn from our colleagues around the world. The United States faces the resurgence of previously eliminated infectious diseases, such as measles,[151] malaria,[152] and even yellow fever.[153] Limited experience with such diseases may translate into delays in diagnosis and access to first-line treatments even at academic hospitals in the United States.[154] In infectious disease, there is a long history of American physicians working abroad, yet it is very difficult for international physicians, especially those from LMIC, to enjoy the same opportunities in the United States. This inequity does not go unnoticed by our international colleagues, and we believe bidirectional exchange to be an important component of international collaboration.[155] Thus, reemergence of infectious diseases in the United States offers an opportunity to reengage international colleagues, especially those from LMIC, as expert consultants in these areas.

NCD management constitutes a significant portion of American medicine, but we still have much to learn. For example, management of myocardial infarction remains bread-and-butter medicine at academic hospitals, and standard practice involves antiplatelet agents, heparin, and referral to the catheterization laboratory for percutaneous coronary intervention.[156,157] Most of the world does not have many (if any) choices of antiplatelet agents, cannot easily monitor an intravenous heparin infusion, and does not have access to a catheterization laboratory. While academic American physicians are aware of the "pharmacoinvasive" options,[156] fewer have actually practiced this way. Our colleagues in Malawi use aspirin, a lower dose of clopidogrel, and enoxaparin, and referral to a catheterization lab means travel to another country.[158] In the clinic, risk stratification for atherosclerotic cardiovascular disease remains bread-and-butter primary care, and standard practice includes modification of risk factors including obesity, sedentary lifestyle, diet, hypertension, dyslipidemia, and smoking.[159] Writing from Nepal, Adhikari articulately describes his patients who walk up and down their mountainous hometowns and continue to suffer atherosclerotic disease at lower body mass index.[160] The traditional risk models derived from the United States do not apply universally, and guideline-recommended doses may not be well tolerated.[160] Whether or not an American medical student will ever practice in Malawi or Nepal is irrelevant; the cognitive flexibility to adapt guidelines to a local context is a fundamental lesson for trainees with a global perspective. Precision medicine may help overcome the limitations of traditional guidelines by using *local* data to identify the ideal interventions for individual patients.

American physicians have even more to learn about health care delivery. While the United States health care system excels at "rescue" medicine,[161] innovation and implementation of cutting-edge technologies, and health care spending, its performance in many core areas remains poor compared to other wealthy countries. Calling health care delivery in the United States a "system" is itself generous, as health care delivery emerges from a patchwork of poorly integrated private, occupational, government, and non-profit programs.[162] Specifically, the United States fails in four key areas: "provid[ing] for universal coverage," "invest[ing] in primary care systems," "reduc[ing] administrative burdens," and "invest[ing] in social services" and is ranked last among 11 HIC on "access to care and equity."[163] Failures of access and equity already plagued health care in

the United States before COVID-19,[164] and the pandemic has only exacerbated these problems, resulting in worse outcomes for underserved populations.[165] In other countries, advanced and comprehensive **community health worker (CHW)**–based programs have succeeded in delivering care for many conditions, including tuberculosis, HIV, and NCDs.[166] In Senegal, for example, expansion of CHWs to detect and treat simple malaria led to increased case detection and decreased symptomatic malaria.[167,168] Leveraging community health programs, Senegal achieved a rotavirus vaccination rate >90% prior to disruptions from supply chain issues and the COVID-19 pandemic, while the United States had still not reached 80% coverage in 2022.[169] While CHWs existed in the United States prior to the pandemic, COVID-19 reemphasized the need for CHWs and reinspired interest in CHW programs.[170,171]

American medicine has much to learn from CHW principles of geographic coverage, proactive case detection, decentralized and home-based care, and social support as key components of a successful health system. CHWs can be the foundation of health systems, supporting disease surveillance, promoting home management of lifelong illnesses, and providing a ready workforce for short-term population health campaigns. Twenty-first-century technologies are redefining the scope of practice of the CHW, and it may prove to be CHWs who leverage these technologies most, both in HIC and LMIC. AI can help guide CHWs in disease surveillance efforts, to utilize and interpret POCT performed in the home or in rural locations, to acquire and interpret POCUS images, and to manage wearable technologies. Trainees must be trained to manage teams outside the clinical environment, including CHWs, mid-level providers, epidemiologists, mobile nursing teams, and data analysts. As a mentor once counseled, "The separation between medicine and public health exists only in small minds." Trainees should have time dedicated to working with federally qualified health centers, local public health offices, mobile health vans, community health fairs, vaccination and health screening campaigns, and contact tracing. To learn from advanced community health models around the world, international electives should be a requirement for all trainees.

Climate and health are inexorably linked, so physicians must learn to understand how climate change affects the health of their patients. The World Health Organization conservatively estimated 250,000 additional deaths "due to climate change" between 2030 and 2050.[172] Among the many effects on health, rising sea levels can displace entire populations; floods and droughts can decrease access to food and increase malnutrition; higher temperatures can expand the geographic risk of vectorborne diseases and prey on vulnerable populations such as neonates and the elderly; higher carbon dioxide levels can decrease the nutritional content of crops; and poor air quality can worsen cardiopulmonary disease.[149] Sadly, LMIC may suffer the most even though they contributed less to climate change.

As an example at the global level, climate change may broaden the areas at risk for malaria, increase the duration of high-transmission seasons, and increase risk of natural disasters that destabilize health systems and displace populations. This may limit and even reverse the reductions in malaria incidence, morbidity, and mortality that have characterized malaria control efforts in recent decades.[173] As an example among underserved patients in the United States, Salas eloquently described the layers of structural violence that connect climate change and a young girl's visit to the emergency department for asthma. The patient lived in a redlined neighborhood close to a major highway and with minimal green space.[174,175] To identify effects of environmental racism and climate change, Salas proposes that the EHR lists the patient's zip code, along with an associated "environmental exposure profile."[174] To mitigate and address issues of air quality, applications "that report [particulate matter], ozone, and pollen levels" can help families avoid high-risk times of day or locations.[174] Further, "prescriptions for home weatherization and air-filtration systems could be made as common as those for albuterol."[174] As discussed earlier, the "exposome" is part of the comprehensive "panoromic" assessment of a patient, and these data can easily be incorporated into AI models.

The academic literature remains exceedingly limited to the experiences of high-income and anglophone countries.[176–178] For example, oncology research funded by the National Cancer Institute, often fails to reflect our country's diversity.[179] Non–English-speaking patients may be excluded from medical research.[180] The English-language academic literature is considered impressive, yet the paucity of diversity and global perspective means that the overwhelming proportion of day-to-day medical experience worldwide remains silenced, hidden, and invisible. Abimbola eloquently summarizes, "[I]f the academic literature to which we give priority does not reflect that local experts are at the forefront of addressing local problems, then there is something deeply wrong with that literature, because it does not reflect reality."[181] Therefore, to optimize the scientific community's fund of knowledge and to bring best practices from around the world to patients who need them, American medical education must empower previously silenced voices around the globe by including international examples from both HIC and LMIC. Discussion of health care around the world should be a longitudinal thread integrated into each block and include perspectives from other HIC, LMIC, and sources in other languages. With its ability to peruse non-English language and

translate among languages, AI models may offer unprecedented ability for multilingual learning.

In summary, trainees must be trained with a global perspective to be adequately prepared for the next epidemics, for the heavy burden of NCDs in populations previously considered lower risk, and for the health sequelae of climate change. As medical education embraces a global perspective, it must acknowledge and address that the roots of the field of "global health" are deeply intertwined with an exploitative, colonialist history.[182–184] While the list of problems with current global health collaborations can be long, there is great promise in equitable collaboration, and there have been many attempts to improve equity in global health collaborations.[155,185] For instance, virtual communities such as the AI-powered platform The Village (https://globalhealthvillage.org/) can help foster equitable collaboration among health professionals from around the globe. Fundamentally, American students and physicians must learn to engage the world without seeking to exploit it.

SECTION 5. EDUCATIONAL NEEDS OF TRAINEES

"Data without interpretation are facts without understanding"[48]
"We spend our days doing the wrong work."[186]

An older faculty member once quipped that he and his co-residents had been able to "know the mechanism of action, pharmacokinetics, and side effects of every medication" used several decades ago, but rapid changes in medical innovation make it impossible for 21st-century trainees to master all medical knowledge at any point during their training. For example, a physician during the mid-20th century could practice a full 50-year career by the time medical knowledge was estimated to double; in contrast, during our four years of medical school, medical knowledge doubled about 19 times.[187] Such evolution in medical knowledge requires ongoing iteration of pedagogy in medical education. In this section, we discuss changes and areas for improvement in undergraduate and graduate medical education (GME).

At the undergraduate level, many schools are reorganizing their curricula. Recent changes include earlier initiation of clinical practicums, reorganizing and shortening the pre-clerkship period, the introduction of problem-based learning and "flipped classroom" models,[188] early integration of the humanities, increased opportunities for research, and changes to the United States Medical Licensing Examination.[189] Despite these changes, there remain clear areas for growth.

Students need study techniques to internalize large amounts of information. Undergraduate medical education currently tumbles as a waterfall onto the student, who is left to gather what drops can be saved in their buckets of memories and notes. Fundamentals of physiology, anatomy, and pathophysiology should be emphasized; esoteric medical trivia should be avoided. To manage the quantity of information, several studies have shown the efficacy of spaced repetition for long-term learning.[190,191] Many medical students have integrated this technique into their study practice by using online spaced-repetition flash cards.[192] Medical schools should incorporate this concept into curriculum design to promote long-term retention. For example, one school created its own spaced-repetition flashcard deck.[193] Others have proposed the implementation of spiral curricula that revisit core principles and deepen knowledge with each reintroduction.[187]

A physician is not simply a knower of facts. The value of a human physician remains in the ability to weigh the relevance and applicability of evidence, to understand the limitations of testing, and to contextualize this knowledge within the patient's psychosocial milieu, goals, and values. For example, we have already seen how providing lay adults with access to the internet does not greatly improve their triage or diagnostic ability.[194] In addition, a large language model called ChatGPT (generative pretrained transformer version 3.5) exceeded expectations on medical standardized testing. The success of AI on standardized tests can be seen as an indictment on the way medical students have been trained. "The framing of medical knowledge as something that can be encapsulated into multiple choice questions," Mbakwe et al. argue, "creates a cognitive framing of false certainty."[195] The strength and value of the physician can no longer be based on "the ability to regurgitate mechanistic models of health and disease."[195] Rather than ask the trainee, "What is the best next step?" which implies a singular answer based on factual knowledge, we might ask trainees to review, interpret, and weigh multiple sources of recommendations.

Students need a foundation in informatics. Clinical informatics is a growing field that focuses on "the analysis, design, and evaluation of information and communication systems to improve patient care, enhance access to care, advance individual and population health outcomes, and strengthen the clinician-patient relationship."[196] Some physicians may evolve into a role of "information specialists," "interpret[ing] the important data, advis[ing] on the added value of another diagnostic test . . . and integrat[ing] information to guide clinicians."[197] The benefits of integrating informatics training with undergraduate medical education include "improving students' skills in handling medical data, enhancing digital infrastructure of the health system, enabling precision medicine, and increasing familiarity with medico-legal and ethical issues with health digitalization."[196] Unfortunately, despite these many benefits, few medical schools have incorporated this training into

their curricula. One study found approximately one-third of students were interested in a career in clinical informatics but unaware of the available training opportunities.[198]

Students need a foundation in precision medicine principles. Precision medicine fellowships are increasing nationwide, but we believe precision medicine should be a methodology used by all physicians, not a separate specialty. The time to change educational paradigms is both now and fleeting. As part of this training, students need a stronger foundation in genetics; otherwise, "the knowledge asymmetry between purveyors of precision health technologies and nongeneticist clinicians [may create] the potential for well-intentioned misapplication of tests…"[72]

Students need a foundation in point-of-care technologies. Previous generations of physicians reviewed patients' peripheral blood smears, and they understood the nuances and limitations of these media. The next generation of physicians must be trained in genetics and principles of predictive modeling, to gain the same insight, respect, and humility using these technologies. Trainees could obtain registered diagnostic sonographer and POCT credentialing during medical school. Since 2018, the Association of Diagnostics and Laboratory Medicine has offered a special certification to credential Certified Point-of-Care Testing Professionals.[199] Some emergency medicine residents may obtain registered diagnostic sonographer certification through a "mini-fellowship" in ultrasound.[83] We believe these resources should be at the disposal of every student physician.

At the GME level, many programs are reorganizing the resident experience. Changes include limitations of work hours, requirements for quality improvement and scholarly projects, opportunities for research and electives, and an ever-increasing variety of Accreditation Council for Graduate Medical Education (ACGME)–approved specialty and subspecialty fellowship training programs. Despite these changes, there remain clear areas for growth. We question several assumptions: (1) trainees learn best by immediate and complete clinical immersion, (2) the historical model of rounding still applies, and (3) documentation is the responsibility of the trainee.

Although the clinical rotations of medical school provide the foundation for residency and clinical immersion in residency builds the foundation for fellowship, the role of the trainee at each stage is unique. Importantly, students and trainees often switch institutions from one phase to the next, and site-specific logistical knowledge can sometimes feel as daunting as the medical knowledge itself. Despite the dramatic adjustments required by trainees at each stage, they often assume the responsibility of being fully functioning in their role during the first few days or weeks. The negative sequelae of this are several, but importantly, clinical care suffers early at the beginning of each academic year.[200,201]

Programs should increase simulation-based learning. Simulation to practice key clinical scenarios and procedures could constitute the majority of time at the beginning of each phase of training. Simulations may test team skills (e.g., running a code),[202] procedural skills (e.g., central lines),[203,204] surgical skills,[205] and overall clinical decision-making. Maintaining a simulation center and designing cases can be time consuming, expensive, and therefore difficult to provide frequently for many trainees, so online simulation tools can offer a more scalable option.[206] For example, an online clinical simulation tool improved students' ability to gather essential information.[207] In our own training, we found online simulations for learning Neonatal Resuscitation Program (https://nrplearningplatform.com/) to be particularly helpful for the opportunity to repeatedly practice before relevant rotations.

Programs should design a smoother transition of responsibility. Incoming and outgoing trainees could overlap such that patients are incrementally transferred to the incoming trainee. The classical structure of graduated autonomy should be reevaluated and structured based on the timing of the academic year, fund of knowledge, or skill set of the trainee.[208] Especially during the beginning of the academic year, hospitals may need to consider lowering patient caps and increasing the number of residents on busy services. The paradigm needs to shift from the question of *What can our trainees survive?* to *How can we optimize the clinical and learning environments to achieve the best patient outcomes?*

Programs should reimagine the process of rounding. For trainees in medical specialties, the process of rounding at academic medical centers can be wildly inefficient and sometimes borders on farce. Challenges include time constraints and the use of EHRs.[209] Chart review and pre-rounding used to be arduous processes which required physically locating and reviewing handwritten records in a paper chart. Thus, the presenting trainee was the only team member who had initially accessed this information. In the 21st century, however, most team members have already reviewed consult notes, results, and imaging on their computer or their phone prior to (or during) rounds and have already acted on these data. Even the family may have already seen new results. Yet, the presenting trainee dutifully reviews data early in the morning and wakes up delirious patients. Team members may ignore the presenter who has already fallen an hour behind the release of new results. The team then moves on to the next patient, and the senior clinicians may return separately to examine the patient themselves at another time, thereby eliminating the possibility of teaching at the bedside. Many teams "round" at a table and never see the patients together at all. When the American Academy of Pediatrics adopted family-centered rounds, it was intended to integrate families into medical decision-making.[210] Family-centered rounds rapidly expanded to other services, but invited criticism for extended duration of rounds, competing demands, burnout, and workflow interference.[210] Furthermore, presenting the plan in front of the family can disempower the presenting resident. For example, the presenting resident may not see new results and miss the opportunity to discuss the plan with the team beforehand.

Modern rounding structure should be adapted to account for the availability of digital information and for the diversity of our patient populations: after brief review to decide the order of rounding, the team could review data, see patients, and discuss plans together. For example, one academic teaching service has eliminated pre-rounding. The senior resident and intern review overnight events, vitals, and lab data together in the morning. With the time saved by eliminating duplicative pre-rounding, the team could spend more time examining the patient together and employ some of the emerging point-of-care technologies discussed above. Such a structure also preserves the opportunity for junior trainees to learn from the master clinicians leading their teams.

Often, interpretation services are needed during rounds, and these services can be difficult to access. As medicine adopts a global perspective, hospital systems must exponentially increase investment for interpretation services for all clinical encounters. Using the best phone interpreter system to which we have access, it regularly takes over a minute to get an interpreter on the phone and ready to interpret in Spanish, the most common language for which we need interpreters. It takes even longer for any other language. AI will also improve its ability to interpret, although this should only be used as a stop-gap measure until an in-person interpreter can be found. Though we recognize that there may be a shortage of in-person interpreters, we maintain that in-person interpretation should be the gold standard of care and hospital systems should invest in robust interpretation departments.

Documentation overwhelmingly falls to trainees and must be reimagined. Outpatient physicians spend twice as much time in the EHR as they do in direct clinical face time with patients,[211] and time spent in the EHR is associated with physician exhaustion.[212] Surgeon author Atul Gawande describes the harrowing account transitioning to a commonly used EHR, including endless clicks for simple tasks, meaningless problem lists, verbose copy-forwarded notes, increased documentation burden, a deluge of in-basket messages, alarm fatigue, and loss of attention to the patient in the room.[213] A succinct condemnation of the current state of the EHR comes from a satire video by celebrity physician Zubin Damania (aka Zdogg MD) who defines the EHR as a "glorified billing platform with some patient stuff tacked on."[214] Many note templates contain copy-forwarded or auto-populated information, thereby leading to duplicative and inaccurate notes.[215] Incorrectly updated notes can have legal consequences.[215] While some have argued for the role of documentation in contextualizing, synthesizing, and tracking data for medical decision-making,[216] we disagree that trainees require documentation to learn and argue that excessive documentation unnecessarily couples their learning to writing. Documentation also simultaneously subverts the learner from direct patient care and didactic learning.

Two broad changes must be made. First, the content of documentation must be questioned. Trainees are taught to satisfy hospital billing and legal departments, rather than to summarize medical information. We recognize that some documentation is a medical necessity, but we consider excessive documentation a "low-value task." We agree that "a holistic system redesign may be needed to reorient incentives and eliminate the need for [these tasks] altogether. Otherwise, AI systems may just efficiently automate low-value tasks, further entrenching those tasks in the culture, rather than facilitating their elimination."[27] Second, we advocate that documentation should be delegated to persons or technologies dedicated to documentation, for example, paid scribes or AI note-writing software. As an example of using humans, the University of Colorado has implemented a program called ambulatory process excellence (APEX), which trains medical assistants to complete many tasks around and during the clinical encounter.[186] Before the visit, the medical assistants initially collect data, perform medication reconciliation, "set the agenda," and screen for preventive care gaps. During the visit, they document while the physician interacts with the patient. After the visit, they provide health education and coaching. The program required a large investment to hire and train medical assistants, but reduced burnout by 75% within 6 months.[186] AI can already do many, if not all, of these tasks. Many AI scribes are now available, and these use speech recognition and natural language processing to transcribe the clinical encounter into a written note.[217] They can listen in multiple languages, learn a provider's note style from past examples, and create notes using a SOAP (subjective, objective, assessment, plan) format.[217] Rather than teaching trainees how to rewrite their notes to respond to billing inquiries, they should be taught how to lead a team of highly valued medical assistants and how to use AI in daily patient care.

In summary, as the practice of medicine changes, the pedagogy of medical education must change. Paranjape et al. describe how "The traditional medical curriculum, which is mostly memorization based, must follow the transition from the information age to the age of AI. Future physicians have to be taught competence in the effective integration and utilization of information from a growing array of sources."[218] Undergraduate medical education must integrate learning techniques that allow for the internalization of large amounts of information and prioritize training in clinical informatics, precision medicine, and point-of-care technologies. Graduate medical education must restructure the transition to greater levels of responsibility, reconceptualize the process of rounding, and revolutionize documentation.

VIGNETTE 2: A 21ST-CENTURY PATIENT ENCOUNTER

Reimagine the clinical encounter described at the start of this chapter. A 57-year-old female presents for a preoperative visit prior to robotic partial colectomy for Stage I colorectal cancer detected on recent colonoscopy. She moved to your area last month, and her local CHW who speaks her language quickly reached out to establish care and to schedule her first colonoscopy. AI software immediately flagged the suspicious area for biopsy, and the diagnosis was made based on the pathology results. Regarding her chronic conditions, she has already completed a "panoromic" assessment. The medications likely to yield the highest benefit have already been discussed, and she started implementing the recommended dietary changes. Based on your first visit with this patient, AI in your practice's scheduling platform has automatically extended the length of this visit and arranged for an in-person interpreter. Prior to the start of the visit, AI in the EHR has pre-populated a note with the requested pre-op information, completed the medication reconciliation, and uploaded a summary of her blood glucose levels and blood pressure recordings from her home devices. Before you can begin, the interpreter opens with the patient's questions: she reports concern about swelling in her legs because her sister was recently diagnosed with a "blood clot in her chest" and she is tearful explaining her younger cousin recently died from a heart attack. She awaits the results of the molecular autopsy to identify any cardiovascular risk factors she may share with her cousin. You review the pre-populated information with her and her risk factors for surgery using the AI-powered risk calculator that is specific to your health system. You determine she does not need an ECG or stress test. You examine her, perform a POCUS of her lower extremities, and she is relieved that there is no evidence of thrombosis. With the extra time, you ask the patient how her family likes their new home and discuss restaurant recommendations. You ensure her address is correct, and then review the environmental risk profile for that neighborhood, which is generated automatically within the EHR. You type nothing during the visit as the ambient AI scribe records the pertinent information from your conversation. With the patient in the room, you review the note and manually make a few modifications together. AI has automatically completed the billing information based on the time, type of visit, and your discussion and routes the necessary information to the surgeon. You instruct the AI scheduling system to schedule a home visit with her CHW after the surgery.

Thought questions
1. How have 21st-century technologies and principles changed this encounter?
2. With what changes do you agree or disagree?
3. What changes will be easier or harder for your health system to implement?

CONCLUSION

Vignette 1 and Vignette 2 demonstrate how the clinical encounter can change from one generation to the next. Medicine of the 21st century must transcend the structural violence of its roots, weave technology and doctoring, embrace global perspectives, and adapt its pedagogy. The future of medicine arrives not tomorrow; it is now. Are we being trained to be the doctors our patients need and expect us to be? As the world changes, so must medicine, and this is for the better. Topol predicts "the digital convergence with biology will definitively anchor the individual [patient] as … the principal driver of medicine in the future."[49] The culmination of civilization's technology leads us right back to where we started: with our focus on the individual patient in front of us.

ACKNOWLEDGMENTS

The authors would like to thank Gifty-Maria J. Ntim, MD, MPH, and Abigail D. Pershing, JD, for their comments on earlier drafts of this chapter.

DISCLOSURES

Daniel Z. Hodson owns stock in Butterfly Network, Inc. Other authors report no disclosures relevant to the content of this chapter.

REFERENCES

1. Possin KL, Tsoy E, Windon CC. Perils of race-based norms in cognitive testing: the case of former NFL players. *JAMA Neurol.* 2021;78(4):377–378. https://doi.org/10.1001/jamaneurol.2020.4763.
2. Hamed S, Bradby H, Ahlberg BM, Thapar-Björkert S. Racism in healthcare: a scoping review. *BMC Public Health.* 2022;22(1):988. https://doi.org/10.1186/s12889-022-13122-y.
3. Cerdeña JP, Plaisime MV, Tsai J. From race-based to race-conscious medicine: how anti-racist uprisings call us to act. *Lancet.* 2020;396(10257):1125–1128. https://doi.org/10.1016/s0140-6736(20)32076-6.
4. Vyas DA, Eisenstein LG, Jones DS. Hidden in plain sight - reconsidering the use of race correction in clinical algorithms. *N Engl J Med.* 2020;383(9):874–882. https://doi.org/10.1056/NEJMms2004740.
5. Braun L. Race correction and spirometry: why history matters. *Chest.* 2021;159(4):1670–1675. https://doi.org/10.1016/j.chest.2020.10.046.
6. Baugh AD, Shiboski S, Hansel NN, et al. Reconsidering the utility of race-specific lung function prediction equations. *Am J Respir Crit Care Med.* 2022;205(7):819–829. https://doi.org/10.1164/rccm.202105-1246OC.
7. Williams WW, Hogan JW, Ingelfinger JR. Time to eliminate health care disparities in the estimation of kidney function. *N Engl J Med.* 2021;385(19):1804–1806. https://doi.org/10.1056/NEJMe2114918.
8. Delgado C, Baweja M, Crews DC, et al. A unifying approach for GFR estimation: recommendations of the NKF-ASN task force on reassessing the inclusion of race in diagnosing kidney disease. *Am J Kidney Dis.* 2022;79(2):268–288.e1. https://doi.org/10.1053/j.ajkd.2021.08.003.
9. Landon MB, Leindecker S, Spong CY, et al. The MFMU Cesarean Registry: factors affecting the success of trial of labor after previous cesarean delivery. *Am J Obstet Gynecol.* 2005;193(3 Pt 2):1016–1023. https://doi.org/10.1016/j.ajog.2005.05.066.
10. Grobman WA, Lai Y, Landon MB, et al. Development of a nomogram for prediction of vaginal birth after cesarean delivery. *Obstet Gynecol.* 2007;109(4):806–812. https://doi.org/10.1097/01.Aog.0000259312.36053.02.
11. Vyas DA, Jones DS, Meadows AR, Diouf K, Nour NM, Schantz-Dunn J. Challenging the use of race in the vaginal birth after cesarean section calculator. *Women Health Iss.* 2019;29(3):201–204. https://doi.org/10.1016/j.whi.2019.04.007.
12. Shahian DM, Jacobs JP, Badhwar V, et al. The society of thoracic surgeons 2018 adult cardiac surgery risk models: Part 1—Background, design considerations, and model development. *Ann Thorac Surg.* 2018;105(5):1411–1418. https://doi.org/10.1016/j.athoracsur.2018.03.002.
13. Tice JA, Miglioretti DL, Li CS, Vachon CM, Gard CC, Kerlikowske K. Breast density and benign breast disease: Risk assessment to identify women at high risk of breast cancer. *J Clin Oncol.* 2015;33(28):3137–3143. https://doi.org/10.1200/jco.2015.60.8869.
14. Lloyd-Jones DM, Huffman MD, Karmali KN, et al. Estimating longitudinal risks and benefits from cardiovascular preventive therapies among medicare patients: the million hearts longitudinal ASCVD risk assessment tool: a special report from the American Heart Association and American College of Cardiology. *Circulation.* 2017;135(13):e793–e813. https://doi.org/10.1161/cir.0000000000000467.

15. Holt HK, Gildengorin G, Karliner L, Fontil V, Pramanik R, Potter MB. Differences in hypertension medication prescribing for Black Americans and their association with hypertension outcomes. *J Am Board Fam Med.* 2022;35(1):26–34. https://doi.org/10.3122/jabfm.2022.01.210276.

16. Rao S, Segar MW, Bress AP, et al. Association of Genetic West African Ancestry, Blood pressure response to therapy, and cardiovascular risk among Self-reported Black Individuals in the Systolic Blood Pressure Reduction Intervention Trial (SPRINT). *JAMA Cardiology.* 2021;6(4):388–398. https://doi.org/10.1001/jamacardio.2020.6566.

17. Vela MB, Erondu AI, Smith NA, Peek ME, Woodruff JN, Chin MH. Eliminating explicit and implicit biases in health care: evidence and research needs. *Annu Rev Public Health.* 2022;43:477–501. https://doi.org/10.1146/annurev-publhealth-052620-103528.

18. Services. USDoHaH. *Fact Sheet: Nondiscrimination in Health Programs and Activities Proposed Rule Section 1557 of the Affordable Care Act.* https://www.hhs.gov/civil-rights/for-providers/laws-regulations-guidance/regulatory-initiatives/1557-fact-sheet/index.html

19. Goodman KE, Morgan DJ, Hoffmann DE. Clinical algorithms, antidiscrimination laws, and medical device regulation. *JAMA.* 2023;329(4):285–286. https://doi.org/10.1001/jama.2022.23870.

20. Shachar C, Gerke S. Prevention of bias and discrimination in clinical practice algorithms. *JAMA.* 2023;329(4):283–284. https://doi.org/10.1001/jama.2022.23867.

21. Phelan SM, Burke SE, Cunningham BA, et al. The effects of racism in medical education on students' decisions to practice in underserved or minority communities. *Acad Med.* 2019;94(8):1178–1189. https://doi.org/10.1097/acm.0000000000002719.

22. Phelan SM, Burke SE, Hardeman RR, et al. Medical school factors associated with changes in implicit and explicit bias against gay and lesbian people among 3492 graduating medical students. *J Gen Intern Med.* 2017;32(11):1193–1201. https://doi.org/10.1007/s11606-017-4127-6.

23. Yousuf Y, Yu JC. Improving representation of skin of color in a medical school preclerkship dermatology curriculum. *Med Sci Educ.* 2022;32(1):27–30. https://doi.org/10.1007/s40670-021-01473-x.

24. Smith DF, Brady PW, Russell CJ. Introducing: health equity rounds. *Hosp Pediatr.* 2023;13(5):459–460. https://doi.org/10.1542/hpeds.2023-007234.

25. Mason BS, Ross W, Chambers MC, Grant R, Parks M. Pipeline program recruits and retains women and underrepresented minorities in procedure based specialties: a brief report. *Am J Surg.* 2017;213(4):662–665. https://doi.org/10.1016/j.amjsurg.2016.11.022.

26. Smith BM, Kuryla CL, Shilkofski NA, et al. Resident perceptions of continuity clinic patient metrics differ from EHR data: pilot use of population health dashboards. *Qual Manag Health Care.* 2023;32(3):155–160. https://doi.org/10.1097/qmh.0000000000000391.

27. Matheny ME, Israni ST, Ahmed M, Whicher D, eds. *Artificial Intelligence in Health Care the Hope, the Hype, the Promise, the Peril.* National Academy of Medicine; 2022.

28. Curtis J. *Medical devices and technology across the years. Yale Medicine Magazine.* The Lane Press; 2019.

29. NEJM Catalyst. *Healthcare Big Data and the Promise of Value-Based Care.* https://catalyst.nejm.org/doi/full/10.1056/CAT.18.0290.

30. Krittanawong C, Zhang H, Wang Z, Aydar M, Kitai T. Artificial intelligence in precision cardiovascular medicine. *J Am Coll Cardiol.* 2017;69(21):2657–2664. https://doi.org/10.1016/j.jacc.2017.03.571.

31. Beam AL, Kohane IS. Big data and machine learning in health care. *JAMA.* 2018;319(13):1317–1318. https://doi.org/10.1001/jama.2017.18391.

32. Obermeyer Z, Emanuel EJ. Predicting the future - Big data, machine learning, and clinical medicine. *N Engl J Med.* 2016;375(13):1216–1219. https://doi.org/10.1056/NEJMp1606181.

33. Gleichgerrcht E, Munsell B, Bhatia S, et al. Deep learning applied to whole-brain connectome to determine seizure control after epilepsy surgery. *Epilepsia.* 2018;59(9):1643–1654. https://doi.org/10.1111/epi.14528.

34. Shin EK, Mahajan R, Akbilgic O, Shaban-Nejad A. Sociomarkers and biomarkers: predictive modeling in identifying pediatric asthma patients at risk of hospital revisits. *NPJ Digit Med.* 2018;1:50. https://doi.org/10.1038/s41746-018-0056-y.

35. Zellweger MJ, Brinkert M, Bucher U, Tsirkin A, Ruff P, Pfisterer ME. A new memetic pattern based algorithm to diagnose/exclude coronary artery disease. *Int J Cardiol.* 2014;174(1):184–186. https://doi.org/10.1016/j.ijcard.2014.03.184.

36. Zellweger MJ, Tsirkin A, Vasilchenko V, et al. A new non-invasive diagnostic tool in coronary artery disease: artificial intelligence as an essential element of predictive, preventive, and personalized medicine. *EPMA J.* 2018;9(3):235–247. https://doi.org/10.1007/s13167-018-0142-x.

37. Mayampurath A, Sanchez-Pinto LN, Hegermiller E, et al. Development and external validation of a machine learning model for prediction of potential transfer to the PICU. *Pediatr Crit Care Med.* 2022;23(7):514–523. https://doi.org/10.1097/PCC.0000000000002965.

38. Davis S, Zhang J, Lee I, et al. Effective hospital readmission prediction models using machine-learned features. *BMC Health Serv. Res.* 2022;22(1):1415. https://doi.org/10.1186/s12913-022-08748-y.

39. Vu E, Steinmann N, Schröder C, et al. Applications of machine learning in palliative care: a systematic review. *Cancers (Basel).* 2023;15(5). https://doi.org/10.3390/cancers15051596.

40. Romero-Brufau S, Wyatt KD, Boyum P, Mickelson M, Moore M, Cognetta-Rieke C. Implementation of artificial intelligence-based clinical decision support to reduce hospital readmissions at a regional hospital. *Appl Clin Inform.* 2020;11(4):570–577. https://doi.org/10.1055/s-0040-1715827.

41. Escobar GJ, Liu VX, Schuler A, Lawson B, Greene JD, Kipnis P. Automated identification of adults at risk for in-hospital clinical deterioration. *N Engl J Med.* 2020;383(20):1951–1960. https://doi.org/10.1056/NEJMsa2001090.

42. Yu K-H, Beam AL, Kohane IS. Artificial intelligence in healthcare. *Nat Biomed Eng.* 2018;2(10):719–731. https://doi.org/10.1038/s41551-018-0305-z.

43. Smith TS. *10 Ways Health Care AI Could Transform Primary Care.* American Medical Association; 2020. https://www.ama-assn.org/practice-management/digital/10-ways-health-care-ai-could-transform-primary-care.

44. Matheny ME, Whicher D, Thadaney Israni S. Artificial intelligence in health care: a report from the National Academy of Medicine. *JAMA.* 2020;323(6):509–510. https://doi.org/10.1001/jama.2019.21579.

45. Hespell R. *Our 10 Biggest AI Moments So Far.* Google Keyword; . https://blog.google/technology/ai/google-ai-ml-timeline/.

46. Sahni NR, Carrus B. Artificial intelligence in U.S. Health Care Delivery. *N Engl J Med.* 2023;389(4):348–358. https://doi.org/10.1056/NEJMra2204673.

47. Kung TH, Cheatham M, Medenilla A, et al. Performance of ChatGPT on USMLE: Potential for AI-assisted medical education using large language models. *PLOS Digital Health.* 2023;2(2):e0000198. https://doi.org/10.1371/journal.pdig.0000198.

48. Haendel MA, Chute CG, Robinson PN. Classification, ontology, and precision medicine. *N Engl J Med.* 2018;379(15):1452–1462. https://doi.org/10.1056/NEJMra1615014.

49. Topol EJ. Individualized medicine from prewomb to tomb. *Cell.* 2014;157(1):241–253. https://doi.org/10.1016/j.cell.2014.02.012.

50. Shademan A, Decker RS, Opfermann JD, Leonard S, Krieger A, Kim PC. Supervised autonomous robotic soft tissue surgery. *Sci Transl Med.* 2016;8(337):337ra64. https://doi.org/10.1126/scitranslmed.aad9398.

51. Gulshan V, Peng L, Coram M, et al. Development and validation of a deep learning algorithm for detection of diabetic retinopathy in retinal fundus photographs. *JAMA.* 2016;316(22):2402–2410. https://doi.org/10.1001/jama.2016.17216.

52. Abràmoff MD, Lavin PT, Birch M, Shah N, Folk JC. Pivotal trial of an autonomous AI-based diagnostic system for detection of diabetic retinopathy in primary care offices. *NPJ Digit Med.* 2018;1:39. https://doi.org/10.1038/s41746-018-0040-6.

53. Lakhani P, Sundaram B. Deep learning at chest radiography: automated classification of pulmonary tuberculosis by using convolutional neural networks. *Radiology.* 2017;284(2):574–582. https://doi.org/10.1148/radiol.2017162326.

54. Rajpurkar P, Irvin J, Zhu K, et al. Chexnet: Radiologist-level pneumonia detection on chest x-rays with deep learning. *arXiv preprint arXiv:171105225.* 2017.

55. Wang S, Patel H, Miller T, et al. AI based CMR assessment of biventricular function: clinical significance of intervendor variability and measurement errors. *JACC: Cardiovascular Imaging.* 2022;15(3):413–427. https://doi.org/10.1016/j.jcmg.2021.08.011.

56. Masutani EM, Chandrupatla RS, Wang S, et al. Deep learning synthetic strain: quantitative assessment of regional myocardial wall motion at MRI. *Radiol Cardiothorac Imaging.* 2023;5(3):e220202. https://doi.org/10.1148/ryct.220202.

57. Esteva A, Kuprel B, Novoa RA, et al. Dermatologist-level classification of skin cancer with deep neural networks. *Nature.* 2017;542(7639):115–118. https://doi.org/10.1038/nature21056.

58. Litjens G, Sánchez CI, Timofeeva N, et al. Deep learning as a tool for increased accuracy and efficiency of histopathological diagnosis. *Sci. Rep.* 2016;6(1):26286. https://doi.org/10.1038/srep26286.

59. Ehteshami Bejnordi B, Veta M, Johannes van Diest P, et al. Diagnostic assessment of deep learning algorithms for detection of lymph node metastases in women with breast cancer. *JAMA.* 2017;318(22):2199–2210. https://doi.org/10.1001/jama.2017.14585.

60. Lång K, Josefsson V, Larsson AM, et al. Artificial intelligence-supported screen reading versus standard double reading in the Mammography Screening with Artificial Intelligence trial (MASAI): a clinical safety analysis of a randomised, controlled, non-inferiority, single-blinded, screening accuracy study. *Lancet Oncol.* 2023;24(8):936–944. https://doi.org/10.1016/s1470-2045(23)00298-x.

61. Kozuka T, Matsukubo Y, Kadoba T, et al. Efficiency of a computer-aided diagnosis (CAD) system with deep learning in detection of pulmonary nodules on 1-mm-thick images of computed tomography. *Jpn J Radiol.* 2020;38(11):1052–1061. https://doi.org/10.1007/s11604-020-01009-0.

62. Conant EF, Toledano AY, Periaswamy S, et al. Improving accuracy and efficiency with concurrent use of artificial intelligence for digital breast tomosynthesis. *Radiol Artif Intell.* 2019;1(4):e180096. https://doi.org/10.1148/ryai.2019180096.

63. Urban G, Tripathi P, Alkayali T, et al. Deep learning localizes and identifies polyps in real time with 96% accuracy in screening colonoscopy. *Gastroenterology.* 2018;155(4):1069–1078.e8. https://doi.org/10.1053/j.gastro.2018.06.037.

64. Voets M, Mollersen K, Bongo LA. Reproduction study using public data of: Development and validation of a deep learning algorithm for detection of diabetic retinopathy in retinal fundus photographs. *PLoS One.* 2019;14(6):e0217541. https://doi.org/10.1371/journal.pone.0217541.

65. Taplin SH, Rutter CM, Lehman CD. Testing the effect of computer-assisted detection on interpretive performance in screening mammography. *AJR Am J Roentgenol.* 2006;187(6):1475–1482. https://doi.org/10.2214/ajr.05.0940.

66. Schupak A. Google apologizes for mis-tagging photos of African Americans. CBS Interactive Inc. Published July 1, 2015https://www.cbsnews.com/news/google-photos-labeled-pics-of-african-americans-as-gorillas/

67. Nicoletti L, Bass D. *Humans Are Biased. Generative AI Is Even Worse. Stable Diffusion's Text-to-Image Model Amplifies Stereotypes About Race and Gender — Here's Why*

That Matters. Bloomberg. https://www.bloomberg.com/graphics/2023-generative-ai-bias/

68. Chan B. Black-box assisted medical decisions: AI power vs. ethical physician care. *Med Health Care Philos.* 2023;26(3):285–292. https://doi.org/10.1007/s11019-023-10153-z.

69. National Research Council Committee on AFfDaNToD. The National Academies Collection: Reports funded by National Institutes of Health. *Toward Precision Medicine: Building a Knowledge Network for Biomedical Research and a New Taxonomy of Disease.* National Academy of Sciences; 2011.

70. Program. NIoHAoUR. *All of Us Research Program Overview.* 2023. https://allofus.nih.gov/about/program-overview

71. Collins FS, Varmus H. A new initiative on precision medicine. *N Engl J Med.* 2015;372(9):793–795. https://doi.org/10.1056/NEJMp1500523.

72. Feero WG. Introducing "Genomics and precision health." *JAMA.* 2017;317(18):1842–1843. https://doi.org/10.1001/jama.2016.20625.

73. Bera K, Schalper KA, Rimm DL, Velcheti V, Madabhushi A. Artificial intelligence in digital pathology – new tools for diagnosis and precision oncology. *Nat Rev Clin Oncol.* 2019;16(11):703–715. https://doi.org/10.1038/s41571-019-0252-y.

74. Zeevi D, Korem T, Zmora N, et al. Personalized nutrition by prediction of glycemic responses. *Cell.* 2015;163(5):1079–1094. https://doi.org/10.1016/j.cell.2015.11.001.

75. Kan MJ, Doudna JA. Treatment of genetic diseases with CRISPR genome editing. *JAMA.* 2022;328(10):980–981. https://doi.org/10.1001/jama.2022.13468.

76. Wong C. UK first to approve CRISPR treatment for diseases: what you need to know. *Nature.* 2023;623(7988):676–677.https://www.nature.com/articles/d41586-023-03590-6

77. Wilkinson E. UK regulator approves "groundbreaking" gene treatment for sickle cell and β thalassaemia. *BMJ.* 2023;383:p2706. https://doi.org/10.1136/bmj.p2706.

78. Aronson JK. When I use a word …. Listening to the patient. *BMJ.* 2022;376:o646. https://doi.org/10.1136/bmj.o646.

79. Fortin VI AH, Dwamena FC, Frankel RM, Smith RC. *Smith's Patient Centered Interviewing: An Evidence-Based Method. 4th ed.* McGraw Hill; 2018.

80. Kleinman A. *The Illness Narratives: Suffering, Healing, and the Human Condition.* Basic Books; 1988.

81. Kleinman A, Eisenberg L, Good B. Culture, illness, and care: clinical lessons from anthropologic and cross-cultural research. *Ann Intern Med.* 1978;88(2):251–258. https://doi.org/10.7326/0003-4819-88-2-251.

82. Kata A. A postmodern Pandora's box: anti-vaccination misinformation on the Internet. *Vaccine.* 2010;28(7):1709–1716. https://doi.org/10.1016/j.vaccine.2009.12.022.

83. Kings County / SUNY Downstate Emergency Medicine. Mini Fellowships. https://clinicalmonster.com/applicants/mini-fellowships/

84. Kreatsoulas C, Shannon HS, Giacomini M, Velianou JL, Anand SS. Reconstructing angina: cardiac symptoms are the same in women and men. *JAMA Intern Med.* 2013;173(9):829–831. https://doi.org/10.1001/jamainternmed.2013.229.

85. Kreatsoulas C. HERMES Study: Using Cardiolinguistics and Artificial Intelligence to Reframe Typical and Atypical Angina. Presentation at ESC Congress; 2019.

86. Wilson PM, Ramar P, Philpot LM, et al. Effect of an artificial intelligence decision support tool on palliative care referral in hospitalized patients: a randomized clinical trial. *J Pain Symptom Manage.* 2023;66(1):24–32. https://doi.org/10.1016/j.jpainsymman.2023.02.317.

87. Lee RY, Brumback LC, Lober WB, et al. Identifying goals of care conversations in the electronic health record using natural language processing and machine learning. *J Pain Symptom Manage.* 2021;61(1):136–142.e2. https://doi.org/10.1016/j.jpainsymman.2020.08.024.

88. Zhang H, Li Y, McConnell W. Predicting potential palliative care beneficiaries for health plans: a generalized machine learning pipeline. *J Biomed Inform.* 2021;123:103922. https://doi.org/10.1016/j.jbi.2021.103922.

89. Cope Z. *The Early Diagnosis of the Acute Abdomen.* Oxford Medical Publications; 1921.

90. Perloff JK. *Physical Examination of the Heart and Circulation.* W.B. Saunders Company; 1982.

91. Simel DL, Rennie D. *The Rational Clinical Examination: Evidence-Based Clinical Diagnosis.* McGraw-Hill Education; 2009.

92. McGee S. *Evidence-Based Physical Diagnosis.* 5th Ed. Elsevier; 2021.

93. Indrasari ND, Wonohutomo JP, Sukartini N. Comparison of point-of-care and central laboratory analyzers for blood gas and lactate measurements. *J Clin Lab Anal.* 2019;33(5):e22885. https://doi.org/10.1002/jcla.22885.

94. García-Fernández AE, Barquín R, Martínez M, Ferrer R, Casis E, Xu C. Performance evaluation of a point of care cartridge of the new GEM Premier ChemSTAT analyzer. *Pract Lab Med.* 2022;31:e00297. https://doi.org/10.1016/j.plabm.2022.e00297.

95. Allardet-Servent J, Lebsir M, Dubroca C, et al. Point-of-care versus central laboratory measurements of hemoglobin, hematocrit, glucose, bicarbonate and electrolytes: a prospective observational study in critically ill patients. *PLoS One.* 2017;12(1):e0169593. https://doi.org/10.1371/journal.pone.0169593.

96. Nichols JH, Christenson RH, Clarke W, et al. Executive summary. The National Academy of Clinical Biochemistry Laboratory medicine practice guideline: evidence-based practice for point-of-care testing. *Clin Chim Acta.* 2007;379(1-2):14–28. https://doi.org/10.1016/j.cca.2006.12.025. discussion 29-30.

97. Abel G, Brugnara C, Saswati D, et al. *Point-of-Care Testing: A "How-To" Guide for the Non-Laboratorian.* 2022. https://www.aacc.org/-/media/Files/Science-and-Practice/POCT-How-To-Guide/POCTGuide_SDx.pdf?la=en&hash=E6A4946FFFE6DDACA275C64BE13A18225422B338

98. Nichols JH, Alter D, Chen Y, et al. AACC guidance document on management of point-of-care testing. *J Appl*

Lab Med. 2020;5(4):762–787. https://doi.org/10.1093/jalm/jfaa059.

99. Kost GJ, Zadran A. Schools of public health should be accredited for, and teach the principles and practice of point-of-care testing. *J Appl Lab Med.* 2019;4(2):278–283. https://doi.org/10.1373/jalm.2019.029249.

100. Garcia-Alamino JM, Ward AM, Alonso-Coello P, et al. Self-monitoring and self-management of oral anticoagulation. *Cochrane Database Syst Rev.* 2010(4):Cd003839. https://doi.org/10.1002/14651858.CD003839.pub2.

101. Heneghan CJ, Garcia-Alamino JM, Spencer EA, et al. Self-monitoring and self-management of oral anticoagulation. *Cochrane Database Syst Rev.* 2016;7(7):Cd003839. https://doi.org/10.1002/14651858.CD003839.pub3.

102. Anderson I, Wool GD, Madden W. The point-of-care INR test for vitamin K antagonist monitoring. *Jama.* 2019;322(21):2129–2130. https://doi.org/10.1001/jama.2019.15720.

103. Pham MD, Agius PA, Romero L, et al. Performance of point-of-care CD4 testing technologies in resource-constrained settings: a systematic review and meta-analysis. *BMC Infect Dis.* 2016;16(1):592. https://doi.org/10.1186/s12879-016-1931-2.

104. Hyle EP, Jani IV, Lehe J, et al. The clinical and economic impact of point-of-care CD4 testing in mozambique and other resource-limited settings: a cost-effectiveness analysis. *PLoS Med.* 2014;11(9):e1001725. https://doi.org/10.1371/journal.pmed.1001725.

105. Ochodo EA, Olwanda EE, Deeks JJ, Mallett S. Point-of-care viral load tests to detect high HIV viral load in people living with HIV/AIDS attending health facilities. *Cochrane Database Syst Rev.* 2022;3(3):Cd013208. https://doi.org/10.1002/14651858.CD013208.pub2.

106. Laksanasopin T, Guo TW, Nayak S, et al. A smartphone dongle for diagnosis of infectious diseases at the point of care. *Sci Transl Med.* 2015;7(273):273re1. https://doi.org/10.1126/scitranslmed.aaa0056.

107. Shokoohi H, Duggan NM, Adhikari S, Selame LA, Amini R, Blaivas M. Point-of-care ultrasound stewardship. *J Am Coll Emerg Physicians Open.* 2020;1(6):1326–1331. https://doi.org/10.1002/emp2.12279.

108. Moore CL, Copel JA. Point-of-care ultrasonography. *N Engl J Med.* 2011;364(8):749–757. https://doi.org/10.1056/NEJMra0909487.

109. Díaz-Gómez JL, Mayo PH, Koenig SJ. Point-of-care ultrasonography. *N Engl J Med.* 2021;385(17):1593–1602. https://doi.org/10.1056/NEJMra1916062.

110. Rozycki GS, Ochsner MG, Schmidt JA, et al. A prospective study of surgeon-performed ultrasound as the primary adjuvant modality for injured patient assessment. *J Trauma.* 1995;39(3):492–498. https://doi.org/10.1097/00005373-199509000-00016. discussion 498-500.

111. Rozycki GS, Shackford SR. Ultrasound, what every trauma surgeon should know. *J Trauma.* 1996;40(1):1–4. https://doi.org/10.1097/00005373-199601000-00001.

112. Kennedy Hall M, Coffey EC, Herbst M, et al. The "5Es" of emergency physician-performed focused cardiac ultrasound: a protocol for rapid identification of effusion, ejection, equality, exit, and entrance. *Acad Emerg Med.* 2015;22(5):583–593. https://doi.org/10.1111/acem.12652.

113. Kimura BJ, Shaw DJ, Amundson SA, Phan JN, Blanchard DG, DeMaria AN. Cardiac limited ultrasound examination techniques to augment the bedside cardiac physical examination. *J Ultrasound Med.* 2015;34(9):1683–1690. https://doi.org/10.7863/ultra.15.14.09002.

114. Lichtenstein DA, Mezière GA. Relevance of lung ultrasound in the diagnosis of acute respiratory failure: the BLUE protocol. *Chest.* 2008;134(1):117–125. https://doi.org/10.1378/chest.07-2800.

115. Huson MAM, Kaminstein D, Kahn D, et al. Cardiac ultrasound in resource-limited settings (CURLS): towards a wider use of basic echo applications in Africa. *Ultrasound J.* 2019;11(1):34. https://doi.org/10.1186/s13089-019-0149-0.

116. Perera P, Mailhot T, Riley D, Mandavia D. The RUSH exam: Rapid Ultrasound in SHock in the evaluation of the critically lll. *Emerg Med Clin North Am.* 2010;28(1):29–56. https://doi.org/10.1016/j.emc.2009.09.010. vii.

117. Seif D, Perera P, Mailhot T, Riley D, Mandavia D. Bedside ultrasound in resuscitation and the rapid ultrasound in shock protocol. *Crit Care Res Pract.* 2012;2012:503254. https://doi.org/10.1155/2012/503254.

118. Heller T, Wallrauch C, Lessells RJ, Goblirsch S, Brunetti E. Short course for focused assessment with sonography for human immunodeficiency virus/tuberculosis: preliminary results in a rural setting in South Africa with high prevalence of human immunodeficiency virus and tuberculosis. *Am J Trop Med Hyg.* 2010;82(3):512–515. https://doi.org/10.4269/ajtmh.2010.09-0561.

119. Heller T, Wallrauch C, Goblirsch S, Brunetti E. Focused assessment with sonography for HIV-associated tuberculosis (FASH): a short protocol and a pictorial review. *Crit Ultrasound J.* 2012;4(1):21. 10.1186/2036-7902-4-21.

120. Kaminstein D, Heller T, Tamarozzi F. Sound around the world: ultrasound for tropical diseases. *Infect Dis Clin North Am.* 2019;33(1):169–195. https://doi.org/10.1016/j.idc.2018.10.008.

121. Bélard S, Tamarozzi F, Bustinduy AL, et al. Point-of-care ultrasound assessment of tropical infectious diseases—a review of applications and perspectives. *Am J Trop Med Hyg.* 2016;94(1):8–21. https://doi.org/10.4269/ajtmh.15-0421.

122. Blaivas M, Lambert MJ, Harwood RA, Wood JP, Konicki J. Lower-extremity Doppler for deep venous thrombosis—can emergency physicians be accurate and fast? *Acad Emerg Med.* 2000;7(2):120–126. https://doi.org/10.1111/j.1553-2712.2000.tb00512.x.

123. Varrias D, Palaiodimos L, Balasubramanian P, et al. The use of point-of-care ultrasound (POCUS) in the diagnosis of deep vein thrombosis. *J Clin Med.* 2021;10(17). https://doi.org/10.3390/jcm10173903.

124. Fischer EA, Kinnear B, Sall D, et al. Hospitalist-operated compression ultrasonography: a point-of-care ultrasound study (HOCUS-POCUS). *J Gen Intern Med.* 2019;34(10):2062–2067. https://doi.org/10.1007/s11606-019-05120-5.

125. Sonko ML, Arnold TC, Kuznetsov IA. Machine learning in point of care ultrasound. *Pocus J*. 2022;7(Kidney):78–87. https://doi.org/10.24908/pocus.v7iKidney.15345.

126. Baum E, Tandel MD, Ren C, et al. Acquisition of cardiac point-of-care ultrasound images with deep learning: a randomized trial for educational outcomes with novices. *CHEST Pulmonary*. 2023:100023. https://doi.org/10.1016/j.chpulm.2023.100023.

127. Narasimhan M, Koenig SJ, Mayo PH. A whole-body approach to point of care ultrasound. *Chest*. 2016;150(4):772–776. https://doi.org/10.1016/j.chest.2016.07.040.

128. Owens DK, Davidson KW, Krist AH, et al. Screening for abdominal aortic aneurysm: US Preventive Services Task Force Recommendation Statement. *JAMA*. 2019;322(22):2211–2218. https://doi.org/10.1001/jama.2019.18928.

129. Blois B. Office-based ultrasound screening for abdominal aortic aneurysm. *Can Fam Physician*. 2012;58(3):e172–e178.

130. Bailey RP, Ault M, Greengold NL, Rosendahl T, Cossman D. Ultrasonography performed by primary care residents for abdominal aortic aneurysm screening. *J Gen Intern Med*. 2001;16(12):845–849. https://doi.org/10.1111/j.1525-1497.2001.01128.x.

131. Mbanjumucyo G, Henwood PC. Focused assessment with sonography for HIV-associated tuberculosis (FASH) case series from a Rwandan district hospital. *Afr J Emerg Med*. 2016;6(4):198–201. https://doi.org/10.1016/j.afjem.2016.07.001.

132. Zhang L, Marcus C, Lin D, et al. A conformable phased-array ultrasound patch for bladder volume monitoring. *Nat. Electron*. 2023 https://doi.org/10.1038/s41928-023-01068-x.

133. Freedman B, Camm J, Calkins H, et al. Screening for atrial fibrillation: a report of the AF-SCREEN international collaboration. *Circulation*. 2017;135(19):1851–1867. https://doi.org/10.1161/circulationaha.116.026693.

134. Perez MV, Mahaffey KW, Hedlin H, et al. Large-scale assessment of a smartwatch to identify atrial fibrillation. *N Engl J Med*. 2019;381(20):1909–1917. https://doi.org/10.1056/NEJMoa1901183.

135. Wyatt KD. A smartwatch to identify atrial fibrillation. *N Engl J Med*. 2020;382(10):975. https://doi.org/10.1056/NEJMc1916858.

136. Qiu J, Wang Y. A smartwatch to identify atrial fibrillation. *N Engl J Med*. 2020;382(10):974–975. https://doi.org/10.1056/NEJMc1916858.

137. Auer J, Primus C. A smartwatch to identify atrial fibrillation. *N Engl J Med*. 2020;382(10):974. https://doi.org/10.1056/NEJMc1916858.

138. Brandes A, Stavrakis S, Freedman B, et al. Consumer-led screening for atrial fibrillation: frontier review of the AF-SCREEN international collaboration. *Circulation*. 2022;146(19):1461–1474. https://doi.org/10.1161/circulationaha.121.058911.

139. Wyatt KD, Poole LR, Mullan AF, Kopecky SL, Heaton HA. Clinical evaluation and diagnostic yield following evaluation of abnormal pulse detected using Apple Watch. *J Am Med Inform Assoc*. 2020;27(9):1359–1363. https://doi.org/10.1093/jamia/ocaa137.

140. Kashou AH, Medina-Inojosa JR, Noseworthy PA, et al. Artificial intelligence-augmented electrocardiogram detection of left ventricular systolic dysfunction in the general population. *Mayo Clin Proc*. 2021;96(10):2576–2586. https://doi.org/10.1016/j.mayocp.2021.02.029.

141. Attia ZI, Kapa S, Lopez-Jimenez F, et al. Screening for cardiac contractile dysfunction using an artificial intelligence-enabled electrocardiogram. *Nat Med*. 2019;25(1):70–74. https://doi.org/10.1038/s41591-018-0240-2.

142. Kannathal N, Acharya UR, Lim CM, Sadasivan P, Krishnan S. Classification of cardiac patient states using artificial neural networks. *Exp Clin Cardiol*. 2003;8(4):206–211.

143. Bhakuni H, Abimbola S. Epistemic injustice in academic global health. *Lancet Glob Health*. 2021;9(10):e1465–e1470. https://doi.org/10.1016/s2214-109x(21)00301-6.

144. Piret J, Boivin G. Pandemics throughout history. *Front Microbiol*. 2020;11:631736. https://doi.org/10.3389/fmicb.2020.631736.

145. Wang Y, Leng P, Zhou H. Global transmission of monkeypox virus-a potential threat under the COVID-19 pandemic. *Front Immunol*. 2023;14:1174223. https://doi.org/10.3389/fimmu.2023.1174223.

146. Hampton LM, Luquero F, Costa A, Legand A, Formenty P. Ebola outbreak detection and response since 2013. *Lancet Microbe*. 2023;4(9):e661–e662. https://doi.org/10.1016/s2666-5247(23)00136-2.

147. Global burden of 369 diseases and injuries in 204 countries and territories, 1990-2019: a systematic analysis for the Global Burden of Disease Study 2019. *Lancet*. 2020;396(10258):1204–1222. doi:10.1016/s0140-6736(20)30925-9

148. Shu J, Jin W. Prioritizing non-communicable diseases in the post-pandemic era based on a comprehensive analysis of the GBD 2019 from 1990 to 2019. *Sci Rep*. 2023;13(1):13325. https://doi.org/10.1038/s41598-023-40595-7.

149. Haines A, Ebi K. The imperative for climate action to protect health. *N Engl J Med*. 2019;380(3):263–273. https://doi.org/10.1056/NEJMra1807873.

150. Romanello M, Napoli CD, Green C, et al. The 2023 report of the Lancet Countdown on health and climate change: the imperative for a health-centred response in a world facing irreversible harms. *Lancet*. 2023 https://doi.org/10.1016/s0140-6736(23)01859-7.

151. Dimala CA, Kadia BM, Nji MAM, Bechem NN. Factors associated with measles resurgence in the United States in the post-elimination era. *Sci Rep*. 2021;11(1):51. https://doi.org/10.1038/s41598-020-80214-3.

152. Network. CHA. Locally Acquired Malaria Cases Identified in the United States. November 20, 2023. https://emergency.cdc.gov/han/2023/han00494.asp

153. Hotez PJ, LaBeaud AD. Yellow Jack's potential return to the American South. *N Engl J Med*. 2023;389(16):1445–1447. https://doi.org/10.1056/NEJMp2308420.

154. Memari M, Domney A, Tee CJ, Stathopoulos AG, Chakraborti C. Barriers to timely diagnosis and treatment of vector-borne diseases in a changing climate: a case report. *Public Health Rep.* 2023;138(3):406–409. https://doi.org/10.1177/00333549221090263.

155. Hodson DZ, Etoundi YM, Parikh S, Boum 2nd Y. Striving towards true equity in global health: A checklist for bilateral research partnerships. *PLOS Glob Public Health.* 2023;3(1):e0001418. https://doi.org/10.1371/journal.pgph.0001418.

156. Byrne RA, Rossello X, Coughlan JJ, et al. 2023 ESC Guidelines for the management of acute coronary syndromes. *Eur Heart J Acute Cardiovasc Care.* 2023 https://doi.org/10.1093/ehjacc/zuad107.

157. O'Gara PT, Kushner FG, Ascheim DD, et al. 2013 ACCF/AHA guideline for the management of ST-elevation myocardial infarction: a report of the American College of Cardiology Foundation/American Heart Association Task Force on Practice Guidelines. *J Am Coll Cardiol.* 2013;61(4):e78–e140. https://doi.org/10.1016/j.jacc.2012.11.019.

158. Health. MMo. *Malawi Stantard Treatment Guidelines.* 6th ed. 2023.

159. Arnett DK, Blumenthal RS, Albert MA, et al. 2019 ACC/AHA Guideline on the Primary Prevention of Cardiovascular Disease: Executive Summary: A Report of the American College of Cardiology/American Heart Association Task Force on Clinical Practice Guidelines. *Circulation.* 2019;140(11):e563–e595. https://doi.org/10.1161/cir.0000000000000677.

160. Adhikari S. Evidence-based medicine in low-income and middle-income countries. *Lancet Glob Health.* 2021;9(7):e903–e904. https://doi.org/10.1016/s2214-109x(21)00144-3.

161. Jecker NS. Rethinking rescue medicine. *Am J Bioeth.* 2015;15(2):12–18. https://doi.org/10.1080/15265161.2014.990169.

162. Moseley III GB. The US Health care non-system, 1908-2008. *AMA J Ethics.* 2008;10(5):324–331.

163. Schneider EC, Shah A, Doty MM, Tikkanen R, Fields K, Willians II RD. *MIRROR, MIRROR 2021. Reflecting Poorly: Health Care in the U.S. Compared to Other High-Income Countries.* 2021. https://www.commonwealthfund.org/publications/fund-reports/2021/aug/mirror-mirror-2021-reflecting-poorly.

164. Dickman SL, Himmelstein DU, Woolhandler S. Inequality and the health-care system in the USA. *Lancet.* 2017;389(10077):1431–1441. https://doi.org/10.1016/s0140-6736(17)30398-7.

165. Magesh S, John D, Li WT, et al. Disparities in COVID-19 outcomes by race, ethnicity, and socioeconomic status: a systematic-review and meta-analysis. *JAMA Netw Open.* 2021;4(11):e2134147. https://doi.org/10.1001/jamanetworkopen.2021.34147.

166. Palazuelos D, Farmer PE, Mukherjee J. Community health and equity of outcomes: the Partners In Health experience. *Lancet Glob Health.* 2018;6(5):e491–e493. https://doi.org/10.1016/s2214-109x(18)30073-1.

167. Linn AM, Ndiaye Y, Hennessee I, et al. Reduction in symptomatic malaria prevalence through proactive community treatment in rural Senegal. *Trop Med Int Health.* 2015;20(11):1438–1446. https://doi.org/10.1111/tmi.12564.

168. Gaye S, Kibler J, Ndiaye JL, et al. Proactive community case management in Senegal 2014-2016: a case study in maximizing the impact of community case management of malaria. *Malar J.* 2020;19(1):166. https://doi.org/10.1186/s12936-020-03238-0.

169. UNICEF. Wa. *Senegal: WHO and UNICEF estimates of immunization coverage: 2022 revision.* 2023. *Immunization country profiles.* https://data.unicef.org/resources/immunization-country-profiles/

170. Peretz PJ, Islam N, Matiz LA. Community health workers and covid-19 - addressing social determinants of health in times of crisis and beyond. *N Engl J Med.* 2020;383(19):e108. https://doi.org/10.1056/NEJMp2022641.

171. Ignoffo S, Gu S, Ellyin A, Benjamins MR. A review of community health worker integration in health departments. *J Community Health.* 2023 https://doi.org/10.1007/s10900-023-01286-6.

172. Organization. WH. *Quantitative risk assessment of the effects of climate change on selected causes of death, 2030s and 2050s.* 2014. https://iris.who.int/bitstream/handle/10665/134014/9789241507691_eng.pdf?sequence=1

173. Samarasekera U. Climate change and malaria: predictions becoming reality. *Lancet.* 2023;402(10399):361–362. https://doi.org/10.1016/s0140-6736(23)01569-6.

174. Salas RN. Environmental racism and climate change - missed diagnoses. *N Engl J Med.* 2021;385(11):967–969. https://doi.org/10.1056/NEJMp2109160.

175. Perera F, Nadeau K. Climate change, fossil-fuel pollution, and children's health. *N Engl J Med.* 2022;386(24):2303–2314. https://doi.org/10.1056/NEJMra2117706.

176. Hommes F, Monzó HB, Ferrand RA, et al. The words we choose matter: recognising the importance of language in decolonising global health. *Lancet Glob Health.* 2021;9(7):e897–e898. https://doi.org/10.1016/s2214-109x(21)00197-2.

177. Roca A, Boum Y, Wachsmuth I. Plaidoyer contre l'exclusion des francophones dans la recherche en santé mondiale. *Lancet Glob Health.* 2019;7(6):e701–e702. https://doi.org/10.1016/s2214-109x(19)30175-5. Plaidoyer contre l'exclusion des francophones dans la recherche en santé mondiale.

178. Boum Y, Mburu Y. Burden of disease in francophone Africa 1990-2017: the triple penalty? *Lancet Glob Health.* 2020;8(3):e306–e307. https://doi.org/10.1016/s2214-109x(20)30040-1.

179. Chen Jr. MS, Lara PN, Dang JH, Paterniti DA, Kelly K. Twenty years post-NIH Revitalization Act: enhancing minority participation in clinical trials (EMPaCT): laying the groundwork for improving minority clinical trial accrual: renewing the case for enhancing minority participation in cancer clinical trials. . *Cancer.* 2014;120(Suppl 7(0 7)):1091–1096. https://doi.org/10.1002/cncr.28575.

180. Frayne SM, Burns RB, Hardt EJ, Rosen AK, Moskowitz MA. The exclusion of non-English-speaking persons from research. *J Gen Intern Med.* 1996;11(1):39–43. https://doi.org/10.1007/bf02603484.

181. Abimbola S. The foreign gaze: authorship in academic global health. *BMJ Glob Health.* 2019;4(5):e002068. https://doi.org/10.1136/bmjgh-2019-002068.

182. Fofana MO. Decolonising global health in the time of COVID-19. *Glob Public Health.* 2021;16(8-9):1155–1166. https://doi.org/10.1080/17441692.2020.1864754.

183. Bump JB, Aniebo I. Colonialism, malaria, and the decolonization of global health. *PLOS Glob Public Health.* 2022;2(9):e0000936. https://doi.org/10.1371/journal.pgph.0000936.

184. Olusanya BO. Systemic racism in global health: a personal reflection. *Lancet Glob Health.* 2021;9(8):e1051–e1052. https://doi.org/10.1016/s2214-109x(21)00147-9.

185. Boum Ii Y, Burns BF, Siedner M, Mburu Y, Bukusi E, Haberer JE. Advancing equitable global health research partnerships in Africa. *BMJ Glob Health.* 2018;3(4):e000868. https://doi.org/10.1136/bmjgh-2018-000868.

186. Wright AA, Katz IT. Beyond burnout - redesigning care to restore meaning and sanity for physicians. *N Engl J Med.* 2018;378(4):309–311. https://doi.org/10.1056/NEJMp1716845.

187. Densen P. Challenges and opportunities facing medical education. *Trans Am Clin Climatol Assoc.* 2011;122:48–58.

188. Prober CG, Khan S. Medical education reimagined: a call to action. *Acad Med.* 2013;88(10):1407–1410. https://doi.org/10.1097/ACM.0b013e3182a368bd.

189. Examination. USML. *USMLE Step 1 Transition to Pass/Fail Only Score Reporting.* https://www.usmle.org/usmle-step-1-transition-passfail-only-score-reporting

190. Rawson KA, Kintsch W. Rereading effects depend on time of test. *J. Educ. Psychol.* 2005;97(1):70–80. https://doi.org/10.1037/0022-0663.97.1.70.

191. Cepeda NJ, Pashler H, Vul E, Wixted JT, Rohrer D. Distributed practice in verbal recall tasks: a review and quantitative synthesis. *Psychol Bull.* 2006;132(3):354–380. https://doi.org/10.1037/0033-2909.132.3.354.

192. Gilbert MM, Frommeyer TC, Brittain GV, et al. A cohort study assessing the impact of anki as a spaced repetition tool on academic performance in medical school. *Med Sci Educ.* 2023;33(4):955–962. https://doi.org/10.1007/s40670-023-01826-8.

193. Jape D, Zhou J, Bullock S. A spaced-repetition approach to enhance medical student learning and engagement in medical pharmacology. *BMC Med Educ.* 2022;22(1):337. https://doi.org/10.1186/s12909-022-03324-8.

194. Levine DM, Mehrotra A. Assessment of diagnosis and triage in validated case vignettes among nonphysicians before and after internet search. *JAMA Netw Open.* 2021;4(3):e213287. https://doi.org/10.1001/jamanetworkopen.2021.3287.

195. Mbakwe AB, Lourentzou I, Celi LA, Mechanic OJ, Dagan A. ChatGPT passing USMLE shines a spotlight on the flaws of medical education. *PLOS Digit Health.* 2023;2(2):e0000205. https://doi.org/10.1371/journal.pdig.0000205.

196. Zainal H, Tan JK, Xiaohui X, Thumboo J, Yong FK. Clinical informatics training in medical school education curricula: a scoping review. *J Am Med Inform Assoc.* 2023;30(3):604–616. https://doi.org/10.1093/jamia/ocac245.

197. Jha S, Topol EJ. Adapting to artificial intelligence: radiologists and pathologists as information specialists. *Jama.* 2016;316(22):2353–2354. https://doi.org/10.1001/jama.2016.17438.

198. Banerjee R, George P, Priebe C, Alper E. Medical student awareness of and interest in clinical informatics. *J Am Med Inform Assoc.* 2015;22(e1):e42–e47. https://doi.org/10.1093/jamia/ocu046.

199. Association for Diagnostics and Laboratory Medicine. *Taking Point-of-Care Testing to New Heights.* https://www.aacc.org/cln/cln-stat/2018/august/16/taking-point-of-care-testing-to-new-heights.

200. Young JQ, Ranji SR, Wachter RM, Lee CM, Niehaus B, Auerbach AD. "July effect": impact of the academic year-end changeover on patient outcomes: a systematic review. *Ann Intern Med.* 2011;155(5):309–315. https://doi.org/10.7326/0003-4819-155-5-201109060-00354.

201. Englesbe MJ, Pelletier SJ, Magee JC, et al. Seasonal variation in surgical outcomes as measured by the American College of Surgeons-National Surgical Quality Improvement Program (ACS-NSQIP). *Ann Surg.* 2007;246(3):456–462. https://doi.org/10.1097/SLA.0b013e31814855f2. Discussion 463-5.

202. Schechter EM, Kaplan L, Hojman H, Bontempo L, Carusone C, Evans LV. Efficacy of a human patient simulator to improve senior residents' skills in functioning as a team leader during trauma resuscitations. *Simul Healthc.* 2006;1(2).

203. Evans LV, Dodge KL, Shah TD, et al. Simulation training in central venous catheter insertion: improved performance in clinical practice. *Acad Med.* 2010;85(9).

204. Leigh VE, Dodge KL. Simulation and patient safety: evaluative checklists for central venous catheter insertion. *Qual Saf Health Care.* 2010;19(Suppl 3):i42. https://doi.org/10.1136/qshc.2010.042168.

205. Azadi S, Green IC, Arnold A, Truong M, Potts J, Martino MA. Robotic surgery: the impact of simulation and other innovative platforms on performance and training. *J Minim Invasive Gynecol.* 2021;28(3):490–495. https://doi.org/10.1016/j.jmig.2020.12.001.

206. Ray JM, Wong AH, Yang TJ, et al. Virtual telesimulation for medical students during the COVID-19 pandemic. *Acad Med.* 2021;96(10).

207. Plackett R, Kassianos AP, Kambouri M, et al. Online patient simulation training to improve clinical reasoning: a feasibility randomised controlled trial. *BMC Med Educ.* 2020;20(1):245. https://doi.org/10.1186/s12909-020-02168-4.

208. Stawicki SP, Firstenberg MS, Orlando JP, Papadimos T, eds. *Contemporary Topics in Graduate Medical Education.* IntechOpen; 2019.

209. Gonzalo JD, Heist BS, Duffy BL, et al. Identifying and overcoming the barriers to bedside rounds: a multicenter

qualitative study. *Acad Med.* 2014;89(2):326–334. https://doi.org/10.1097/acm.0000000000000100.

210. Patel SJ, Khan A, Bass EJ, et al. Family, nurse, and physician beliefs on family-centered rounds: A 21-site study. *J Hosp Med.* 2022;17(12):945–955. https://doi.org/10.1002/jhm.12962.

211. Sinsky C, Colligan L, Li L, et al. Allocation of physician time in ambulatory practice: a time and motion study in 4 specialties. *Ann Intern Med.* 2016;165(11):753–760. https://doi.org/10.7326/m16-0961.

212. Adler-Milstein J, Zhao W, Willard-Grace R, Knox M, Grumbach K. Electronic health records and burnout: time spent on the electronic health record after hours and message volume associated with exhaustion but not with cynicism among primary care clinicians. *J Am Med Inform Assoc.* 2020;27(4):531–538. https://doi.org/10.1093/jamia/ocz220.

213. Gawande A. The Upgrade. Why doctors hate their computers. *The Atlantic.* 2018.

214. Damania Z. *EHR State of Mind.* https://zdoggmd.com/ehr-state-of-mind/.

215. Siegler EL, Adelman R. Copy and paste: a remediable hazard of electronic health records. *Am J Med.* 2009;122(6):495–496. https://doi.org/10.1016/j.amjmed.2009.02.010.

216. Bowker D, Torti J, Goldszmidt M. Documentation as composing: how medical students and residents use writing to think and learn. *Adv Health Sci Educ Theory Pract.* 2023;28(2):453–475. https://doi.org/10.1007/s10459-022-10167-x.

217. McFarland A. *10 Best AI Medical Scribes.* Unite AI; 2023. https://www.unite.ai/best-ai-medical-scribes/

218. Paranjape K, Schinkel M, Nannan Panday R, Car J, Nanayakkara P. Introducing artificial intelligence training in medical education. *JMIR Med Educ.* 2019;5(2):e16048. https://doi.org/10.2196/16048.

10

Building a Diverse and Equitable Future
The Role of Geographic Information Systems, Spatial Analysis, and Social Justice in Medical Education

Anand Gourishankar, Kendrick Davis, and Kristen S. Kurland

SUMMARY

Medical education and knowledge are expansive and increasingly complex beyond human capacity, emphasizing a futuristic approach. This chapter reimagines medical education through diversity, equity, and social justice. Inspired by **geographic information systems** (GIS) and spatial analysis, we explore innovative methods to promote inclusivity and reduce health care inequities. More importantly, we attempt to show how GIS can transform medical curricula by combining cutting-edge technology with social justice, highlighting foundations, progression of the field, and advancements. We examine how geospatial analysis helps identify health care access, inequities, resource distribution, and social determinants of health. Thus this chapter allows the study of how space-related factors affect health and shows how GIS in medical education can improve cultural and social competence. Our discussion extends to GIS educators' and researchers' challenges and offers insights into the future landscape of incorporating GIS in medical education. Therefore, this chapter lays the groundwork for a diverse and equitable future in medical education, reflecting the moral imperative of our time.

INTRODUCTION

GIS technology, developed in the 1960s, has been utilized for land-use planning, cartography, and natural resource management.[1] Simply put, GIS is a computer system with location-based data shown on a map, but GIS is far more than visualizing data on a map. It uses advanced tools to analyze multiple "layers" of information. In the 1970s and 1980s, GIS advanced significantly, developing computer-based mapping, modeling, and spatial analysis systems. We began to see the application of GIS in the health sector in the 1980s, initially focused on epidemiology and disease mapping, helping in disease surveillance and outbreak investigations.[1] In the early 1990s, GIS became more accessible, thanks to advancements in software and hardware. Educational institutions started integrating GIS into related disciplines, including environmental health, urban design and planning, public health, and disaster management.

Today, many academic, governmental, and private organizations use GIS to analyze the equity and social justice impact of public policies, laws, regulations, projects, and programs. With the help of health and other sciences, GIS can help understand why things are placed where they are and how they are connected. For example, GIS technology enables us to examine and visualize data that provide insights into determinants of health and health care inequities.

By incorporating medical (health) geography involving fields such as GIS, **spatial analysis**, population health, and **social justice** into medical education, we can obtain insights into the connection between places, health, and disease. These fields of study allow us to grasp how environmental factors influence health and equip decision-makers with the skills to address health care inequities—an impetus to reimagine education methods.

The need to reimagine education in all health-related fields is crucial to address critical challenges facing health care organizations. Many existing medical education programs rely on teaching methods and curricula that do not adequately prepare students (here onwards, any learner types) for the rapidly changing health care landscape. Institutions must embrace innovative technical approaches in medical education to bridge this gap. By doing so, we can better equip students with the skills and knowledge needed to tackle real-world health-related challenges. Over more than two decades, educators and researchers have acknowledged GIS and spatial perspectives across various disciplines, especially the significance of analyzing educational phenomena via a spatial lens.

Geospatial analysis using GIS is one area of innovation in reimagining medical education. Integrating technologies, like GIS with an equity lens, into medical education empowers health care professionals and policymakers to understand and tackle injustices affecting decision-making processes and improve health outcomes. We greatly enhance student engagement and motivation by incorporating learning strategies and leveraging geospatial applications. When integrated effectively, such tools and technologies can provide learning experiences, access to up-to-date information, and visualizations that enrich our students' educational journey while improving long-term outcomes for underserved communities.

By examining and understanding data related to multiple factors contributing to poor health, students can identify areas with disadvantages and understand how these elements contribute to inequities in health. GIS uses multiple approaches necessary to understand the impact of social injustice. For example, GIS can help pinpoint areas where access to health care is limited or nonexistent. Students can identify underserved regions that require health care resources by mapping the locations of health care facilities, public transportation, drive times, and population demographics such as poverty. This knowledge can guide targeted interventions and policies to address these inequities and promote societal fairness.

As medical providers in partnership with policymakers, we can use this information to develop strategies that promote and improve access to health care services, ensuring that everyone, regardless of their status or where they live, has opportunities for quality care. GIS also enables the analysis of how environmental factors impact health outcomes. Students can map hazards such as air pollution, poor water quality, or inadequate green spaces to understand how these are associated with health inequities. If adequately supported by local governments and policymakers, this study may assist advocacy efforts to achieve justice that creates healthier communities for all residents. Moreover, health geography mapping allows professionals from health care specialties to collaborate effectively by visualizing and analyzing data.

With this understanding and geospatial toolsets at their disposal, future health care professionals can address health care inequities and champion justice within our system. We must fully embrace GIS as an educational resource as we strive toward creating a more equitable and just health care system for all individuals. To ensure future health professionals can develop an understanding and use of GIS toolsets, we must build upon education that promotes medical or health geography.

WHAT IS MEDICAL OR HEALTH GEOGRAPHY LITERACY?

Geography lessons start in elementary school, and this subject of study continues throughout middle and high school. Middle and high schools, universities, and colleges increasingly adopt GIS and geospatial technologies in geography curricula. Under President Obama's ConnectED initiative, elementary and secondary schools in the United States had freely available GIS software (ArcGIS Online, Esri, Inc.).

Medical geography involves examining how health and disease are distributed in geographic locations. Medical geography (also known as health geography) literacy includes spatial thinking, skills, and information needed to understand and solve health-associated problems related to location or place. Hence, it includes examining the provisioning of diseases, environment, and health care in different geographical areas and knowing how these affect one another. It utilizes GIS and spatial analysis to explore the connections between health and the surrounding environment (natural, built, and social), considering a range of factors.

The field of medical geography is valuable for addressing health care inequities, promoting justice, and informing medical education. Geospatial data can come from retrospective sources, such as the US Census Bureau, and other data sources obtained from verified sites, such as Data.gov. For prospective data collection, GIS requires location data such as ZIP codes or longitude and latitude to enter GIS applications. For example, data such as disease, socioeconomic status, health behaviors, and environmental or physical conditions connected to geographic locations are collected and entered into a computer system (in the case of GIS) for mapping, modeling, applying geostatistics, and various spatial analysis methods. Therefore, in today's world of medical geography, GIS is an integral tool.

A unique capability of GIS is its ability to store related graphic features in separate collections of files called map layers. Two common types of map layer formats are **vector** and **raster**. Vector-based maps have point, line, and polygon features. A point has x and y coordinates. A line has start and end points that might have additional shape vertices in between for bends in the lines. A polygon has three or more lines joined to form a closed area. Most graphic features in a GIS that have analytic values (attributes), like population or accidental overdose deaths, are vector-based thematic maps. Each map layer has data records associated with each vector feature. A second kind of GIS data is a raster map, a checkerboard of small squares with a solid color fill (pixels). Raster data can be physical features such as land use or satellite imagery. GIS can also generate raster maps from vector data for advanced analysis. In an obesity study, a point feature could be a patient address with medical record data showing increases or decreases in a patient's BMI, a line feature could be a street or sidewalk showing walkability near a patient's home, and a polygon feature could be a park showing access to green space. A raster map for such a study could be an aerial image showing land use for a park.[2]

Although resources for data or spatial databases are exhaustive, consider the project's accuracy, completeness, cost, license, and scale. We obtain data from many sources, including electronic health records from a health care organization; local city and county governments (physical features such as streets, parks, or public transportation); state and local health departments; federal agencies such as the US Census Bureau (population demographics), the US Geological Survey, Environmental Protection Agency, National Oceanic and Atmospheric Administration, US

Department of Transportation, GPS satellite imagery (land use, water, environmental data); National Cancer Institute, Centers for Disease Control and Prevention (health survey data); commercial sources (Esri, Google Earth Engine, Maxar, HERE Technologies, Pitney Bowes); nonprofit organizations (Natural Earth data, OpenStreetMap Foundation, World Resources Institute, Environmental Defense Fund); community organizations (local community development corporations, environmental justice organizations, neighborhood associations); and academic institutions (for example, the University of Wisconsin Area Deprivation Index).

Using GIS technology, medical geographers can investigate the availability and accessibility of health care services, including hospitals, clinics, and pharmacies, and identify populations with limited access to care. Researchers can pinpoint neighborhoods with high rates of diseases and investigate environmental factors that could contribute to these rates. Medical geography studies the spatial spread of infectious diseases and the physical factors contributing to their transmission.

Through its approach, medical geography provides an understanding of health and disease by teaching students about social and environmental influences on community well-being while equipping them with the skills to tackle health care inequities. For example, biological, behavioral, and social factors affect pediatric asthma. GIS can illustrate the association between places with higher asthma morbidity and **social factors** (e.g., social determinants of health). In Fig. 10.1 we classified the percentage of adults with high school diplomas (shades of magenta) into quintiles. Next, we geocoded addresses, aggregated data at the census tract level in the District of Columbia and overlaid the emergency department encounter map layer on top of the adult education layer. This **choropleth map** aids visualization of disparate rates of higher emergency department visits in higher areas of adults with high school diplomas.[3]

In summary, medical and health geography literacy is comprehending and applying geographic principles and techniques to studying health and health care. It is vital in advancing our understanding of the complex interplay between location, environment, and public health. It leads to more effective health policies and interventions—a geospatial approach toward reimagining medical education and promoting health and well-being.

PROMOTING HEALTH EQUITY THROUGH MEDICAL GEOGRAPHY

Promoting **health equity** through medical geography is a multidisciplinary/interdisciplinary approach that combines geographic analysis to reduce health inequities among populations. It recognizes that where people live, work,

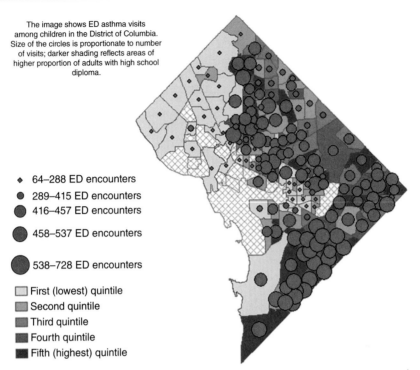

The image shows ED asthma visits among children in the District of Columbia. Size of the circles is proportionate to number of visits; darker shading reflects areas of higher proportion of adults with high school diploma.

- ◆ 64–288 ED encounters
- ● 289–415 ED encounters
- ● 416–457 ED encounters
- ● 458–537 ED encounters
- ● 538–728 ED encounters

- First (lowest) quintile
- Second quintile
- Third quintile
- Fourth quintile
- Fifth (highest) quintile

Fig. 10.1 Emergency department (ED) visits per 1000 children (ED encounters, rates proportional to the size of circles) with asthma emerged from electronic health records from the hospital. (From Tyris J, Gourishankar A, Ward MC, Kachroo N, Teach SJ, Parikh K. Social determinants of health and at-risk rates for pediatric asthma morbidity. *Pediatrics*. 2022;150(2):e2021055570.)

and play can significantly impact their health outcomes. By understanding the spatial distribution of health resources, environmental factors, and social determinants of health, medical geography helps policymakers, health care providers, and researchers develop strategies to address inequities in health care access and health outcomes. Therefore, using visual aids and geographical analysis, medical geographers can identify and understand the root causes of health inequities. We can develop more targeted and effective interventions that ensure everyone has an equal opportunity to achieve good health and well-being, regardless of where they live.

Graphically presenting social and economic data superimposed on health outcomes maps makes it possible to visualize patterns and trends, communicating vital information to a broader audience. For instance, geographical maps can highlight inequities in health outcomes and lack of access to health care services or showcase equity and social justice problems such as poor air quality, contaminated water, or lack of food availability compared to at-risk populations. This map visualization is a powerful way to enhance clarity and facilitate a comprehensive understanding of complex

health issues to enable policymakers and health care professionals to pinpoint areas of need and more effectively target interventions (e.g., policy maps).

Similarly, combining maps with charts and graphs can illustrate inequities in income, education, or other health determinants, helping to uncover the root causes of studying and guiding policy decisions. Promoting health equity involves more than creating maps for research and analysis by medical and health professionals. It involves stakeholders at all levels, including patients and citizens. GIS story maps and dashboards are two geospatial tools for sharing geospatial health data.

Story maps are a dynamic and interactive way to convey geographical information and narratives by combining maps, text, images, and other media to tell a compelling spatial story. GIS story maps enable users to explore geographic data, patterns, and stories through a user-friendly interface, making complex information accessible to a broad audience. Whether used for educational purposes, environmental advocacy, urban planning, or historical documentation, they provide an engaging and informative platform for presenting location-based information and fostering a deeper understanding of the world. GIS-based dashboards and advanced geospatial analytics allow stakeholders to explore data and metrics in statistical, spatial, and temporal forms. It also enables the functionality to manage the data, for example, add and edit new data. Geovisualization and visual analytics have broad applicability, including web-based approaches for end-users. Also, GIS promotes and informs health care professionals by displaying various equity indices and metrics to facilitate action.

By collecting on-the-ground field data and community feedback for use in a GIS project, medical education learners can witness the lived experiences of communities' social justice. This practice has long been in place in fields such as urban planning. In essence, this approach is a way to recognize differences in health care access and may aid changes in policies and distribution of resources that prioritize marginalized communities. For example, consider an intervention to improve health care accessibility in a marginalized community. Various strategies can be implemented to achieve this goal, such as setting up a clinic, providing transportation services for clinic visits, and offering assistance to ease the burden of health care expenses. Another intervention could focus on improving the environment in a neighborhood. For example, GIS could track clinic usage, services received, and patients' locations. This tracking helps evaluate clinic effectiveness and identify areas requiring more services. Transport services can be evaluated by tracking the number of people using them, their travel distances, and their appointments.

Some strategies to address health equity include creating parks and green spaces, reducing air pollution, and ensuring access to healthy food options. With the help of public and private data, GIS can identify and map areas with a high prevalence of medical conditions such as asthma or obesity, areas lacking green spaces, healthy food options, and clean air. We could create maps and dashboards to visualize and communicate findings to stakeholders.

In Chicago, a study discovered a link between the presence of food stores and low obesity rates.[4] As a result, a program initiated the establishment of food stores in neighborhoods historically lacking access to resources. Similarly, research conducted in Los Angeles showed that proximity to parks is associated with reduced asthma rates.[5] Similar studies can inform agencies to initiate programs to establish parks and green spaces in marginalized neighborhoods.

GIS can promote health equity by addressing population characteristics to obtain a sense of community demographics, health inequities, and trends; provide insight into community health that is actionable (e.g., hot spots of high lead levels in children and allocate resources to replace lead pipes); provide beneficial information to the community (maps of parks, food markets, services); and empower

citizens and stakeholders with tools such as dashboards monitoring progress and performance of the program in their community. With a focus on using GIS for projects addressing health inequities, we equip learners with the ability to address unfair and unjust distributions of wealth, opportunities, and privileges that inevitably adversely impact health in disadvantaged communities.

SOCIAL JUSTICE AND MEDICAL EDUCATION

Social justice means treating all individuals equitably regardless of race, religion, gender, sexual orientation, or other personal attributes. The realm of social justice intertwines with education in many ways. For instance, aspiring doctors must learn about social determinants or economic factors that impact health outcomes. Moreover, they should be well versed in recognizing and addressing bias, unconscious prejudice, and discrimination. Medical institutions can actively incorporate principles of justice into their curricula and training programs to combat racism and biases. Furthermore, integrating geography with a focus on social justice values encourages medical students to be sensitive to marginalized community needs and advocate for health care equity. This approach also recognizes the importance of diversifying the health care workforce, ensuring that it reflects the diverse backgrounds and experiences of the patient population.

Area health education center networks, such as the Health Resources and Services Administration's Council on Graduate Medical Education, strategize with the Department of Health and Human Services on health care shortages using GIS and spatial analysis.[6] The distribution of health care professionals can directly impact access to health care services and contribute to health inequities. Communities suffer poor health outcomes with uneven distribution of physicians, especially in underserved or rural areas. Applying GIS to assess the distribution of primary care providers can address diversity and health care deserts. GIS can play a crucial role in promoting social equity in medical education by identifying and addressing health care inequities. Such tools aid in creating a more equitable health care system.

Location-based demographic data are a key indicator of disadvantaged segments of a community when viewed with a social justice lens. Does where you live matter to health? GIS allows us to understand the relationship between people, where they live, and their health. Many inequities exist in society, but race, poverty, and place are key predictors of inequity. We recognize health status differences by class, race or ethnicity, gender, and geography. Learners must study health inequities in theory and methodology with GIS use. Fig. 10.2 provides a schematic approach to health conditions and inequity (social injustice) with the individual context of genetic, behavioral, and biological attributes intersecting with the geographical context.

From a geography standpoint, we can visualize the phenomenon of interest through maps across various spatial contexts. GIS addresses health problems on multiple levels, considering context, spatial dependency, and **spatial heterogeneity**. **Spatial dependency** (spatial autocorrelation) measures the similarity between values of variables at nearby locations. It can identify areas where risk factors are clustered or health outcomes are clustered—demonstrating their relationships.

Using the principles in Fig. 10.2, a county-level study of the United States examined high rates of low birthweight in US counties clustered in the southeastern US, particularly for Black infants—an inequity linked to education levels in counties.[7] A study of this kind enables medical students to familiarize themselves with the service territory and the health care requirements of the inhabitants in the surrounding areas. GIS brings attention to social injustice by illustrating inequities in health care. Spatial regression can model the relationship between risk factors and health outcomes (suppose social injustice) while controlling for the spatial relationships between various factors. It can account for the potential confounding effects of spatial factors. **Spatial regression** models include geographic weighted regression, multiscale geographic weighted regression, spatial error or lag model, and similar extensions of these models. Details of these models are beyond the scope of this chapter. By iterative processes of map making, geostatistical and geospatial analysis, and modeling, GIS will help move beyond the superposition of two variables on a map and show interactions and spatial connections. Methods such as qualitative research are useful to understand the conditions experienced in different spatial contexts and literature review to identify potential mechanisms by which space (location or place) could influence the condition.

For example, a study on inequities in cardiovascular health used GIS to examine the relationship between poverty and heart disease.[8] The study found that people living in areas with high poverty rates were likelier to have heart disease. The study also found that the spatial distribution of heart disease cases was similar to the spatial distribution of poverty rates. However, the study also found that the relationship between poverty and heart disease varied depending on the racial/ethnic composition of the area. African Americans were more likely to have heart disease, even after controlling for the poverty rates in their area. This information suggests an interaction between poverty, race/ethnicity, and heart disease. By teaching medical students such examples of how to use GIS to identify and address inequities in cardiovascular health, we can help prepare

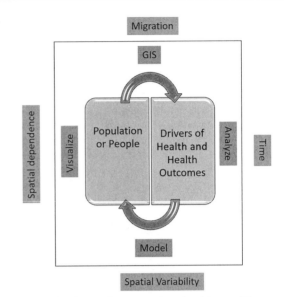

Fig. 10.2 A schematic approach to health conditions and inequity (social injustice) with the individual context of genetic, behavioral, and biological attributes intersecting with the geographical context.

them to become more effective and socially just physicians. A direct example of a location or place (geographical space) directly affecting health is the proximity to superfund toxic sites. These hazardous sites are known to be associated with diabetes, cancer, and respiratory illness.

GIS supports the integration of social justice into medical education, ensuring that medical students better understand the landscape of their service regions with a lens toward illuminating various social and structural determinants of health that contribute significantly to health disparities and inequities.

GEOGRAPHIC INFORMATION SYSTEMS AND SPATIAL ANALYSIS FOR HEALTH EQUITY IN MEDICAL EDUCATION

As previously noted, students are exposed to geospatial thinking and the "science of where" well before medical school. In high school, we learn about geography and its subdisciplines, including physical, human, and environmental geography. All these are foundational in human health and medical education. Physical geography explores the Earth's physical features and processes, including climate and natural disasters. Human geography focuses on populations, cultures, and society. Examples such as population growth, demographics, and urbanization (for example, the analysis of cities, urban planning, and the challenges of urban growth) relate directly to health concerns. Political geography and geopolitical conflicts often lead to migration or food and water scarcity. Environmental geography focuses on the interactions between humans and the environment in regard to important issues such as pollution, deforestation, and climate change.

From the student's perspective, medical and health geography literacy and geospatial analysis technologies provide multiple educational benefits at various levels. Students learn computer technology and applications while addressing health equity and social justice issues. They learn to manipulate and analyze health-related data to improve health outcomes. Students gain a deeper understanding of various research concepts and principles while exercising analytical and modeling skills. Lastly, students experience a sense of satisfaction through first-hand experiences learning about the communities in which they will serve.

We can tailor the knowledge depth and skills students experience to the learner's needs and the program's requirements. For example, at its core, GIS provides students with a comprehensive overview of geospatial principles and applications and hands-on training in GIS software. This approach would best suit students who plan to use geospatial technologies extensively in their future careers, such as public health physicians, epidemiologists, and health policy researchers. On the other hand, as an adjunct to teaching about a particular subject, GIS could teach students about, for example, the epidemiology of infectious diseases, the social determinants of health, or the impact of climate change on health. This approach would best suit students who do not need to become GIS experts but could benefit from using GIS to enhance their understanding of a particular topic. Whether or not every medical student or health care professional needs to have the facility with geospatial data and analysis is a matter of debate.

Students' education using GIS can provide descriptive maps, show an association between factors, and sometimes establish causality with an iterative process and other tools. Here are some specific examples: (1) Epidemiology: map the distribution of diseases, identify clusters of cases, and track the spread of outbreaks; (2) **Social determinants of health**: map the distribution of social and environmental factors that affect health, such as poverty, crime, and access to health care; (3) Health policy: analyze the impact of health policies on different populations and geographic areas; (4) Climate change and health: map the distribution of climate-sensitive diseases, such as malaria and dengue fever. GIS can also assess different populations' vulnerability to the health impacts of climate change.

How can we successfully introduce GIS and spatial analysis for health equity in the medical education curriculum?

We cannot simply teach a GIS software application and expect successful outcomes or changes to communities based on one map or study. Geospatial projects use multiple "layers" of information and sometimes big data. While some students are comfortable with spreadsheets and databases, many require support from IT professionals, statisticians, librarians, or GIS experts.

Issues related to health equity that may use GIS are often complicated and require a multidisciplinary approach and critical thinking. For example, GIS can identify problems, but interventions and solutions often require external collaboration. If a childhood obesity study identifies that lack of green space results in high BMI scores, local governments would need to enact policies to add more green space to a city, including the involvement of mayors, city councils, city planners, or architects. If lack of clinics or access to health care facilities is the issue, transportation experts may need to be involved to devise and implement a viable solution. By harnessing expertise and resources, interdisciplinary projects help to ensure that geospatial projects are successful and that their communities benefit from the power of GIS. GIS projects can use qualitative and quantitative perspectives and data from patients and citizens.

When should GIS be taught in medical schools? In the first 2 years of medical school, students learn about the foundations of medicine, medical ethics, pathology, microbiology, or immunology. The school introduces them to clinical skills, research, and patient care. During this time, medical students can be exposed to geospatial "awareness," but it is unlikely that many will have time to dive deeply into its capabilities. In the last 2 years of medical school, medical students are busy with clinical rotations, career planning, transitions to residency, and specializations, so it might be difficult to integrate geospatial technology into medical education fully. However, during these years, medical students should learn about health equity and geographic factors that contribute to poor health outcomes and the possibility of how GIS technologies and spatial analysis can improve those poor health outcomes.

Some instances where the medical school can teach GIS in the early years are: (1) During the pre-clerkship years, teach students the basics of GIS, such as collecting, analyzing, and visualizing spatial data. Students could learn how to use GIS to solve real-world problems in health care, such as identifying areas with high rates of chronic diseases or tracking the spread of infectious diseases. (2) During the clerkship years, students could learn "how" to use GIS to support clinical decision-making and improve the quality of patient care. For example, students could use GIS to identify patients at high risk for complications or develop integrated treatment plans.

We have found that GIS fits nicely in residency programs for multiple reasons. Residents and medical students are introduced to various data types, from national to local and retrospective to prospective data. Our residents and fellows are trained in understanding, accessing, and using various data types that are powerful when mapped for analysis. Quality improvement projects also contribute to social justice and health equity topics.

Given that the Accreditation Council for Graduate Medical Education (ACGME) recognizes the need for diverse programs to prepare physicians for several roles, including scientists, this organization expects scholarly activities to align with the missions of said schools and the needs of their service communities. Dashboards became an integral part of the COVID-19 pandemic to monitor factors like outbreaks, clusters, spreading, rates, and percentages of citizens with and without COVID-19 (web-based COVID dashboard created by the Johns Hopkins University)[9]; similarly, dashboards can be employed for numerous quality improvement interventions.

Here are a few examples of how GIS is currently used in medical schools to address health equity issues. This work often explores multidisciplinary approaches to understanding environmental, social, population health, and geographic factors influencing health for data-driven decisions to improve patient care and public health outcomes. Data such as crime, education, access to food, poverty, language barriers, and neighborhood characteristics can help visualize areas of concern and, with advanced spatial analytic tools, offer insights for solutions and intervention.

One project involved medical students, residents, fellows, and attendings at the University of Pittsburgh Children's Hospital of Pittsburgh in conjunction with the Health Care Policy and Health Care Analytics facility and students at Carnegie Mellon University (CMU). At the heart of the project was identifying chronic conditions (including asthma, diabetes, and mental health) where school nurses could aid in caring for students.

In the first phase, using advanced GIS tools, a medical fellow/PhD student taking a Health GIS course at Carnegie Mellon University created the following maps (Fig. 10.3) to identify areas for asthma interventions. The map on the left identified factors that contributed to asthma exacerbation, including poor air quality (obtained from Environmental Protection Agency air monitors), housing complaints (obtained from the local county public health department), and smoking prevalence (obtained from a tobacco smoking study). Using multivariate data-mining clustering tools, we created a map showing the concentrations of all three factors (map on the left). The center map used GIS networking tools to show drive time accessibility to pediatric and primary care sites and populations with poor access. The right-side map showed the use of GIS intersection tools to identify "intervention areas."

GIS physical features could also be overlaid with physical and socioeconomic data to help health care providers understand where asthma issues occur and tell policymakers where to focus on built environment solutions such as increasing green space, tree canopies, or addressing permeable surfaces. In collaboration with the School of Architecture at Carnegie Mellon University, medical students and researchers at Children's Hospital of Pittsburgh are conducting related projects and changes to city neighborhoods. Other GIS components of this project involved a University of Pittsburgh

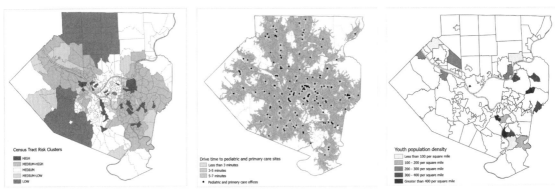

Fig. 10.3 The map on the left identifies factors that contribute to asthma exacerbation, including poor air quality, housing complaints, and smoking prevalence. Multivariate data-mining clustering tools create a map showing the concentrations of all three factors (map on the left). The center map used GIS networking tools to show drive time accessibility to pediatric and primary care sites and populations with poor access. The right-side map shows the use of GIS intersection tools to identify "intervention areas."

medical student and a CMU health policy student who spent a summer exploring school nurse and student ratios for the entire state of Pennsylvania compared to education outcomes such as test scores. In addition, a medical fellow in adolescent medicine, who studies mental health issues and violence, is also part of the project and could help decide where school nurse participation should occur.

Health care policy and health analytics students continue working with the Children's Hospital team to identify specific schools to target based on readmission data from the hospital's emergency department database and county health department data. Fig. 10.4 is an example of a dashboard using publicly available data that analyzes asthma emergency department visits and hospitalizations. This interactive dashboard created from the medical fellow/PhD student project is currently used in a textbook to educate medical students and health professionals.[10]

Future designs of the school nurse collaboration project and chronic conditions include using GIS, advanced data analytics, machine learning, and other data sources, such as social media, to measure the success of school nurse

involvement with patients, families, clinicians, and community organizations.[11]

Another example of interagency interactions is where Children's National Hospital partners with George Washington University, Howard University College of Medicine, and the District of Columbia's Department of Health. The community health needs assessment identifies key community health priorities accounting for geographic locations.[12] The medical students, residents, and fellows take courses on GIS and are productive in scholarly work. Children's National Hospital's IMPACT DC asthma clinic created a dashboard and continues to provide targeted services and research using GIS tools.

At a community-distributed medical school, such as the University of California, Riverside, the locations of facilities, patients, and health-related resources are spread inequitably across the region. GIS can be a powerful science and set of tools for framing scholarly activities, particularly quality improvement research projects. An example of GIS's role in medical education is our integrated GIS Quality Improvement research training curriculum at

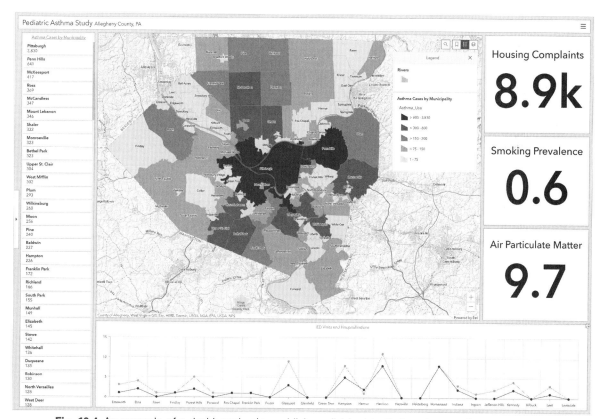

Fig. 10.4 An example of a dashboard using publicly available data that analyzes asthma emergency department visits and hospitalizations. Used herein with permission. © 2024 Esri. All rights reserved.

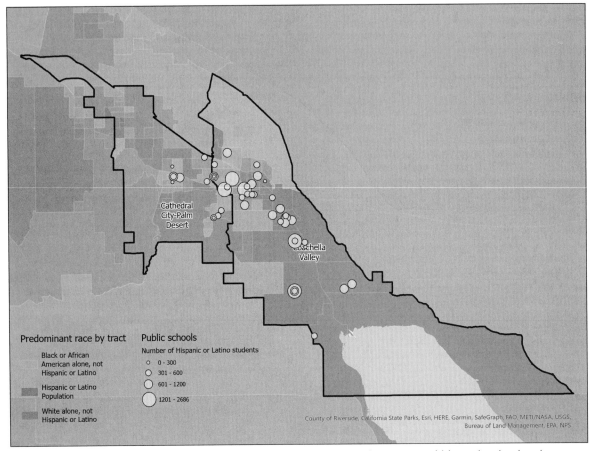

Fig. 10.5 GIS is used to explore the relationship between various races within each school and the communities in which they reside.

our Psychiatry & Neurosciences residency program at the University of California, Riverside, School of Medicine.

Quality improvement/GIS curriculum immerses residents throughout their 4 years of residency. Teams of residents assemble to actively participate in GIS/quality improvement projects rooted in the surrounding service community and geared toward health improvements. One such project, "Safe and Unsafe Routes to and from Schools," is in partnership with the City of Palm Desert and the Palm Desert School District and is designed to be expanded to the larger Coachella Valley region of nine cities.

Palm Desert is located 122 miles east of Los Angeles, with a population of over 50,000, of which over 30% of the population is Hispanic, Asian, or Black. Desert Sands Unified School District (DSUSD) serves the City of Palm Desert. DSUSD enrolls 26,000 students across 34 school sites, of which 16% are Hispanic, 3% are Asian, and 2% are Black. By contrast, Coachella Valley, a neighboring city of

Palm Desert, has a population of over 45,000, of which over 96% are Hispanic. Coachella Valley Unified School District (CVUSD) services the City of Coachella Valley. CVUSD enrolls over 16,000 students across 22 school sites, of which over 97% are Hispanic students. GIS is used to explore the relationship between various races within each school and the communities in which they reside (Fig. 10.5).

The poverty rate in Palm Desert is 12.7%, with a median family income greater than $64,000, versus Coachella Valley's poverty rate of 18.9%, with a median family income of just under $34,000. GIS is also used to explore these poverty rates (Fig. 10.6).

Representing this initial demographic data in GIS enables our psychiatry residents to familiarize themselves with the landscape of their service region, identify structural or social determinants of health inequities in and across communities, begin to collect additional relevant data, analyze those data, and employ GIS dashboards and

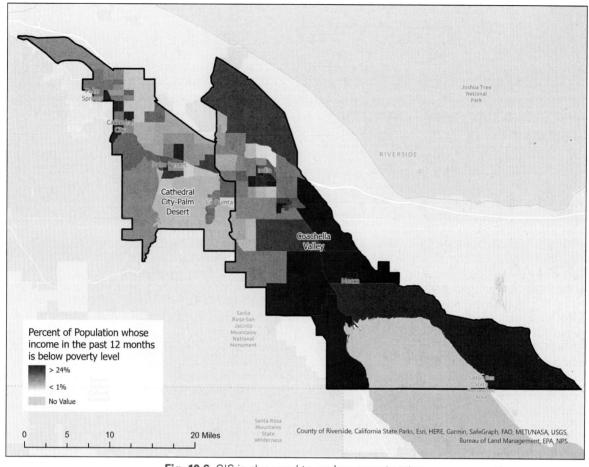

Fig. 10.6 GIS is also used to explore poverty rates.

story maps for health improvement interventions. Story maps have become a unique and effective method to showcase digital narratives that illustrate the physical, social, and economic landscape. This exercise allows our residents to further connect with the regions they serve. The residents collaborate with local governments, making GIS necessary for informed decision-making. Ultimately, GIS becomes a critical tool in identifying health care inequities to best aid residents in capturing the community's needs.

The comprehensive and interconnected structure of geospatial technologies provides robust analytical capabilities. Agencies and organizations participating in GIS projects provide platforms and resources to further the cause. Here are a few examples of how the GIS approach serves people:

- The National Cancer Institute GIS portal mentions surveillance programs and research to reduce cancer health inequities.[13]

- GIS effectively identifies areas in Los Angeles County to meet the population-to-physician ratio in primary care shortage areas.[14]
- The health department monitors blood lead levels in children in the municipality.[15]
- The Centers for Disease Control and Prevention (CDC) identified high-risk communities for COVID-19. The CDC uses demographic data, social determinants of health, and more to provide effective vaccine delivery.
- The National Association of Counties (NACo) provides help in counties with high rates of diabetes.
- The Environmental Protection Agency's AirNow website provides real-time data on air quality in the United States, which helps monitor the impact of air pollution control interventions, such as vehicle emission standards and power plant regulations.
- The National Oceanic and Atmospheric Administration's (NOAA) Coral Reef Watch website helps monitor the

health of coral reefs by conservation interventions, such as marine protected areas and sustainable fishing practices.

- The United States Geological Survey's (USGS) National Earthquake Hazards Reduction program monitors the impact of earthquake preparedness and mitigation efforts.

OVERCOMING CHALLENGES AND FUTURE DIRECTIONS

Universities that are reducing support for geography departments are harming their role in scholarship and education despite technology's growing importance.[16] We must protect geography as a tech-enhanced tool (including GIS) for solving current issues.

We must address the challenges of implementing GIS into medical education effectively. Both medical students and residents have limited time to devote to GIS projects. Building collaborative support from researchers, librarians, and IT specialists is critical. We must build sufficient time for learning to support GIS project implementation. We provide our trainees with research support by working with interdisciplinary partners to form research teams. There is a benefit in incentivizing and promoting GIS projects with trainees' forums that showcase projects and credit and recognize the trainees' work. Lastly, funding for GIS programming and projects is essential for an effective and sustainable program. Implementing geography, GIS, spatial analysis, and social justice in medical education comes with challenges. First, it is often perceived as unconventional in the curriculum and requires more support from faculty and administrators. Additionally, these fields demand skills and knowledge that may need to be more readily available in schools, making it difficult to find qualified instructors for these courses.

Further research is needed to assess the effectiveness of integrating geography, GIS, geospatial analysis, and social justice into education. This research should primarily focus on how these fields impact student learning, patient care, and overall health outcomes. Collaboration between educators, geographers, GIS specialists, and social justice advocates is crucial to developing and implementing educational programs. To advance health equity and promote justice through medical geography and education in the future, we must:

1. Implement educational programs incorporating medical geography alongside GIS technology, spatial analysis techniques, and principles of social justice
2. Research to evaluate the effectiveness of these programs
3. Advocate for policies addressing health determinants while striving toward achieving health equity

4. Foster partnerships with community organizations to address existing health inequities

Furthermore, it is crucial to address the following aspects:

1. Enhance the knowledge and understanding of geography, GIS, spatial analysis, and social justice among students, faculty members, and administrators
2. Execute training programs for health care professionals focusing on these subjects
3. Develop resources and tools that enable professionals to integrate these topics into their practice
4. Promote research to evaluate the effectiveness of these interventions
5. Advocate for health care policies prioritizing geography, GIS, spatial analysis, and social justice

GIS in medical education can significantly enhance physicians' capabilities by providing them with spatial awareness and analytical skills crucial in health care. Understanding the geographical distribution of diseases, patient demographics, and health care resources allows physicians to make informed decisions. GIS enables health data mapping, helping physicians identify patterns, clusters, and disease trends. This spatial perspective aids resource allocation, outbreak management, and personalized patient care. By integrating GIS into medical education, physicians can better navigate complex health landscapes, optimize public health interventions, and ultimately contribute to improved health care outcomes for individuals and communities.

Reimagining medical education using the geographic lens and addressing health inequity involves understanding GIS and geospatial principles, foundations, and applications in health care. We recommend appropriate curriculum development, implementation, and improvisation for the learners' educational requirements. Some suggestions, but not limited to these, are taking a GIS course and embedding geospatial data and technologies into the medical curriculum in epidemiology, public health, and clinical medicine programs. It also provides students opportunities to apply real-world problems to understand better the geographic distribution of diseases, risk factors for diseases, and the impact of interventions on diseases, improving health and health equity. GIS can be valuable for fostering connections between medical education, health equity, social justice, and other related domains.

TAKE-HOME POINTS

1. GIS can be valuable tools in health care for mapping the distribution of diseases, social determinants of health,

and the impact of health policies on different populations and geographic areas.

2. Integrating GIS with an equity lens into medical education can better equip students with the skills and knowledge needed to tackle real-world health-related challenges and address health inequities.

3. To ensure that future health professionals can develop an understanding and use of GIS toolsets, we must build upon education that promotes medical or health geography and advocate for health policies prioritizing geography, GIS, spatial analysis, and social justice.

ANNOTATED BIBLIOGRAPHY

- Cromley EK, McLafferty SL. *GIS and Public Health*. 2nd ed. The Guilford Press; 2011.

This book continues to be widely regarded as a seminal work concerning utilizing geographic information systems (GIS) in public health. Specifically designed for professionals in the health care industry, this academic publication offers a current analysis of GIS methodologies. The authors provide state-of-the-art approaches for arranging and assessing critical health records, encompassing demographic data, medical occurrences, risk factors, and the contact information of health care providers. The authors present these methods by utilizing their profound expertise in the respective fields. This edition illuminates the function of GIS in public health, rendering it an exceptional resource for researchers and professionals in this domain. Its status as a seminal work in the field is a testament to its profound influence and widespread recognition. For individuals investigating health inequities or spatial epidemiology, this book continues to be a vital reference for professionals whose fields intersect with public health and GIS. The companion website contains lab exercises with data available for download, catering to academic and personal purposes.

- Cobb CD. Chapter 4. *Geospatial Analysis: A New Window Into Educational Equity, Access, and Opportunity*. Review of Research in Education; 2020.

This chapter comprehensively reviews the literature on using geographic information systems (GIS) in education research. The author thoroughly searched various literature databases and identified 60 research articles related to GIS and education. The author recorded key features of each study, such as research topic, publication year, context, equity concepts, GIS techniques used, and the role of geospatial methods in the study. The data were assembled into a data matrix and analyzed using an iterative coding process. The author also discusses the limitations of the search process and the need for more research on the use of GIS in education. Overall, this chapter provides a comprehensive overview of educational GIS research and highlights the potential of geospatial methods for promoting educational equity and access.

- Gatrell AC. *Geographies of Health*. Wiley; 2001.

This book examines the many links between health and geography. It thoroughly examines how geographical perspectives aid health research. The book carefully examines many studies that link health outcomes to the complex interaction between social and physical environments. Gatrell's writing makes it easy to follow as they discuss important theoretical perspectives, research methods, and findings. Also, international research is included in the book to help readers learn. Gatrell provides information-filled text boxes, suggested readings at the end of each chapter, a complete list of sources, and a guide to useful websites. This book is easy to understand and focuses on people, making it a good resource for learning about the complex relationship between geography and health.

REFERENCES

1. Musa GJ, Chiang PH, Sylk T, et al. Use of GIS mapping as a public health tool- from cholera to cancer. *Health Serv Insights*. 2013;6:111–116. https://doi.org/10.4137/HSI. S10471. Published 2013 Nov 19.
2. Kurland KS. *GIS Jump Start for Health Professionals. Chapter 1: Introducing GIS for health*. Esri Press; 2022.
3. Tyris J, Gourishankar A, Ward MC, Kachroo N, Teach SJ, Parikh K. Social determinants of health and at-risk rates for pediatric asthma morbidity. *Pediatrics*. 2022;150(2): https:// doi.org/10.1542/peds.2021-055570. e2021055570.
4. Huang H. A spatial analysis of obesity: interaction of urban food environments and racial segregation in Chicago. *J Urban Health*. 2021;98(5):676–686. https://doi.org/10.1007/ s11524-021-00553-y.
5. Douglas JA, Archer RS, Alexander SE. Ecological determinants of respiratory health: examining associations between asthma emergency department visits, diesel particulate matter, and public parks and open space in Los Angeles, California. *Prev Med Rep*. 2019;14:100855. https:// doi.org/10.1016/j.pmedr.2019.100855. Published 2019 Mar 27.
6. U.S. Department of Health and Human Services. *HHS Invests $11 Million to Expand Medical Residencies in Rural Communities*. 2023. https://www.hhs.gov/about/ news/2023/07/26/hhs-invests-11-million-expand-medical-residencies-rural-communities.html
7. Brown CC, Moore JE, Felix HC, Stewart MK, Tilford JM. Geographic hotspots for low birthweight: an analysis of counties with persistently high rates. *Inquiry*. 2020;57. https://doi.org/10.1177/0046958020950999. 46958020950999.
8. Mensah GA, Mokdad AH, Ford ES, Greenlund KJ, Croft JB. State of disparities in cardiovascular health in the United

States. *Circulation.* 2005;111(10):1233–1241. https://doi.org/10.1161/01.CIR.0000158136.76824.04.

9. Ahasan R, Alam MS, Chakraborty T, Hossain MM. Applications of GIS and geospatial analyses in COVID-19 research: a systematic review. *F1000Res.* 2020;9:1379. https://doi.org/10.12688/f1000research.27544.2. Published 2020 Nov 27.

10. Kurland KS. *GIS Jump Start for Health Professionals. Chapter 5: Creating health GIS dashboards.* Esri Press; 2022.

11. *School Nurse Engagement Project, Heinz College Systems Synthesis,* 2022–2023.

12. Children's National. *DC Health Matters Collaborative.* 2022. https://www.childrensnational.org/in-the-community/advocacy-and-outreach/community-initiatives-and-partnerships/dc-health-matters-collaborative.

13. National Cancer Institute. *GIS Portal for Cancer Research.* 2022. https://gis.cancer.gov/research/health_disparities.html.

14. Juarez PD, Robinson PL, Matthews-Juarez P. 100% access, zero health disparities, and GIS: an improved methodology for designating health professions shortage areas. *J Health Soc Policy.* 2002;16(1–2):155–167. https://doi.org/10.1300/j045v16n01_13.

15. Cuyahoga County Board of Health. *Lead Poisoning Prevention.* 2022. http://ccbh.net/lead-poisoning/.

16. AAG. *The State of Geography: Data and Trends in Higher Education.* 2022. https://www.aag.org/the-state-of-geography-data-and-trends-in-higher-education/

PART IV

Case Studies: Admission, Selection, Pathways, and Pipelines

11

The Mission-Based Program Model
A Programmatic Framework to Drive Diversity and Health Equity in Medical Education

Khanh-Van Le-Bucklin, Candice Taylor Lucas, Carol Major, Charles Vega, and Julie Youm

SUMMARY

Physicians hold the great privilege of impacting health outcomes from the level of an individual patient to that of a population. Developing a health workforce that reflects the composition of our diverse communities and societal realities requires an intervention by the institutions of medical education to create the necessary pathways toward this end. The mission-based program (MBP) model was developed at the University of California, Irvine School of Medicine to recruit and advocate for physician leaders who will focus on areas of health care for which a specific need has been identified. In this chapter, we share the structure of the MBP model, successful outcomes from our current programs, and valuable lessons learned. We offer this approach as an evidence-based intervention for improving the future diversity of the health workforce and, ultimately, equitable patient outcomes.

INTRODUCTION

Mission-based programs (MBPs) are designed to support the professional growth of talented future physicians with demonstrated skill and passion for addressing the health needs of historically marginalized and systematically excluded communities at increased risk of health inequities. MBPs foster inclusive spaces for learning, support community-engaged experiential learning opportunities, and sponsor opportunities for impactful service. A diverse workforce with unique knowledge, compassion, and abilities is needed to realize better health outcomes for communities disproportionately impacted by **systemic racism**, **intergenerational inequity**, and trauma. This chapter outlines how academic medical institutions can use MBPs to achieve this goal.

BACKGROUND

The Association of American Medical Colleges (AAMC) projects that the United States could face a shortage of up to 124,000 physicians by 2034, with both primary and specialty care fields impacted.[1] The growing shortage of physicians is becoming a threat to health care accessibility for low-income populations. Medical schools across the country have looked for various ways to tackle the threat of health care inaccessibility of underrepresented diverse populations. As medical schools work to address this workforce shortage, it is imperative that institutions consider and respond to regional and national health needs as they strive to foster **health equity** for patients, families, and communities. Several studies have identified that physicians who are **underrepresented in medicine** are more likely to care for patients from underserved populations. Thus, recruiting diverse medical learners may be helpful to the goal of improving health equity. The decision by the US Supreme Court to enact a policy against considering race and ethnicity in admissions has led institutions of higher education to look for new ways to achieve diverse bodies of learners.

Mahdavynia et al. stated that "Social accountability can help cultivate a healthy and skilled medical workforce and be effective in improving health services provided to the people."[2] MBPs are one way to achieve this accountability by providing structural guidelines for academic medical centers to produce diverse physician advocates who address the health needs of underrepresented and underresourced communities and champion health equity.

The University of California, Irvine School of Medicine (UCISOM) created its first MBP, the Program in Medical Education for the Latino Community (PRIME-LC) in 2004, in recognition of the unique health inequities experienced by underresourced Latino communities. This effort was led by Dr. Alberto Manetta and supported by then University of California Irvine (UCI) Chancellor Michael Drake, who was instrumental in securing support from the University of California (UC) Office of the President and the California State Legislature to make PRIME-LC a reality. PRIME-LC also secured critical grant funding in its early years from the California Endowment and the UniHealth Foundation to move the program forward.

More than 20 years later, PRIME-LC is a well-established program and academic model of inclusive excellence. PRIME-LC provides medical learners with a curriculum tailored to train physicians to be skilled clinicians and advocates who provide culturally and linguistically responsive care to Latino communities. In complement to the success of the PRIME-LC program's purpose of addressing the health needs of underserved Latino communities, Drs. Carol Major, Khanh-Van Le-Bucklin, and Kaosoluchi Enendu founded the Leadership Education to Advance Diversity-African, Black, and Caribbean (LEAD-ABC) program in 2019 in awareness of the distinct need to produce physician leaders skilled in tackling issues introduced by the intersectionality of anti-Blackness and health inequities disproportionately affecting ABC communities.[3] The UC Office of the President acknowledged the value of this MBP by adding LEAD-ABC to the UC PRIME consortium and granted state support for the program in 2022. The program is now known as PRIME-LEAD-ABC. Additionally, California sponsored the creation of an affiliate program at UC Riverside School of Medicine.

We present MBPs here as a replicable and vital tool for sustaining and strengthening socially accountable medical schools. To successfully achieve this, programs must focus on (1) creating a mission-aligned curriculum, (2) intentionally recruiting talented medical learners, (3) growing a community of peer and faculty mentors, and (4) ensuring sustainable administrative and funding support.

THE CORE CURRICULAR PILLARS OF A MISSION-BASED PROGRAM

The MBP model was developed to recruit and advocate for physician leaders who will focus on areas of health care for which a specific need has been identified. MBPs at UCISOM[4] are structured as 4-year programs with longitudinal courses designed to expand learners' knowledge, abilities, and confidence in addressing the health care needs of mission-based patients and communities. Each program supports learners' professional development and identity formation as physician leaders through mission-focused clinical training, mentorship, and community engagement.

We find that to best prepare learners for service in a mission area, they need a holistic and integrated academic exposure. Accordingly, we identified four core pillars that create the curricular foundation for an MBP (Fig. 11.1):
1. Preclerkship phase seminar series
2. Mission-based clinical preceptorships
3. Clinical phase electives
4. Scholarly capstone project

Pillar 1: Preclerkship Phase Seminar Series

Learners receive early exposure to the significant issues in patient care, health equity, and **social determinants of health** that challenge a mission-based population through a longitudinal seminar series that runs across each year of

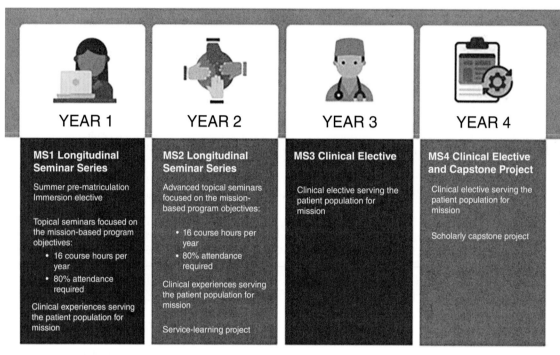

Fig. 11.1 Mission-based programs model.

the preclerkship phase. The seminar series is comprised of a minimum of ten curricular hours during each preclerkship year. The seminar series is carefully curated by the MBP directors, and seminars are taught by expert faculty in each content area. Examples of content covered in the MBPs at UCISOM include "Chicano-Latino Studies" sessions that focus on important issues regarding Latino culture and health care for PRIME-LC learners and "Community Engagement and Capacity Building" for PRIME-LEAD-ABC learners.

Activities to support community development between faculty, learners, and staff within each MBP are also conducted as early as the summer prior to matriculation to the medical school. These activities range in implementation including:

- A formal summer immersion program for PRIME-LC that starts 1 month prior to the start of the first year with the goals of exposing learners to health conditions in California's Latino communities through a collaboration

with the UCI Department of Chicano/Latino Studies, UCI outreach clinics, and community partners. Education community engagement is delivered through real-world experiences where PRIME-LC learners:
  - ° Visit the state capitol in Sacramento to advocate for addressing health care inequities and learn about health care policy.
  - ° Visit the US–Mexico border to learn about immigration politics and regulation.
  - ° Learn about rural health care by interviewing migrant farmworkers as well as shadowing physicians at rural clinics.
- An elective opportunity for incoming first-year PRIME-LEAD-ABC learners to meet with program directors and other PRIME-LEAD-ABC learners 1 week prior to the start of the first-year orientation.
- A pre-first-year orientation workshop and social event for program directors and new cohorts in the MBP to begin community building.

Further, at UCISOM, learners apply their learning from the seminar series to a mission-based **service-learning** project that is a school requirement for graduation.

Pillar 2: Mission-Based Clinical Preceptorships

Early clinical experiences have been a vital part of the pre-clerkship curriculum for over two decades with successes reported from the start of their integration into medical school curriculum.[5] The MBP framework extends the integration of early clinical experiences during the preclerkship phase in two important ways:

- First, learners are assigned to faculty preceptors during their clinical skills foundation courses who have direct patient care experience in their respective mission-based communities. These preceptors provide clinical skills training with an emphasis on the specific health care needs of the patients they will serve. For example, learners in the PRIME-LEAD-ABC program are assigned as a cohort in their longitudinal clinical foundations course with preceptors who have experience addressing the diverse and unique health needs of Black communities. Clinical skills development maintains the lens of this mission throughout their academic training.
- Second, learners are placed at clinical sites where they can gain a first-hand, immersive experience with their mission-based patient population. For example, learners in the PRIME-LC program are assigned to clinics serving the Latino community where they can see patients alongside experienced faculty as they gain exposure to cultural factors and socio-economic determinants of health that influence this population.

Pillar 3: Clinical Phase Electives

During the clinical phase, the MBP framework includes elective rotations that focus on mission-based learning in the clinical setting. These electives occur at clinical sites selected to provide further first-hand, immersive experiences with specific patient populations and community engagement. Clinical elective offerings include mission-based patient-care experiences, a longitudinal seminar series fostering reflection and professional identity formation, and an international rotation to compare the physician-patient relationship and health care systems between the United States and other countries.

Pillar 4: Scholarly Capstone Project

A scholarly project represents the capstone of an MBP. Learners are mentored and supported in the design and completion of scholarly work that is intended to be disseminated to a broad audience and advance efforts in addressing the health care needs and inequities related to a mission. Scholarly projects include peer-reviewed publications, conference presentations, development of digital resources, and service-learning projects.

Graduation with Distinction

All learners in an MBP complete the requirements for the MD degree. By completing the requirements outlined through the four curricular pillars of an MBP, learners are qualified to receive a graduation with distinction for the MBP. This distinction is intended to highlight and differentiate those who have the skills to become physician leaders in service to their respective mission-based patients and communities.

In total, the four core curricular pillars of the MBP provide a roadmap for institutions that want to develop a program with a mission-based focus to address regional and national health needs. There are strong implications from the multi-program implementation of MBPs at UCISOM for the feasibility and transferability of the MBP model to other academic institutions.

OUTREACH AND RECRUITMENT

Beyond the curriculum, our MBPs could not thrive without the right learners in place for this special training. Therefore, we have taken a systematic approach to the recruitment of medical learners whose career goals are to practice where they are needed most and promote health equity. Recruitment starts at the level of junior high school and follows learners through the post-baccalaureate period.

Successful outreach and recruitment require a combination of activities in the community along with events on campus. UCISOM features many medical student organizations which provide mentorship and instruction on medical school admissions, and most of their efforts focus on underrepresented in medicine (URiM) populations. These organizations bring in faculty and residents as well as admissions staff to guide learners on their path to medical school, and they receive support from the UCISOM Office of Belonging, Equity, and Empowerment (BEE). Mentorship and guidance sessions are both in-person and virtual, and there are group and individual sessions available.

One challenge to this approach is determining outcomes. Moreover, while it is important to get qualified mentors to the communities that need them, many of the families we serve have never set foot on a college campus. To address these issues, we created Open Medical School (OMS). OMS is held quarterly on campus, and it includes junior high/high school and college/post-baccalaureate tracks for invited learners.

Learners in our longitudinal mentorship programs are invited to attend OMS, along with their families. We offer them an immersive 1-day experience in medical education, from patient simulation to dissection to point-of-care ultrasound and inspiring speakers who reflect the learners' backgrounds.

Our outreach programs, tied together by OMS, also address another critical need in mentorship by using technology to promote an ongoing relationship with mentees. Mentees can reach out to learners and faculty through email, social media, and online meetings. UCISOM also follows mentees in a database. This allows us to promote ongoing communication with mentees, and it serves as a conduit to survey mentees regarding their progress toward medical careers and their satisfaction with SOM programs. Specifically, junior high and high school learners are queried regarding their attitudes and progress toward post-secondary education and careers in health care, while college and post-baccalaureate learners answer questions about their attitudes, challenges, and progress toward careers in health care.

The results of these surveys allow us to track mentees at individual and group levels and help us estimate the effectiveness of our outreach efforts. The BEE office follows these results and works on quality improvement efforts during quarterly meetings with representatives at the learner and faculty levels.

Since 2018, our outreach efforts have been further enhanced through the UCISOM Academies. These week-long on-campus programs run during the summer quarter and are divided into two groups:

1. A high school academy focused on all interested learners at the high school level. This academy offers need-based scholarships.
2. PRIME-LC and PRIME-LEAD-ABC Academies that focus on prospective learners for MBPs, with a preference for learners closer to the time of application for medical school. All learners receive scholarships to attend these academies without tuition.

The MBP Academies include instruction on the medical school application and interview skills. The Academies are under the direction of two UCISOM faculty, with a staff coordinator and six paid medical student directors. Four of these medical students are from MBPs, which allows for the opportunity to get to know the potential applicants better. All MBP Academy learners meet with faculty leaders of the MBP during the summer. Thus, the academy not only helps learners with their application to medical school, but it allows the MBP to get to know potential applicants better prior to the interview season. In 2023, 61 learners completed the MBP Academy.

Each MBP also has a series of recruitment events associated with local or national nonprofit educational organizations or universities throughout the year, and the MBPs contribute to general outreach efforts to prospective medical students. However, with all of these outreach activities,

overstretching and burnout are real concerns. The MBPs work with the BEE office to balance responsibilities and find the most efficient course for our learners and faculty.

When applicants to MBPs arrive on campus for their interviews, they receive special attention with student and faculty interviews by individuals associated with the programs. They have the opportunity to meet the MBP directors and have social time with students and faculty to ask questions and discover the sense of family within the MBPs. In addition, PRIME-LC requires a third student interview in Spanish to assess the applicant's ability with the language. All students entering PRIME-LC must have competent skills in Spanish.

Further, MBPs are featured on UCISOM's website, and we act on all opportunities to advocate for health equity among people of color. MBPs have frequently been featured in media stories about health training and equity.[6,7] PRIME-LC learners complete media training as part of their pre-first-year summer immersion program, which prepares them to share their stories and messages for the community.

In 2020 the COVID-19 pandemic was highly disruptive to our outreach efforts due to restrictions on in-person events. We compensated with more online contacts and actually forged several new partnerships using video-conferencing technology. This perseverance and our multimodal model were recognized in 2023 with a $3.6 million grant from the California Department of Health Care Access and Information to identify and prepare more college undergraduates with a mission of service for a career in medicine.

COMMUNITY BUILDING

Community building is central to sustaining MBPs. Interdisciplinary campus partnerships strengthen curriculum development and growth, enhance mentorship opportunities, and anchor MBPs in historic and current events. Critical partnerships between PRIME-LC and the UCI Department of Chicano/Latino Studies and PRIME-LEAD-ABC and the UCI Department of African American Studies establish a foundation for learner understanding about historic and recurrent events impacting the health of minoritized communities. Faculty allies from the UCI Schools of Public Health and Nursing further strengthen mentorship and guidance as learners strive to understand and address the structural determinants of health.

Community partnerships with regional health advocates, community physicians, nonprofit organizations, local minority-owned businesses, and faith-based institutions are also vital as they foster clinical and service-learning experiences for learners and enable opportunities for community-partnered outreach programs and scholarship. Such partnerships also enhance learners' awareness of patient and community narratives and foster cultural humility through learning about community members' real-life experiences. In an attempt to reduce barriers to equitable care, learners in our MBP, along with their faculty mentors, lead community-based initiatives that are able to blend neighborhood voices and research endeavors. Our learners frequently serve as liaisons between the medical world and the community.

In acknowledging the value of community building on and off campus, it is imperative that we emphasize the importance of mentorship on multiple levels. Mentorship, coaching, and sponsorship provide valuable support systems for MBP learners. Interdisciplinary faculty mentorship further strengthens the development of successful physician leaders by facilitating meaningful reflection as trainees grow in their professional identities as physician advocates and change agents and providing guidance in the creation and implementation of service programs and scholarly projects. Peer mentorship and coaching also build community in medical education by nurturing a culture of collaboration, communal growth, belonging, and well-being.[8–11]

Faculty sponsorship of learners, by nominating learners for curricular or service opportunities and facilitating networking through warm introductions, elevates the visibility of MBP-affiliated learner contributions to the medical school and surrounding community. Sponsorship and acknowledgment of students' accomplishments demonstrates value for learners and confirms institutional support for the MBPs' core mission and vision. In enabling learners who are underrepresented in medicine to be fully seen for their strengths and talents, MBPs establish spaces for belonging and professional growth where student potential is optimized.

In focusing on community building as a core component of MBPs, institutions can foster inclusive environments for underrepresented learners in medicine and learners broadly with similar areas of passion and expertise. MBPs can contribute to the successful recruitment, retention, and success of medical student leaders and scholars who are dedicated to enhancing their understanding of the driving socio-cultural and environmental forces maintaining health inequities and committed to working to find solutions to eradicate these connections. Thus, in supporting MBPs, academic institutions can adopt structural programs with great potential to optimize health outcomes for underresourced and minoritized communities at greatest risk of facing barriers in access to health care and health-related resources.

ADMINISTRATION AND FUNDING

The administration of an MBP requires an institutional commitment of resources. From a people perspective, it is important for the following roles to be established: program leadership, key personnel, and core faculty instructors and mentors.

Program directors should be leaders who are highly knowledgeable in the MBP area of focus. Ideally, these faculty have significant experience in curriculum and program development. Beyond curriculum design and implementation, core duties for MBP directors include recruitment and selection of MBP scholars, student counseling and mentorship, and community outreach. Institutions should allocate sufficient protected time for program directors to carry out their responsibilities. We recommend a minimum of 20% protected time with incremental increases based on program size.

Key personnel include a program coordinator who can provide administrative support to the program directors. We recommend a minimum of 50% time allocated for the coordinator to support the program. For larger programs, a full-time coordinator may be necessary. Expansion of student success services, such as academic advising, may be warranted based on learner utilization.

A dedicated core group of faculty is critical to the success of the MBPs. While serving as instructors, these faculty also serve as role models and mentors for learners. We recommend developing partnerships with faculty from across disciplines. For example, at UCISOM, we partner with faculty in the Chicano/Latino Studies and African American Studies departments. Protected time is provided to faculty who direct a core course or thread within the programs.

In addition to faculty and personnel support, other resource considerations include facilities needs, program activities, and scholarship support. Space requirements include offices for the program directors and coordinator and instructional facilities. Budgets should include support for program activities such as orientation, graduation, recruitment, outreach, field trips, mentorship functions, community service events, and travel to conferences. Finally, scholarship funding is critical to the success of the MBPs. Because a significant percentage of learners in MBPs come from economically disadvantaged backgrounds, limiting their debt burden contributes to the successful recruitment and retention of these learners. All learners in our PRIME-LC and PRIME-LEAD-ABC programs receive scholarships. Scholarship and program funding sources include state support, grants, tuition, clinical revenues, and philanthropic donations.

DIVERSIFYING THE PHYSICIAN WORKFORCE

The MBP model has demonstrated great success since its first implementation in 2004 through PRIME-LC. During this time, PRIME-LC has graduated 160 alumni. PRIME-LC has done well in the residency match, with the majority of learners matching into one of their top three programs. Approximately 70% have chosen a primary care discipline. Nearly 80% of PRIME-LC alumni who completed postgraduate training are practicing in California, and 95% report working in federally qualified health centers (FQHCs), FQHC look-alikes, or county health facilities. Nearly 70% see a majority of low-income Latino patients in their practice, and over 60% report other leadership roles in health equity outside of their clinical practice. Such work includes teaching and mentorship; community health education; and contributions to local or national programs for Latino health. PRIME-LC has invested in an alumni network to promote connections and opportunities for its ever-growing cohort of physician leaders, and connections with alumni are a great advantage for current PRIME-LC learners as well.

Similarly, the PRIME-LEAD-ABC program graduated its first medical student scholars in 2021 and has since grown to a full 4-year cohort of learners. While there were no Black medical students who graduated in the UCISOM Class of 2020, the incoming class that matriculated in August 2020 included 12% Black learners. This percentage has since been sustained for three consecutive years at a level that is more than two times that of Black physicians in the United States (5%), and six times the local population of Black residents (2%). The program currently has 46 diverse medical student scholars across all years with a common passion for addressing the health needs of ABC communities.

All PRIME-LEAD-ABC medical student scholars enter medical school with strong backgrounds in leadership, service, scholarship, and advocacy and continue to excel as medical student leaders. In 2023 PRIME-LEAD-ABC had 10 alumni training in postgraduate programs at top institutions of their choosing; 80% are in primary care fields that include family medicine, internal medicine, psychiatry, and emergency medicine, and 20% in surgical specialties—orthopedics and otolaryngology. Additionally, 50% of PRIME-LEAD-ABC alumni stayed in the state of California for residency training, and in comparison to the Black/African American population of Orange County (2.3%), each alum has chosen to do their training in areas with Black/African American populations ranging between 5% and 52%, representing cities across the United States from San Francisco to Washington, DC.

ENVISIONING THE FUTURE

The MBP model serves as an effective programmatic framework to establish pathway programs for physician leaders who aim to address racial and socio-economic inequities in health care. We envision the adoption of MBPs across medical schools as an opportunity to address a greater number of minoritized and marginalized patient populations. However, systemic barriers to implementation of an MBP are likely in academic medical centers where a lack of diversity persists. These barriers include finding faculty who are trained and experienced within the mission area, identifying the clinical sites where MBP rotations can occur, and allocating sufficient funding to support the infrastructure and administration of the MBP. Some of these barriers could be addressed by shifting local resources and priorities, while other barriers could be addressed by creating affiliations with partner institutions. The potential impact of an MBP beyond those involved in the program to the greater student body, institutional culture, and community is considerable and one which we suggest is worth the effort of adopting the MBP model.

The alumnus perspective below summarizes the transformational effects of MBP programs at the individual and system levels:

> "PRIME-LC became my home and family, where I received the support and training to achieve my dream to serve my community. With the skills and connections I developed—both as a medical student and in the PRIME-LC Family Medicine Residency Program—I've helped to develop the Health Scholars Program, a health professionals pipeline program mentoring more than 100 students in clinical and service-oriented projects in the highest-need areas of Orange County. I put my training to work every day and help support the next generation of PRIME-LC students forge their own paths."

> —*Marco Angulo, MD, MSS, PRIME-LC*
> *Class of 2011.*
> *Director of Education, AltaMed.*

SUMMARY

In this chapter, we shared the structure of the MBP model, successful outcomes from the current UCISOM programs, and valuable lessons learned. We offer this approach as an evidence-based intervention for improving the future diversity of the health workforce and, ultimately, equitable patient outcomes. In closing, we share this reflection by PRIME-LEAD-ABC Co-Director, Dr. Candice Taylor Lucas on the current and future impact of PRIME-LEAD-ABC scholars:

Seen

We see your promise
We see your strength
We see your wisdom as you travel great lengths
You are thoughtful
You are caring

You are treasured and often daring
We need your talent
We need your drive
We celebrate you as you strive
You are noticed
You are seen
You are the manifestation of Martin Luther King's dream

REFERENCES

1. AAMC. *AAMC Report Reinforces Mounting Physician Shortage.* 2021https://www.aamc.org/news/press-releases/new-aamc-report-confirms-growing-physician-shortage
2. Mahdavynia S, Larijani SS, Mirfakhraee H, et al. The impact of socially accountable health professional education: systematic review. *J Family Med Prim Care.* 2022;11(12):7543–7548. https://doi.org/10.4103/jfmpc.jfmpc_835_22.
3. Major C, Taylor Lucas C, Enendu K, Youm J, Worsham U, Le-Bucklin KV. Leadership Education to Advance Diversity-African, Black and Caribbean (LEAD-ABC): a mission-based model approach to addressing racial diversity and inclusive excellence in medicine. *Acad Med.* 2021;96(11S):S199–S200. https://doi.org/10.1097/ACM.0000000000004300.
4. UCI School of Medicine. *Mission-based Programs.* https://medschool.uci.edu/education/programs/medical-education/mission-based.
5. O'Brien-Gonzales A, Blavo C, Barley G, Steinkohl DC, Loeser H. What did we learn about early clinical experience? *Acad Med.* 2001;76(4 Suppl):S49–S54. https://doi.org/10.1097/00001888-200104001-00010.
6. Enendu K. *Because You Can Breathe, You Must Speak* https://students-residents.aamc.org/attending-medical-school/because-you-can-breathe-you-must-speak
7. UCI. *UCI Podcast: The Promise and Success of PRIME-LC.* 2022https://news.uci.edu/2022/09/16/uci-podcast-the-success-of-prime-lc/
8. Afghani B, Santos R, Angulo M, Muratori W. A novel enrichment program using cascading mentorship to increase diversity in the health care professions. *Acad Med.* 2013;88(9):1232–1238. https://doi.org/10.1097/ACM.0b013e31829ed47e.
9. Yemane L, Kas-Osoka O, Burns A, Blankenburg R, Prakash LK, Poitevien P, et al. Upholding Our PROMISE: underrepresented in medicine pediatric residents' perspectives on interventions to promote belonging. *Acad Med.* 2023;98:1434–1442. https://doi.org/10.1097/ACM.0000000000005443.
10. Roberts LW. Belonging, respectful inclusion, and diversity in medical education. *Acad Med.* 2020;95(5):661–664. https://doi.org/10.1097/ACM.0000000000003215.
11. Lane-McKinley K, Turner-Essel L. How to Cultivate a Culture of Belonging in Academic Medicine. In: Roberts L, eds. *Roberts Academic Medicine Handbook.* Springer; 2020. https://doi.org/10.1007/978-3-030-31957-1

12

Re-imagining Clinical Interviewing

Bridging the Gap Between Theory and Practice for Equitable Care

Nataliya Pilipenko and Nancy M. Chang

SUMMARY

Although many students enter medical training with strong medical knowledge, humanistic values, and antiracist attitudes, the clinical practice of medicine does not consistently deliver patient care aligned with these values. While communication skills are recognized as a central medical competency, current training is missing clear, unified, and operationally defined components. This results in persistent gaps converting theory and curriculum to real-world patient care. While current antiracist work is an important step forward, practical guidance for its implementation in patient care is needed. Additionally, current clinical interviewing efforts leave learners with limited practical preparation to confront the complex multidimensional demands of modern clinical practice. In this chapter, we review existing approaches to communication training and provide guidance to advance a more equitable, collaborative, and patient-centered approach. We address the following communication tasks: informed consent, tasks for the start of the visit, agenda setting, interviewing techniques, electronic health record integration/documentation, working with interpreters, working with companions, culturally informed interviewing, and steps for completing the interview. Each task includes specific skills, the rationale behind these skills, and illustrations.

INTRODUCTION: UNDERSTANDING THE CARE GAP

Despite disproportionately high spending on health care, the US lags behind other high-income countries in advancing health equity.[1] Structural racism and inequities are embedded within health and education systems propagated by policies, guidelines, curricula, and technology. In this context, physicians often struggle to operate from a collaborative, antiracist, and antioppressive position of cultural and structural humility. As the chasm between physicians' humanistic values and patients' experiences of care widens, educators must address communication training. This chapter reviews existing approaches and provides guidance to advance toward a more equitable, collaborative, and **patient-centered clinical interview**.

PROFESSIONALIZATION AND POWER DIFFERENTIALS IN HEALTH CARE

All learners undergo a process of **professionalization**. Medical students and residents are socialized to the culture of medicine which is an "integrated pattern of learned beliefs and behaviors … styles of communicating, ways of interacting, views on roles and relationships."[2] Self-awareness of **professionalization** (i.e., acculturation into medicine) and personal background factors are central to understanding the differences between physicians' and patients' views and experiences of medical care and illness.

Professionalization and power are intrinsically linked. Specifically, power operates via mechanisms such as wealth, whiteness, citizenship, patriarchy, heterosexism, and others. Within a caregiving relationship, an asymmetry of power is held and potentially exacerbated by a myriad of (perceived) differences between the patient and the physician. While growing efforts focus on expanding diverse representation in health care, medical learners are entering training with knowledge and attitudes grounded in the ideals of equity, inclusion, and humanism. However,

gaps in patient communication remain pervasive and compromised by biases[3,4] as physicians continue to struggle in identifying and addressing contextual factors (e.g., finances, access, social support, abilities).[5] Thus individualized care delivery is not purely knowledge or values driven.

THE CURRENT STATE OF CLINICAL INTERVIEWING TRAINING

Communication skills have been long recognized as a central competency in medical education and clinical practice.[6,7] However, integration and application of these skills within clinical care remains an ongoing challenge.[8] While several models of communication, including the Calgary-Cambridge guide[7,8] and Smith Model[9] were proposed and some positive contributions noted,[10,11] due to complexity and the need for further operationalization, extensive uptake and systemic implementation of these models remain limited.

Additionally, real-world medical training must incorporate structured in vivo observation, feedback, and assessment of patient care encounters. While important work incorporating patients' perspectives into learner feedback is in the literature, implementing these best practices[12,13] requires further integration. There remains a lack of clearly defined standards for goals of care, learner conduct, and approaches to clinical interviewing that effectively integrate both patient and faculty perspectives.

Following the discontinuation of the United States Medical Licensing Examination (USMLE) Step 2 Clinical Skill Exam in 2020,[14] no certifying platform for independent assessment of performance-based communication skills of graduating US medical students exists. Despite efforts to enhance workplace-based patient communication assessments, the uptake has been limited. The standards as well as faculty training have also not been well defined.[15] In addition, simulation training using standardized patient encounters, fails to capture the complexity, nuance, and high stakes of clinical care. Thus, the current training system lacks overarching, operationally defined guidelines against which performance is assessed while specific assessments may lack rigor and ecological validity.

Overall, the existing state of medical education requires re-imagining. Gaps in the literature and a dearth of implementation research limit the field's ability to advance clinical interviewing training. Moreover, embedding antiracism and equity into clinical interviewing is challenging without practical and evidence-informed guidance. Medical educators and institutions must appraise and address educational gaps between simulation and real-world patient care delivery.

CURRENT TRAINING IN EQUITABLE/ANTIRACIST CLINICAL CARE

Both stereotyping and racial bias negatively impact communication across all patient groups, with a disproportionately negative impact noted for Black patients.[3] Johnson and colleagues[16] note that lack of engagement and participation from health professionals, rather than time spent with the patient, explains such inequities. In addition, ableism, sexism, and other forms of discrimination and stereotyping remain common, although their impact is often overlooked. Overall, poor communication is common and affects every patient, however, minoritized and marginalized patients are disproportionately affected.

Current medical education paradigms and training efforts[17] focus on raising awareness about system-level issues as well as various forms of bias, privilege, diversity, equity, inclusion, and racism. These efforts are supported by systematic reviews[18] indicating that bias against racially minoritized patients is common and significantly impacts communication and outcomes. Existing training tends to offer education focused on awareness raising and addressing systemic issues.[17,19-22] Such training is vital to paving the way toward equitable care. However, this work is often limited to awareness raising and lacks a focus on skill development. Also, such curricula are implemented mostly in the preclinical curriculum with fewer opportunities for real-world patient interactions.[17,19,23] While these efforts address insight enhancement and group processes, research is needed to assess translation and sustainability of these trainings in clinical practice.

WHERE DO WE GO FROM HERE?

Learners entering clinical settings without a cohesive and clear framework for equitable and **patient-centered clinical interviewing** are prone to self-created communication pitfalls. For example, failing to effectively elicit a patient's goals for the visit and then becoming frustrated when a patient continues to bring up concerns throughout the visit. Thus, to promote equitable care, all learners must develop strong clinical interviewing foundations. However, it is not sufficient to tell learners to practice antiracist, equitable, patient-centered care. We must clearly define how this is to be done by articulating specific interviewing behaviors.

BRIDGING ACROSS THE COMMUNICATION GAP

Patient-physician communication affects both care satisfaction and medical regimen adherence, synergistically leading to improved health outcomes for historically disadvantaged populations.[24] Overall, patient-centered care requires integration of two interconnected processes: provision of medical care and **socialization** of patients to the care delivery. In this context, **socialization** is the orientation to the visit's parameters as well as physicians' professional responsibilities and constraints. **Socialization** thus buttresses shared understanding of the visit supporting transparent and egalitarian relationships. Physicians who establish illness management care goals must achieve and maintain bilateral understanding between themselves and patients. Unilateral understanding is not enough—understanding must be effectively communicated by the physician back to the patient. Additionally, the physician must balance and align expectations to protect both patient and physician from frustration, burnout, and mutual distrust.

When working with patients who experience complex psychosocial circumstances, steeped in a history of racism, prejudice, and system mistrust, physicians are at risk of becoming overwhelmed by areas outside of their expertise. As physicians report limited preparation in addressing psychosocial concerns,[25] issues of interprofessional work require integration within medical training. Currently, interprofessional education (IPE) is largely in preclinical settings and focuses on physicians' roles, with over 90% of IPE collaboration forged with nursing training programs.[26] However, advancing IPE requires identification of interprofessional competencies and common language, addressing interprofessional stereotyping through intergroup contact, building students' inclusive social identities, and fostering pro-diversity beliefs.[27]

Although medical students report interest and openness to interprofessional work training,[28] mounting evidence indicates overarching challenges for interprofessional integration/collaboration work in clinical settings. Specific challenges include physicians "lack of time and training, poor role definition, professional identity concerns, and poor communication with interdisciplinary team members are systemically noted."[29] Van Duin and colleagues[30] encapsulate challenges as follows: "junior doctors struggle to bridge the gap between themselves and the interprofessional team, preventing … integrative process." Therefore, skills in effective and collegial work with IPEs must become fundamental to training. If overlooked, lack of IPE bridging will most adversely affect patients with interlocking, minoritized identities, who already navigate multiple stressors and confront barriers to health care access.

MAPPING CLINICAL ENCOUNTERS

A detailed overview of the clinical components and techniques relevant to starting, navigating, and wrapping up communication within a clinical visit is summarized in the next few sections of this chapter. While these domains may be familiar from other sources, we aim to integrate and highlight these as vehicles toward collaborative and antioppressive clinical care. In re-imagining medical education, we must consider the currently overlooked and poorly integrated armamentarium of clinical interviewing skills and build learners' understanding of underlying principles as well as self-efficacy utilizing these techniques. Each step of a clinical interview is an opportunity to integrate both existing best practices and a more collaborative and antioppressive approach with different steps complimenting each other.

Step One: Informed Consent

The process of **informed consent** is an ethical and legal obligation central to equitable and high-quality care delivery. **Informed consent** is a key opportunity to socialize the patient to the encounter while promoting trust, clarity of goals, and building rapport for the remainder of the visit. Patients should be explicitly informed about the process/procedure, goals, outcomes, and anticipated follow-up. At the initial visit, lack of established connection and possible history of suboptimal experiences should be acknowledged, while patients' questions and feedback are explicitly sought.

Example: "Today is our first visit, and we do not yet know each other, which can be stressful. I am here to make sure things go as well as possible for you so that your goals for this visit are met. I am also here to answer any questions that you might have."

Informed consent is critical when serving patients who may have experienced mistrust due to their past care experiences, those who experience challenges navigating the intricacies of the health care labyrinth. The following vignette illustrates a scenario when consent is overlooked.

Vignette 1*

Mary is a medical student working under the guidance of a faculty physician who asks her to complete an interview with Mrs. A who is a 74-year-old, monolingual French Creole-speaking female. When Mary enters the exam room, she sees a patient sitting next to a woman. The following conversation ensues:

Mary: Hi! I'm Mary, a medical student. I'll ask you some questions before you see the doctor. Is this your daughter? Will she translate for you?

Patient: [Looks confused but nods and smiles.]

Mary: Ok! Let's get going! I have a lot of questions for you today. The doctor tells me you are having some memory problems, right?

Patient's companion [To Mary]: I'm her neighbor, but I can help. She spends a lot of time at my home. She asked me to drive her here today. I need to go to work, but I can stay a little to help.

Patient [to companion]: Is she asking you to stay?

Companion [to patient]: Don't worry, I can help you.

Mary: Ok! Let's get started.

Mary proceeds with the visit, asking multiple questions about personal and medical history (including sexual history) which the companion translates partially since she is confused about some terms which Mary uses, but she is embarrassed to ask for clarifications. The companion often tries to help by interjecting her knowledge and opinions of Mrs. A's functioning. Mary also completes cognitive screening. She completes the interview by saying:

Mary: Thank you! It was nice to meet you. I'll go and talk to the doctor, and we will let you know the plan for you when we come back.

In Vignette 1, opportunities for adequate socialization and the informed consent process are missed. Mary fails to realize and address that the patient's lack of comprehension prevents her from understanding and therefore consenting to the care plan or questioning it. Mary does not elicit the patient's concerns, and the patient is provided with no information about the visit, leading to potential embarrassment when deeply personal questions are asked in front of the neighbor. This vignette illustrates how power asymmetry in health care can play out. Mary (being in a position of more power) does not seem aware of potential gaps in communication, while the patient is unable to self-advocate from a potentially vulnerable position. This is compounded by the patient's language needs.

Step Two: Starting the Visit

Implicit bias is more likely to be activated under stressful work conditions.[18] Therefore, following a set of standard guidelines at the beginning of the visit paves the way to improved care delivery via increased participation in care, enhanced rapport, and decreased risk of preventable errors. Essential tasks, as outlined here, are discrete components of clinical interviewing that help mitigate bias.

Essential Tasks

Self-identify by name, role, and any supervisory relationship(s).

Example: "Hello, I am Mary, a medical student working with Dr. Jade today. I was hoping to speak with you and gather information for Dr. Jade before she meets with you today. Do you have any concerns about me being a part of your team today?"

Identify the patient by full name and date of birth.

Example: "Can you please confirm your full name and your date of birth, for me?'"

Preferred name and pronouns should be established.

Example(s): "Do you prefer to be called Maria, Mrs. A, or by another name? How do you prefer to be called? What is/are your preferred pronouns/do you have a preferred pronoun: do you prefer he, she, they, or another pronoun?"

Acknowledge delays: **If care has been delayed**, explicitly acknowledge, and apologize for the wait. This demonstrates respect for the patient and acknowledges discomfort, supporting rapport building.

Example: "I am very sorry to keep you waiting."

When using telehealth:

1. Ensure that the patient is in the state/territory where care can be medico-legally delivered.
2. The patient is in a private setting.
3. Companions are appraised.

Example: "Which state are you located in as we speak? Do you have privacy for this visit? Is there anyone else in the room? Can you introduce us?"

Ensure comfort: Explicitly addressing patient comfort both helps to build collaboration and trust and may mitigate reminders connected to a history of trauma or suboptimal care. Consider asking: "Is there anything that you need before we get started today?" Please see *Working with Companions* and *Working with Interpreters* sections for further specifics.

Steps 1 and 2 outline central considerations for establishing trust and transparency necessary for patient-centered communication when working with any patient group. Given the absence of training focused on these domains, however, medical learners often lack cognitive schemas and practical skills in performing these tasks in a time-efficient manner. Most affected by this gap in training are historically minoritized patients who may struggle to self-advocate in situations when these foundational tasks are missed.

Step Three: Collaborative Agenda Setting

Agenda setting serves as a critical roadmap for clinical visits. It is at the heart of patient-centered, antiracist inquiry as patient and physician engage in collaborative discussion aimed at understanding the patient's goals as well as physician's needs. Despite the importance of agenda setting, this crucial step is seldom completed adequately,[31] leading to unmet expectations and dissatisfaction. The following six tasks integrate published research[32-34] and outline the key components for agenda setting. While these may appear prescriptive, each task is central to establishing clarity about expectations and ensuring a clear visit plan is established.

Agenda Setting in Six Specific Tasks

Task 1: Introduce patient to collaborative **agenda setting**

Why? This step is central to **informed consent** and helps to avoid confusion as it clearly states the physician's request of creating a "problem list" before engaging in prioritization and exploration.

Example: "I was hoping we can start our visit by setting a plan for ourselves. Can we start by naming all the problems or concerns that you have about your health before we proceed?"

Task 2: Elicit or confirm initial concern

Why? It is important to avoid overly vague/nonspecific inquiry (e.g., "How is it going?" "What brings you here?") and focus on the patient's goals, concerns, or expectations.

Example: "How were you hoping I could help you today?" "I understand you are coming in to follow up on your diabetes management, is this correct?"

When receiving a nonspecific response (e.g., "I had a follow-up appointment" or "They told me to come in"), further **clarifications** are needed: "What do we need to take care of today to best help you?" or "What was the plan from the last visit?" These questions demonstrate forthcoming intention to understand the patient's complex situation, while maintaining active focus on goals of care from the patient's perspective.

Task 3: Elicit additional concerns

Why? Due to prior negative experiences with health care, anxiety, or other factors, patients may not initially bring up their most important concern. Therefore it is important to elicit concerns fully and to proactively seek feedback to ensure that all questions and issues are known and addressed.

Example: "Anything else that we should talk about? Any other concerns we should address today?"

Task 4: State own agenda

Why? Outlining one's own agenda is central to a physician's ability to deliver health care in line with practice standards. It is important to avoid vague and nonspecific statements such as "health care maintenance," "standard care," or "follow up on labs" as patients cannot consent to these due to lack of understanding. If the patient's and physician's agendas are aligned, this should be explicitly noted to promote collaborative care and establish trust.

Example: "I was hoping to discuss your blood sugar results, vaccine for COVID, and follow up on the referral to ophthalmology from our last visit."

Task 5: Summarize agenda items and set a collaborative agenda

Why? List all agenda items brought up and explicitly ask which item is most important for the patient to address during the visit. This step allows the patient to clarify agreement and openly express preferences as it controls for the provider's biases and enforcement of physician-centered agendas.

Example: "You are hoping to talk about your back pain and the work leave paperwork. I am hoping to talk about vaccines for COVID and flu. Which problem do you think is the most important to address today? Where would you like to begin?"

Task 6: Inform patient about time limits

Why? To act as a partner in the visit, the patient needs to understand the visit's parameters. Any problem can be described in a lengthy or succinct way. Knowledge of time available is central to the amount of elaboration to be provided. Being transparent about such limits can also foster trust.

Example: "We have about 30 minutes today and I will need to step away to talk to my supervisor, which will take about 10 minutes. We might not get through all the issues, but I will document them in my note, and we can prioritize these for the next visit, which we can set up today."

Agenda setting in medical care remains largely overlooked and poorly performed.[31] This section presents an overarching framework for agenda setting and specific steps—currently missing in medical education and at the bedside. The following section outlines key interviewing techniques that are necessary to master for implementation of agenda setting as well as other patient-centered communication tasks outlined in this chapter.

Step Four: Interviewing Techniques

Given the complexity of intersectional minoritized identities, extensive medical visit agendas, and time constraints, having a strong repertoire of interviewing techniques is necessary. Moreover, physicians must understand the goal and purpose of these techniques which current training fails to clearly outline and integrate. This section presents key techniques, the rationale behind each technique's use, and practice recommendations. Vignette 2 illustrates these techniques within a patient care interview example.

Open-ended questions: Allow for data collection in an elaborated, open format. However, not all open-ended questions are equally effective. For example, both "How is it going?" and "How are you hoping I can help you today?" are open-ended questions. The first question gives no clarity about the interviewer's intention and can result in a nonspecific answer leading to inefficient use of time and bidirectional frustrations. The second question inquires about specific goals thus bridging understanding between the patient's goals and the physician's understanding of these goals. Overall, an interview based on open-ended questions requires the patient to understand and match the physician's conceptualization and priorities, that is, understand goals behind the question rather than provide a literal answer. When working with diverse patients, open-ended questions need to be mindfully constructed by the physician to identify the central component of the inquiry. Moreover, open-ended questions must be supported by other active interviewing techniques including reflections, summaries, and redirection to maintain bilateral understanding and goal-directedness within the interview.

Clinical Practice Recommendation: Challenge yourself to formulate open-ended questions clearly and intentionally.

Interruptions/Redirection

A frequently cited study[35] reported that on average physicians redirected patients' opening statement after 23.1 seconds, and if not interrupted, patients would continue speaking for only 6 seconds more (on average). Despite the methodological limitations of this work and recent divergent findings,[36] results are frequently used to portray interruptions as purely negative and to be avoided. Guidance in situations when a patient provides an extended narrative which the physician struggles to understand is lacking, and it is impossible to pace an interview or achieve goals of the visit without tactful interruptions.[37] If an interruption is made, it is important to state the intention behind the interruption and emphasize the goal of understanding the patient clearly to be most effective. Examples:
- "Let me make sure that I understand…"
- "Can I interrupt you for a moment? I want to make sure that I understand what you are saying."
- "Can I ask you a question about …?"

Following an interruption with a summary and a clarification can maintain the momentum of the interview without negatively impacting the rapport. Furthermore, acknowledging time limits of the visit for obtaining a full historical picture of the presenting problem may be helpful.

Example: "You have been dealing with [concern] for a long time, and there are many important details to your story. Since our time is limited today, I am hoping to ask a few clarifying questions to make sure that I am not missing any dangerous symptoms."

Clinical Practice Recommendation: Interruptions can be minimized via the use of active interviewing techniques (reflections, summaries, empathy statements) such as active engagement in dialogue, communicating an understanding of what the physician comprehends, and being transparent and sensitive about interruptions when they occur.

Reflections

Reflections, repeating or mirroring back information stated by the patient, are brief (one or few words) and ensure that the interviewer both correctly understands (hears) and communicates this understanding back to the patient. Reflections are particularly critical when utilizing interpreter services.

Summaries

Summaries, repetition of the narrative stated by the patient, are selective (i.e., focus on the key components of the storyline) and aim to achieve shared understanding of the events, antecedents, maintaining factors, etc. Summaries are critical to establishing a shared understanding of the problem. Additionally, **summaries** are effective turning points for the interview—summarizing the statement of the presenting concern allows us to agree on its specifics, fill in any gaps in the storyline, correct misunderstandings, and ask for corrections.

Continuers

Continuers, verbal or nonverbal communications of the physician encouraging patients to keep speaking,[33] can include nodding and statements such as "ok," or "I see." Utilization of **continuers** is central to maintaining patient's disclosure; however, a physician who wishes to clarify, redirect, and refocus is unlikely to achieve these tasks by relying on **continuers**—continuer utilization would be analogous to pressing gas in a car when wishing to stop or turn. **Reflections**, **summaries**, and **empathy** statements need to be utilized for this purpose.

Affirmations

Affirmations, statements that explicitly recognize a patient's efforts to address the problem, utilize "you" rather than "I," focus on specific behaviors, and are not compliments.

Example: "You are determined to improve your diabetes control and take multiple steps to do so—you set reminders to take medications daily and track calories." Follow up with "What do you see as the next steps?" or "How can I help you?" to engage patients as partners in care and proactively plan treatment.

While statements such as: "Congratulations on quitting smoking! I am so proud of you," are common and aim to support the patient, these demonstrate physician's appraisal and value judgment of the patient's behaviors.

Empathy Statements

The term **empathy** is often misused as a synonym for "being nice" or confused with sympathy. At its core, **empathy** means "feeling with rather than feeling for."[38] Communication of **empathy** is critical to antiracist, patient-centered communication. While physicians may not share a patient's experiences, feelings of sadness, grief, and anger are universally understood. Naming a patient's emotions promotes deeper understanding and fosters trust.

Literature in psychotherapy, including trauma-specific therapies, highlights the importance of recognizing, naming, and processing emotions as key steps in symptom management. It is important to note that an **empathy** statement explicitly names the emotion which the physician recognizes and allows for the patient to correct any misunderstanding.

The following examples illustrate statements that are not **empathetic**:

"I am so sorry!" and "This is great! I am proud of you!" Both statements focus on the speaker's appraisal and emotions, not the patient's emotional reaction.

"It sounds like you have been through a lot/like a challenging experience." Both statements validate experience and communicate alignment however emotion is not explicitly named.

Empathy statements can include: "You are anxious about your upcoming appointment," "I understand that you are worried about the test results," and "I can see that you were angry about not getting a timely response to your question."

Clarifications

An extensive body of literature highlights differences between patients' and physicians' use of medical terminology, emphasizing the need to address these discrepancies to promote patient-centered decision-making. Differences in terminology drive illness-related behaviors among minoritized patients.[39,40] It is therefore critical to elicit the patient's illness understanding and beliefs, before providing education.

Example: "You mentioned suffering from hypertension. Can you tell me how you understand this illness? How does it affect your body? What do you do to control symptoms?"

Example: "Your child was prescribed daily antisteroid medication for asthma. Sometimes parents are concerned about these daily medications. What is your understanding of why the medication was prescribed to be taken every day?"

Vignette 2*

Physician: I am hoping we can start by setting up a plan for our visit today. We have about 20 minutes. Can we start by first naming the issues that we are both concerned about? [*socialization to agenda setting, open-ended question*]

Patient: Yes, there is that back pain which I was telling you about. Still bothering me although I have been going to physical therapy.

Physician: So back pain [*reflection*] is on our agenda for today. What other concerns do you have? [*open-ended question*]

Patient: Meds. Let's look at the meds. They also called me about that sleep apnea machine and were telling me that I am not covered for it. I told them that I was!

Physician: I am hearing medication review and sleep apnea machine [*reflection*], correct?

Patient: Yes! And a rash. It's on my back and I have been putting Aveeno on it. Last time it happened it helped but now it's not going away. I thought maybe a steroid cream or maybe something homeopathic.

Physician: Sorry to cut you off! [*interruption*] Sounds like you are worried [*empathy*] about the rash, not sure why Aveeno is not helping [*reflection*]. I am putting rash on our list but just want to make sure we have our agenda. Is this ok? [*socialization*]

Patient: Sure! I get it. It's a lot!

Physician: It sounds like you are taking many steps to address your concerns—going to appointments with physical therapy, staying on top of meds, tackling the rash [*affirmation*].

Patient: I am doing my best.

Physician: I was hoping we can talk about your referral to a smoking cessation specialist. Would that be, ok? [*physician's agenda is stated*]

Patient: Yes, that's ok.

Physician: Here is our agenda as I understand: back pain, medications review, sleep apnea machine, rash, smoking cessation referral [*summary*]. Is there anything else?

Patient: No! That's plenty!

Physician: Sounds good! If we do not have time to get through all these concerns today, which one should we tackle first? Which one is most important? [*prioritizing agenda collaboratively*]

Patient: Sleep apnea machine. Back pain is not getting better if I cannot sleep.

In summary, active and mindful utilization of interviewing skills lays the foundation for patient-centered interviewing. Setting standards for teaching and utilization of these techniques are currently absent, contributing to a lack of clear assessment parameters and learner support.

Step Five: Electronic Health Record Integration

The EHR is a tool for care delivery, communication, and protection of both patients and physicians. Unfortunately, to date, EHR integration techniques are largely overlooked in training. Such skill deficits may adversely impact the care of all patients, as physicians are unable to balance patient-centeredness with documentation requirements. Implementation of the 21st Century Cures Act and the Health Insurance Portability and Accountability Act (HIPAA) Access Right[41] results in improved access. However, whether increased transparency will translate into improved care and care experiences for all patients remains to be seen and will likely be contingent on providers' overall ability to communicate in patient-centered and effective ways.

In addition to the EHR integration challenges, concerns of stigmatizing, biased, and stereotype-driven language are important to address as poor visit documentation can compromise an established therapeutic alliance.[42] More specifically, clinical notes that convey doubt lead to misunderstanding and inappropriate decision-making,[42] with up to 10% of patients reported being surprised or offended by what they see in clinical documentation.[43] Also, studies observe more skepticism and negative description included in the records of certain patient groups.[44,45] With wider implementation and growing tolerance of "copy and pasting" of physicians' own and borrowed content within the medical record[46] there is a potential risk of rapid propagation of misunderstanding and stereotyping within medical records.

Although a comprehensive discussion of documentation practices is outside the scope of this chapter, ongoing training and increased awareness aimed at eliminating language which confers judgment or perpetuates stereotyping (e.g., noncompliant) is an important part of a physician's lifelong learning.[44,45] Physicians at all levels of training need to work toward improved familiarity with guidelines advising on best practices for inclusive and antiracist language.[47]

Integrating the EHR into the clinical interview is central to efficiency and should be incorporated into medical students' training to support transition between simulated and real-world patient interactions. The following steps are based on work of Duke and colleagues.[48]

EHR introduction: in line with **informed consent** principles, patients must be offered a brief introduction to the EHR at the start of the visit—providing key information and framing the EHR as a tool to patient-centered care. Given the extensive history of adverse experiences within medicine, for multiple patient groups, clarity and transparency are key to fostering trust.

Triadic relationship: facilitate shared engagement with the EHR by positioning the screen within view of both patient and physician, forming a triangle where patient, physician, and EHR are positioned in the corners. This setup facilitates eye contact and engagement.

Signposting: is an explicit statement informing patients about a physician's actions in the EHR such as accessing data, lab results, and tests. **Signposting** acts as a conduit to the shared understanding of the visit processes.

Reading back: **reading back** while typing accomplishes the goals of summarizing while allowing patients to make corrections to data entered into the record and manage power differentials. **Reading back** allows physicians to focus on the narrative of the patient's experience without becoming overwhelmed by concurrent tasks of listening and typing.

EHR Integration Example

Physician: Before we get started, please give me one second to log into your medical record.

Patient: [nods] Ok.

Physician: To make sure I provide you with the best care and do not forget anything, I will type as we speak, and my note will become a part of your chart. Once the visit is over, you will have a copy of the note in your patient portal. If you have any questions about the note, I will be happy to talk to you about it.

Patient: So, our meeting today is going to be in my record?

Physician: Yes! In fact, I am going to share the screen with you so that you can see exactly what I am typing [*turns screen to allow for a* **triadic relationship**]. Can you see the screen?

Patient: Yes, I can see it now.

Physician: As we speak, we can also look at some important information like your test results and list of medications.

Patient: Yes, I was hoping you can explain the MRI scan again. They called me and talked about it, but I didn't understand exactly what I need to do now.

Physician: Absolutely! I am going to make a note right now about this. Will put it on our agenda.

[*types and reads back*—Review MRI results and next steps]. What questions or concerns do you have about the EHR?

Patient: I think it makes sense. I'll ask you if something concerns me.

Patient and physician proceed with **agenda setting**. The physician types the agenda items while **reading back** each item to the patient. Patient identifies MRI results review as top priority for the visit.

Physician: Sounds good. Let's begin with the MRI result review. It sounds like you are quite worried about these. Let me open the MRI report [*signposting*] and I will summarize what I am seeing.

Step Six: Working With Interpreters

Growing numbers of US residents report limited English proficiency[49] with almost two-thirds of Spanish-speaking immigrants self-identifying English literacy as "below basic."[50] Providing interpreter services in medical settings is regulated under federal law, with provisions outlined in the 2003 Department of Health and Human Services guidance.[41] Although competence in working with interpreter services is central to the modern-day equitable practice of medicine, this communication competency is largely overlooked in physicians' training, contributing to challenges in learner transitions into clinical settings.

Working With Interpreters: Common Errors

Not engaging in appropriate consent procedures for medical interpreter use: In line with **informed consent** principles, to decline medical interpreter services, patients need to understand scope (confidential service), goals (provision of full translation), risks (possible discomfort), and benefits (ability to provide information, including sensitive information). Patients must consent or decline interpreter use while

the interpreter is already present to allow for an appropriate consent process. Vignette 1 illustrates failure to recognize the core of the consent process.

Provider "getting by" on limited proficiency: This practice illustrates both disregard toward a commitment to best practices but also may exacerbate power asymmetries in care. Among other documented examples of the potential catastrophic consequences of such practice is the work of Price-Wise[51] which describes the case of 18-year-old Willie Ramirez. In this account, "mistranslation, medical malpractice, and prejudice" significantly contributed to misunderstanding of the patient's presentation, resulted in delay in appropriate medical procedures, and culminated in the patient's lifelong disability. Medical education should appraise learners to narratives of patients affected by poor practice to raise awareness of power dynamics and its implications.

Utilizing unqualified individuals as interpreters: Using unqualified persons to act as interpreters results in errors of omission and commission. While a patient may be comfortable arriving to the visit with a companion, this comfort is unlikely to extrapolate to discussion of sexual health, physical functioning, and emotional health issues which are routinely discussed in medical care. Physicians should not assume that patients anticipate such inquiry.

Asking an interpreter to function outside of capacity. Examples include requests to confirm the physician's grammar or confirming "that the patient understood." While interpreters may step outside of their role on occasions when misunderstanding due to cultural differences occurs, this is an exception for situations whereby medical error appears likely. Interpreters function in a narrowly defined role that offers protection to both patient and physician and carries a specific set of responsibilities. An interpreter is not there to coach a physician, nor should they be asked to play a role in the visit's dynamics.

Several excellent guidelines and publications are available to support physicians in improving competence when working with interpreter services.[52] The following communication strategies can provide overarching support for patients and physicians.

Providing instructions and information to the interpreter. Visits should begin with a physician's self-identification with name and other relevant information. Names should be spelled out to avoid inaccurate pronunciation. Additionally, the following may be requested. Example: "Please translate everything that I say to the patient and everything that the patient says to me. Please translate in short segments as I will be documenting during the visit."

***Socializing** patients to the process of care delivery via interpreter service.* While interpreters will inform patients about confidentiality and privacy, it may be helpful to

socialize patients to the use of interpreter services. Example: "We are working with an interpreter today, so I will speak in short phrases to help with translation. I want to ask you to do the same, pause after one to two statements so that the interpreter can translate everything. This will help me understand you and not miss anything."

Step Seven: Working With Companions

The impact of a companion's attendance on medical visit outcomes is a complicated area of inquiry given the diversity of settings, patient populations, and patient companion relationships (which may or may not be familial). Wolf and Rotter[53] note that "despite a broad appreciation that families matter, specific knowledge regarding which actions and behaviors undertaken by family members are most helpful, or efficacious in improving health, is limited." Overall, findings on the impact of a companion's presence are equivocal, however some note improvement in patient-centered communication for accompanied Black patients.[54] Overall, there needs to be further investigation concerning whether companions' presence affects health care outcome versus a visit's satisfaction. That stated, it is also important to build alliances with families and seek guidance from patients on their preferences related to family/caregiver involvement.

Based on a systematic review, Laidsaar-Powell and colleagues[55] propose the following preliminary strategies for working with companions: (1) companions should be encouraged and involved; (2) helpful companion behaviors should be acknowledged; and (3) role preferences of patient/companions should be agreed upon and clarified. At this point, the medical education system does not prepare learners for addressing the complexity of accompanied visits, thus learners entering clinical care may be oblivious to important practices and potential concerns.

The following scenario illustrates integration of patient companions. Ms. Johnson is a 35-year-old Black/African American female presenting for a second-trimester prenatal care visit with an adult male companion and a young child. As the physician enters the room, the patient is sitting on the exam table located behind the physician's chair, the companion is sitting on the chair facing the EHR screen and the child is walking around the room.

Identification of Patient and Companion(s)

Upon entering the room, companions must be acknowledged and greeted. Relationships between the patient and their companions must be assessed and documented and never assumed. Consider directly asking about the plan for the companion's involvement in the visit.

Example:

Physician: Hello Mrs. Johnson! It's nice to see you today. I see you have company today. Please introduce us!

Patient: [pointing at the child] This is my niece, Grace. I had to bring her with me because her mother, my sister, is working.

Physician: [looking at the child] Hello, Grace! It's nice to meet you!

Patient: This [pointing at the adult companion] is my partner, Troy.

Physician: It's nice to meet you, Troy. I am Dr. First.

Companion: It's nice to meet you, doctor.

Physician: It's great that you are coming in together today. Are we anticipating that Troy will be able to stay for the whole visit?

Patient: Yes, I think it's important that he is involved.

Physician: I agree. Troy, to make sure I have my documentation in order, can I get your full name for the records? How do you prefer to be called?

Capacity Considerations and Focus on the Patient

Medico-legal considerations dictate that adult patients with capacity for decision-making are primary actors in said decision-making. Tactfully focusing on the patient while acknowledging roles and importance of companions is central. This is particularly important when working with older adults with limited English proficiency who may be at increased risk of being infantilized. Examples may include the following companion statement: "I understand that you are concerned about your [parent's] care but in order to help you both best, I need to ask them direct questions and hear their own answers. This will help us best understand [parent's] needs and experiences."

Example [continued]:

Physician: Mrs. Johnson, before we begin, can I ask you and Troy to change places? I want to make sure that you and I can both see the screen as I document.

Patient: Oh! Right! Let's look at those labs. [Changes position to allow for **triadic relationship** with EHR.]

Physician: Just to ensure that we are on the same page–it is best practice that today we follow up on last visit's labs and test results, talk about red flags during pregnancy, and do a physical exam. Troy, I am hoping to start by asking Mrs. Johnson some questions. I also want to address any concerns that you may have and hear your opinion about anything we might have missed before we finish today. How does this sound?

Importance of Privacy

Over 10 million people residing in the US are affected by family or partner violence with women, particularly pregnant women, being disproportionately victimized.[56] Furthermore, the US Department of Justice reports that at least 10% of adults over the age of 65 will experience at least one form of elder abuse (neglect, financial exploitation, physical or psychological abuse) in a course of 1 year, noting underreporting of elder abuse overall in rural and tribal areas.[57] Moreover, several large-scale studies highlight the disproportionate impact of elder abuse on Black patients.[58,59] Overall, violence and abuse within the home are both pervasive and widely underrecognized. Physicians need to be mindful about risk to any patient and avoid stereotyping as related to home violence. To begin assisting victims by identifying mistreatment through screening and discussion, physicians must proactively ensure the patient's privacy during accompanied visits is ensured.

Outside of safety considerations (in line with the principle of consent and **socialization** to care) it is important to remember that neither patients nor companions may anticipate inquiry and examinations which may take place. For example, while the patient in Vignette 1 might be satisfied with her neighbor being involved in medication discussions, she might not wish for her neighbor to be privy to her sexual health information. Given the asymmetry of power and possible risks of victimization at the hands of a companion, patients should not be expected to self-advocate for privacy in medical visits.

Example [continued]:

Physician: Whenever patients come with companions, I always make sure that I spend 5 minutes with the patient alone. It's best practice for all patient care to make sure that we have a chance to explore any problems in full.

Ensuring a Comfortable Environment for Patients and Companions

Although often overlooked, logistics and ergonomics of the care delivery are important both for patient comfort as well as management of a physician's fatigue and work-related burden. All persons present (including children) need to have a comfortable place for the duration of the visit. It is also important to consider the engagement of children while in the visit, while minimizing noise and disruptions which can negatively affect a physician's ability to concentrate.

Example [continued]:

Physician: Before we get started, I just want to make sure that everyone is comfortable. Since this is a 20-minute visit and that can be long for a child, can we give Grace a toy or a book to keep her busy?

Patient: She likes to play a game on my phone.

Physician: Great! Is it possible to give her earphones or adjust the volume? Sometimes those games come with sound effects!

Patient: Yes! That noise gives me a headache too.

Successful integration of companions across patient care can be a great asset for patient-centered care. It is important to note that given the complexity of minoritized identities and acculturation, physicians should suspend reductionistic perspectives which can be dictated by conceptualization along the individualistic-collectivistic continuum. Proactive integration of companions in line with principles of **informed consent** while maintaining awareness of possible power dynamics and abuse risks is critical. Future medical education efforts must bridge these constructs to support both learners and patients.

Step Eight: Culturally Informed Interviewing

In clinical practice, patients present with interlocking, minoritized identities in the context of navigating stressors within and outside of the health care system. Limiting the patient's experiences to a singular identity is reductionistic, however long-standing tradition in medicine (as well as other helping professions) emphasizes a focus on group identity characteristics regardless of acculturation and other complexities.

Research focusing on communication in medical care highlights the importance of recognition and integration of minoritized patients' preferences and life experiences to support health care and life choices. Understanding of the patient's unique experience is central to collaboration and key to disrupting tendencies toward reductionism and stereotyping.

Culturally informed interviewing may be considered an extension of biopsychosocial-grounded inquiry. Smith's Model[60] and the 4 Habits Model[33] are two succinct models of biopsychosocially informed interviewing. Both models provide operationally defined steps toward biopsychosocially informed interviewing.

However, culturally informed assessment needs to go beyond biopsychosocial conceptualization and engage in direct inquiry, eliciting a patient's view of illness and treatment. Based on the work by Kleiman and colleagues, Betancourt[2] proposed the ESFT model, outlined as specific inquiry questions allowing for culturally informed assessment of a patient's unique view of illness and illness management.

E: stands for explanatory model and includes questions focusing on a patient's understanding of symptom etiology, treatment preferences, quality of life impact, clarification of symptom-related concerns, and efforts for symptom management.

S: focuses on social and environmental factors with a focus on medical care, including inquiry about medication access and affordability.

F: identifies fears and concerns about a medical regimen, including acquired knowledge and beliefs about treatment and side-effects.

T: stands for therapeutic contracting (or treatment) focusing on understanding a patient's medication-related knowledge.

ESFT offers clear and succinct questions which offer an opportunity to bridge the gap between patient-physician illness understanding. As inquiry utilizes **open-ended** yet focused questions that address tendencies toward directive communication. Although there are other models, ESFT provides a focused, strategic, and structured approach to a culturally informed interview for all patients.

Step Nine: Completing the Visit

The final minutes of each visit should focus on the goal of care and treatment planning discussion. Such discussion can be enhanced and strengthened via a **summary** of each agenda item, discovery, and proposed treatment. For example, the 4 Habits Model[33] proposed by Frankel and Stein, provides clear and specific guidelines for visit wrap-up behaviors. This process strengthens bilateral understanding and offers the patient control in revising the narrative. Such a summary can also facilitate efficacy and hope as progress toward goals and mutual commitment to change are strengthened.

Beck[37] suggests that the final step of the patient encounter should involve eliciting a patient's feedback about the visit via specifically asking for perceptions about the visit. Eliciting feedback helps to maintain rapport, reestablishes patients' central role and control in the visit, and allows for any negative interactions or miscommunication to be addressed.

Example: [after summary]

Physician: Before we finish, I want to ask for your opinion about the visit today.

Patient: I think it was ok. Now I understand why you are recommending physical therapy. Plan for my rash also makes sense, and I will pick up medications this afternoon.

Physician: Happy to hear that we made progress. Was there anything that bothered you about today's visit? Anything that I did not understand or should do better?

Patient: I do wish we had more time, but I think you are doing your best. I am always happy to see you.

Physician: Having more time can help and I do wish we could have more! I want to make sure though, that if there is anything that bothers you about what I am saying, you let me know. Do you think you can tell me if anything like that comes up?

Patient: Sure! I think you are great, but I will let you know.

CONCLUSION

Structural inequities are magnified by physicians' struggles with consistent implementation of care using humanistic, collaborative, and antiracist communication. Current efforts to advance training in antiracism and equity, while an important step, have not yet demonstrated a tangible impact on physicians' behaviors in patient care. At the same time, the impact of **professionalization** and power asymmetry in health care delivery require further attention. The medical education system currently lacks overarching standards and certification of communication competencies. This offers a unique opportunity in re-imagining medical education to meet the highest standards of care for collaborative and antiracist interpersonal communication. In doing so, both the new strategies and known (but overlooked) techniques must be amalgamated to create a unified view of the training standards to enhance humanistic and equitable care. This chapter outlines routine tasks and techniques and offers the rationale behind specific recommendations, reviews common pitfalls, and identifies opportunities for change.

*Note: All names and personal information have been fictionalized. Vignettes are based on authors' observations/reviews of patient care visits and can include an amalgamation of observations across different interviews.

DISCLOSURE

Material presented in this chapter was utilized by N. Pilipenko PhD, ABPP, for implementation of the teaching grant *Clinical Interviewing in Primary Care Setting* supported by the Provost Innovative Course Design Grant, Columbia University.

REFERENCES

1. Schneider EC, Shah A, Doty MM, Tikkanen R, Fields K, Williams II RD. *Mirror, Mirror 2021. Reflecting Poorly: Health Care in the U.S. Compared to Other High-Income Countries.* The Commonwealth Fund. 2021. https://www.commonwealthfund.org/sites/default/files/2021-08/Schneider_Mirror_Mirror_2021.pdf

2. Betancourt JR. Cultural competency: providing quality care to diverse populations. *Consult Pharm.* 2006;21(12):988–995. https://doi.org/10.4140/tcp.n.2006.988.

3. Cooper LA, Roter DL, Carson KA, et al. The associations of clinicians' implicit attitudes about race with medical visit communication and patient ratings of interpersonal care. *Am J Public Health.* 2012;102(5):979–987. https://doi.org/10.2105/AJPH.2011.300558.

4. Johnson RL, Roter D, Powe NR, Cooper LA. Patient race/ethnicity and quality of patient-physician communication during medical visits. *Am J Public Health.* 2004;94(12):2084–2090. https://doi.org/10.2105/ajph.94.12.2084.

5. Weiner SJ, Schwartz A, Weaver F, Goldberg J, Yudkowsky R, Sharma G, et al. Contextual errors and failures in individualizing patient care: a multicenter study. *Ann Intern Med.* 2010;153(2):69–75. https://doi.org/10.7326/0003-4819-153-2-201007200-00002. 20.

6. Kavic MS. Competency and the six core competencies. *JSLS.* 2002;6(2):95–97.

7. Kurtz SM. Doctor-patient communication: principles and practices. *Can J Neurol Sci.* 2002;29(Suppl 2):S23–S29. https://doi.org/10.1017/s0317167100001906.

8. Kurtz S, Silverman J, Benson J, Draper J. Marrying content and process in clinical method teaching: enhancing the Calgary-Cambridge guides. *Acad Med.* 2003;78(8):802–809. https://doi.org/10.1097/00001888-200308000-00011.

9. Fortin VI AH, Dwamena FC, Frankel RM, Lepisto B, Smith RC, eds. *Smith's Patient-Centered Interviewing.* 4th ed. McGraw Hill; 2018.

10. Dewi SP, Wilson A, Duvivier R, Kelly B, Gilligan C. Perceptions of medical students and their facilitators on clinical communication skills teaching, learning, and assessment. *Front Public Health.* 2023;11 https://doi.org/10.3389/fpubh.2023.1168332. 1168332. Published 2023 Jun 26.

11. Rasenberg E, Brand G, van Weel-Baumgarten E. Integrating medical and practical skills in communication skills training: do students feel it supports them with transfer from classroom to practice? *PEC Innov.* 2023;2:100158. https://doi.org/10.1016/j.pecinn.2023.100158. Published 2023 Apr 25.

12. Zabar S, Ark T, Gillespie C, et al. Can unannounced standardized patients assess professionalism and communication skills in the emergency department? *Acad Emerg Med.* 2009;16(9):915–918. https://doi.org/10.1111/j.1553-2712.2009.00510.x.

13. Zabar S, Hanley K, Watsula-Morley A, et al. Using unannounced standardized patients to explore variation in care for patients with depression. *J Grad Med Educ.* 2018;10(3):285–291. https://doi.org/10.4300/JGME-D-17-00736.1.

14. United States Medical Licensing Examination (ESMLE). *Work to Relaunch USMLE Step 2 CS Discontinued.* 2021. www.usmle.org/work-relaunch-usmle-step-2-cs-discontinued

15. Kogan JR, Hauer KE, Holmboe ES. The dissolution of the step 2 clinical skills examination and the duty of medical educators to step up the effectiveness of clinical skills assessment. *Acad Med.* 2021;96(9):1242–1246. https://doi.org/10.1097/ACM.0000000000004216.

16. Johnson RL, Roter D, Powe NR, Cooper LA. Patient race/ethnicity and quality of patient-physician communication during medical visits. *Am J Public Health.* 2004;94(12):2084–2090. https://doi.org/10.2105/ajph.94.12.2084.

17. Boutin-Foster C. R.E.A.C.T: A framework for role modeling anti-racism in the clinical learning environment. *Med Teach.* 2022;44(12):1347–1353. https://doi.org/10.1080/0142159X.2022.2094231.

18. Hall WJ, Chapman MV, Lee KM, et al. Implicit racial/ethnic bias among health care professionals and its influence on health care outcomes: a systematic review. *Am J Public Health.* 2015;105(12):e60–e76. https://doi.org/10.2105/AJPH.2015.302903.

19. Falusi O, Chun-Seeley L, de la Torre D, et al. Teaching the teachers: development and evaluation of a racial health equity curriculum for faculty. *MedEdPORTAL.* 2023;19:11305. https://doi.org/10.15766/mep.

20. Medlock M, Weissman A, Wong SS, et al. Racism as a unique social determinant of mental health: development of a didactic curriculum for psychiatry residents. *MedEdPORTAL.* 2017;13:10618. https://doi.org/10.15766/mep_2374-8265.10618.

21. Holm AL, Rowe Gorosh M, Brady M, White-Perkins D. Recognizing privilege and bias: an interactive exercise to expand health care providers' personal awareness. *Acad Med.* 2017;92(3):360–364. https://doi.org/10.1097/ACM.0000000000001290.

22. Godkin M, Ferguson W, Diop D. A required inter clerkship on multiculturalism for third-year medical students. *Acad Med.* 2002 May;77(5):469.

23. Tarleton C, Tong W, McNeill E, Owda A, Barron B, Cunningham H. Preparing medical students for anti-racism at the bedside: teaching skills to mitigate racism and bias in clinical encounters. *MedEdPORTAL.* 2023;19:11333. https://doi.org/10.15766/mep_2374-8265.11333.

24. Betancourt JR, Carrillo JE, Green AR. Hypertension in multicultural and minority populations: linking communication to compliance. *Curr Hypertens Rep.* 1999;1(6):482–488. https://doi.org/10.1007/BF03215777.

25. Astin JA, Soeken K, Sierpina VS, Clarridge BR. Barriers to the integration of psychosocial factors in medicine: results of a national survey of physicians. *J Am Board Fam Med.* 2006;19(6):557–565. https://doi.org/10.3122/jabfm.19.6.557.

26. West C, Graham L, Palmer RT, et al. Implementation of interprofessional education (IPE) in 16 U.S. medical schools: common practices, barriers and facilitators. *J Interprof Educ Pract.* 2016;4:41–49. https://doi.org/10.1016/j.xjep.2016.05.002.

27. Kauff M, Bührmann T, Gölz F, et al. Teaching interprofessional collaboration among future healthcare professionals. *Front Psychol.* 2023;14:1185730. https://doi.org/10.3389/fpsyg.2023.1185730. PMID: 37303913; PMCID: PMC10250594.

28. Zechariah S, Ansa BE, Johnson SW, Gates AM, Leo G. Interprofessional education and collaboration in healthcare: an exploratory study of the perspectives of medical students in the United States. *Healthcare (Basel).* 2019;7(4):117. https://doi.org/10.3390/healthcare7040117. Published 2019 Oct 15.

29. Rawlinson C, Carron T, Cohidon C, et al. An overview of reviews on interprofessional collaboration in primary care: barriers and facilitators. *Int J Integr Care.* 2021;21(2):32. https://doi.org/10.5334/ijic.5589. Published 2021 Jun 22.

30. van Duin TS, de Carvalho Filho MA, Pype PF, et al. Junior doctors' experiences with interprofessional collaboration: wandering the landscape. *Med Educ.* 2022;56(4):418–431. https://doi.org/10.1111/medu.14711.

31. Robinson JD, Tate A, Heritage J. Agenda-setting revisited: when and how do primary-care physicians solicit patients' additional concerns? *Patient Educ Couns.* 2016;99(5), 718–723. doi: 10.1016/j.pec.2015.12.009

32. Epstein RM, Mauksch L, Carroll J, Jaén CR. Have you really addressed your patient's concerns? *Fam Pract Manage.* 2008;15(3):35–40.

33. Frankel RM, Stein T. Getting the most out of the clinical encounter: the four habits model. *J Med Pract Manage.* 2001;16(4):184–191.

34. Kowalski CP, McQuillan DB, Chawla N, et al. The hand on the Doorknob: visit agenda setting by complex patients and their primary care physicians. *J Am Board Fam Med.* 2018;31(1):29–37. https://doi.org/10.3122/jabfm.2018.01.170167.

35. Marvel MK, Epstein RM, Flowers K, Beckman HB. Soliciting the patient's agenda: have we improved? *JAMA.* 1999;281(3):283–287. https://doi.org/10.1001/jama.281.3.283.

36. Plug I, van Dulmen S, Stommel W, Olde Hartman TC, Das E. Physicians' and patients' interruptions in clinical practice: a quantitative analysis. *Ann Fam Med.* 2022;20(5):423–429. https://doi.org/10.1370/afm.2846.

37. Beck JS. *Cognitive Behavior Therapy: Basics and Beyond.* 3rd ed. Guilford Press; 2021.

38. McWilliams N. *Psychoanalytic Diagnosis: Understanding Personality Structure in the Clinical Process.* 2nd ed. Guilford Press; 2011.

39. Heurtin-Roberts S, Reisin E. The relation of culturally influenced lay models of hypertension to compliance with treatment. *Am J Hypertens.* 1992;5(11):787–792. https://doi.org/10.1093/ajh/5.11.787.

40. Arcoleo K, Marsiglia F, Serebrisky D, Rodriguez J, Mcgovern C, Feldman J. Explanatory model for asthma disparities in latino children: results from the Latino Childhood Asthma Project. *Ann Behav Med.* 2020;54(4):223–236. https://doi.org/10.1093/abm/kaz041.

41. Morgan S, Moriarty L. 21st Century CURES ACT & the HIPAA Access Right. U.S. Department of Health and Human Services Office for Civil Rights. The Office of the National Coordinator for Health Information Technology. https://www.healthit.gov/sites/default/files/2018-12/LeveragingHITtoPromotePatientAccess2.pdf.

42. Goddu A, O'Conor KJ, Lanzkron S, et al. Do words matter? Stigmatizing language and the transmission of bias in the medical record. *J Gen Intern Med.* 2018;33(5):685–691. https://doi.org/10.1007/s11606-017-4289-2. Epub 2018 Jan 26. Erratum in: *J Gen Intern Med.* 2019 Jan;34(1):164. PMID: 29374357; PMCID: PMC5910343.

43. Fernández L, Fossa A, Dong Z. Words matter: what do patients find judgmental or offensive in outpatient notes? *J Gen Intern Med.* 2021;36(9):2571–2578. https://doi.org/10.1007/s11606-020-06432-7.

44. Beach MC, Saha S, Park J, et al. Testimonial injustice: linguistic bias in the medical records of black patients and women. *J Gen Intern Med.* 2021;36(6):1708–1714. https://doi.org/10.1007/s11606-021-06682-z.

45. Sun M, Oliwa T, Peek ME, Tung EL. Negative patient descriptors: documenting racial bias in the electronic health record. *Health Aff.* 2022;41(2):203–211. https://doi.org/10.1377/hlthaff.2021.01423.

46. Steinkamp J, Kantrowitz JJ, Airan-Javia S. Prevalence and sources of duplicate information in the electronic medical record. *JAMA Netw Open.* 2022;5(9):e2233348. https://doi.org/10.1001/jamanetworkopen.2022.33348.

47. Williams J, Andreou A, Castillo E, et al. Antiracist documentation practices-shaping clinical encounters and decision making. *N Engl J Med.* 2023;389:1238–1244. https://doi.org/10.1056/NEJMms2303340.

48. Duke P, Frankel RM, Reis S. How to integrate the electronic health record and patient-centered communication into the medical visit: a skills-based approach. *Teach Learn Med.* 2013;25(4):358–365. https://doi.org/10.1080/10401334.2013.827981.

49. Zeigler K, Camarota SA. *67.3 Million in the United States Spoke a Foreign Language at Home in 2018.* Center for Immigration Studies. 2019. https://cis.org/Report/673-Million-United-States-Spoke-Foreign-Language-Home-2018.

50. Richwine J. Immigrant literacy: Self-assessment vs. reality. Center for Immigration Studies. Published June 21, 2017. https://cis.org/Immigrant-Literacy-Self-Assessment-vs-Reality.

51. Price-Wise G. *An Intoxicating Error: Mistranslation, Medical Malpractice, and Prejudice.* Center for Cultural Competence, Inc. 2015.

52. Juckett G, Unger K. Appropriate use of medical interpreters. *Am Fam Physician.* 2014;90(7):476–480.

53. Wolff JL, Roter DL. Family presence in routine medical visits: a meta-analytical review. *Soc Sci Med.* 2011;72(6):823–831. https://doi.org/10.1016/j.socscimed.2011.01.015.

54. Otto AK, Reblin M, Harper FWK, et al. Impact of patients' companions on clinical encounters between black patients and their non-Black oncologists. *JCO Oncol Pract.* 2021;17(5):e676–e685. https://doi.org/10.1200/OP.20.00820.

55. Laidsaar-Powell RC, Butow PN, Bu S, et al. Physician-patient-companion communication and decision-making: a systematic review of triadic medical consultations. *Patient Educ Couns.* 2013;91(1):3–13. https://doi.org/10.1016/j.pec.2012.11.007.

56. Huecker MR, King KC, Jordan GA, Smock W. Domestic violence. In: *StatPearls.* StatPearls Publishing. 2023. https://www.ncbi.nlm.nih.gov/books/NBK499891.

57. Steinman KJ, Burnett J, Hoffman R. Racial/ethnic group differences in older adults' involvement with adult protective services. *J Gerontol Soc Work.* 2023:1–10. https://doi.org/10.1080/01634372.2023.2191118.

58. Li M, Dong X. Identifying the incidence and factors associated with the risk of elder mistreatment. *JAMA Netw Open.* 2021;4(8):e2119593. https://doi.org/10.1001/jamanetworkopen.2021.19593.

59. Steinman KJ, Burnett J, Hoffman R. Racial/ethnic group differences in older adults' involvement with adult protective services. *J Gerontol Soc Work.* 2023:1–10. https://doi.org/10.1080/01634372.2023.2191118.

60. Fortin A, Dwamena F, Frankel RM, Smith RC. *Smith's Patient Centered Interviewing: An Evidence-Based Method.* 3rd ed. McGraw-Hill; 2012.

PART V

Case Studies: Community Partnerships

13

Community-Directed Graduate Medical Education as a Pathway to Improved Health Equity and Social Justice

Kate Rowland, Deborah Edberg, Lucia A. Flores, Steven K. Rothschild, and Lisa Sanchez-Johnsen

SUMMARY

Separating health care, health services, clinicians, and clinician training from the communities for whom they care drives inequity. Improving the distribution of clinicians increases equitable access, distribution of services, and reduces disparities, resulting in improved health. We propose three concrete steps graduate medical education (GME) can take to reduce this separation and address health care inequities. First, GME must evolve from its current emphasis on hospital-based training to training that takes place in communities. New physicians must train, in whole or in part, in the communities they intend to care for. Community needs, health disparities, and existing inequities in health care outcomes must be considered when

creating and funding future training programs. Next, GME must collaborate with communities and share power in decision-making and direction-setting. Physicians graduating from community-directed residencies will complete training more aligned with their patients and with a better understanding of their patients' needs, as voiced by the patients and communities themselves. We present a framework for creating community-directed GME programs based on principles from community-based participatory research. Finally, GME must be transparent and accountable. GME programs are not, by and large, responsible to society or their local communities for the positive or negative impacts they have on health, even though the majority are funded by public dollars. We propose new metrics, such as clinical outcomes, equity outcomes, and workforce outcomes, that will more accurately assess the impact of the public funds spent on GME.

SECTION 1: THE ORIGINS AND CONSEQUENCES OF HOSPITAL-BASED GRADUATE MEDICAL EDUCATION

How Communities Matter to Health

Community can be defined as a group of people joined by a commonality in which they feel a sense of membership or unity. Geography is one of the most common ways of describing a community, but communities are not strictly defined in terms of location.[1] In the United States, many people self-define as part of a community based on their racial or ethnic identity. Community often includes overlapping concepts of culture, such as shared beliefs, ideas, and spiritual practices. Communities exist within communities. For example, within geographic communities, communities of identity arise, such as mothers of small children living in a certain neighborhood or intensive care nurses working in a particular hospital.

In the United States, health is a local phenomenon. A person's neighborhood influences their opportunity for health and their likelihood of experiencing inequitable health care and health outcomes. Communities provide the social, political, and economic infrastructure that contribute to health outcomes. Each of the US Department of Health and Human Service's five categories of social determinants of health are connected to the community where a patient lives: economic stability, education access and quality, health care access and quality, the neighborhood and the built environment, and the social and community context.[2] In medicine, the concept of social determinants is often used to describe barriers to health such as food or housing insecurity. This conceptualization minimizes the powerful and positive force that community determinants contribute to health. Communities, community identity, and community resources contribute to individual health, healing, and resilience.[3,4] The factors that create a community infrastructure and the factors that have led to inequitable distribution of resources within communities are beyond the scope of this chapter but will be familiar to many readers.

The Institute of Medicine (renamed the National Academy of Medicine in 2015) in its report on the *Future of the Public's Health in the 21st Century*[5] asserted that a healthy community is one in which its members have a leadership role in the health care of that community. However, in most communities, health is not fully participatory. Health care systems provide services and incentives based on generalized and assumed formulas rather than

based on the needs of the communities they provide care for.[3] Medical education is one facet of medicine that has contributed to the continuation of this systemic impediment to healthy communities. This chapter describes how the disconnect between communities and health care began, the implications of perpetuating it, and suggestions for how to incorporate community direction into graduate medical education (GME). When we think about reducing inequity and increasing social justice in health care and medical education, the solutions must begin at the community level.

The Word We Will Not Use in This Chapter

In discussing community-led GME, we will not discuss "empowerment" or "empowering" community members. The word empowerment perpetuates the myth that the problem we seek to solve is due to a lack of knowledge or resources by community members. The work we are insisting on is that of removing the barriers to participation that we as medical educators have ourselves put into place. This chapter describes a movement toward community expertise in medical education, acknowledging the historic privileging of academic knowledge over lived experience.

The Evolution of Graduate Medical Education in the United States

To understand why GME is not creating a just and equitable health care environment, it is helpful to understand the history of medical education and the deliberate decisions that have been made and continue to be reinforced.

Modern residency training in the United States evolved alongside hospitals. For centuries, people were cared for at home. Hospitals were few and reserved for those without means or family to take care of them. People were born, played, worked, aged, and died at home.[6] Physicians may have attended school outside of the local area, but more frequently, they participated in an apprenticeship model that allowed them to train and transition to practice within their own community.

Beginning after the US Civil War and continuing into the start of the 20th century, local training disappeared in favor of university-based medical schools. Many factors contributed to this movement, but the American Medical Association (AMA)-backed Flexner report (1910) detailing the state of medical education in the United States is the most noteworthy and perhaps the most flawed. The Flexner report assessed the worthiness of each school by the strength of its research potential and the size of its endowment. Even at the time the report was published, the focus and conclusions of the Flexner report were directly opposed by advocates who held that people's needs and welfare should be centered in medical education, rather than the creation of new scientific knowledge. The report was effective in marginalizing whole groups of people, centralizing training in urban centers, and undermining primary care. The racism, ethnic bias, and anti-Semitism written into the Flexner report continue to impact medical training opportunities and have contributed to health inequities observable today.[7–9]

In codifying research output and endowment size as two central metrics for medical schools, the Flexner report institutionalized the physician-as-scientist paradigm in US medical education. To achieve these metrics, medical schools consolidated training in universities, and then universities aligned with teaching hospitals. In doing so, the first academic medical centers were created. These university medical centers and teaching hospitals were almost exclusively urban institutions run by specialists. Research and researchers were centered instead of patients, and many private practitioners, particularly generalist physicians, were excluded from teaching students at all. Because generalist physicians were the physicians who spent the most time caring for people in communities, students had little access to community-based education or role models, and the number of rural and primary care physicians plummeted.[10,11] Most modern specialties were founded in this era, with the earliest specialty boards founded in 1933 and 16 more founded in the next decade.[12] Thus most modern specialty training programs originated, and have not deviated significantly, from a model of care based on Flexner's original ideal of a physician-scientist, whose primary goal was less about patient care and more about the pursuit of research.

Graduate Medical Education in the United States Today

Our current GME policy consistently produces physician shortages in rural areas and areas with high social deprivation, where the effects of lack of care are compounded by social determinants of health. As of 2022 there were more than 150,000 medical residents in Accreditation Council for Graduate Medical Education (ACGME)–accredited programs, rotating at more than 8600 individual training sites. Of the more than 3100 counties in the United States, only 525 are home to a graduate medical training program.[13] Over 83 million Americans live in federally designated **health professional shortage areas** (HPSAs). In our home state of Illinois alone, the Health Resources and Service Administration (HRSA) designates more than 750 medically underserved areas.[14]

The US has no national or policy-driven method of adjusting physician training to meet population needs. Nationally, about 60% of US physicians train in the south and northeast regions, and forecasting by the Association of American Medical Colleges suggests that by 2030, the east region will be oversupplied with physicians, while the west region will not have enough physicians to meet population needs.[15] Approximately 80% of the US population lives in an urban area, defined by the US Census Bureau as an area with a population greater than 50,000 people. Nearly 98% of medical residents train in urban areas and 89% of physicians from all specialties practice in urban areas. These numbers are slightly better in primary care; approximately 77% of family physicians practice in urban areas, compared with 90% of general internists and 91% of general pediatricians.[16,17]

Physicians who train at **academic medical centers**, as opposed to community-based training programs, are more likely to be specialists who stay in or close to urban settings.[18] These shortages are particularly profound with specialty care, in part because of the very low rates of specialty training available in rural settings.[10] Robust and accessible primary care is a necessary and central component for creating a healthy population,[19] and primary care reduces inequity in health care at a greater rate than specialty care. However, the rate of primary care physicians per person in the US is shrinking rather than growing[18] as we train physicians who do not practice primary care at a much more rapid pace.[16]

Physicians who train in communities are more likely to practice in communities.[20–24] Graduates of **Teaching Health Center GME** programs (THCGME), community-based GME programs designed to close the workforce gaps in rural and underserved communities, are more likely to practice in rural locations compared with residents from programs with other kinds of funding. They are also more likely to provide care in underserved communities, with about 35% of THCGME graduates practicing in **medically underserved areas** compared with 18.6% of graduates from other programs. Graduates of these programs are also more likely to stay within 5 miles of training to practice.[14,20] We discuss THCGME in more detail later in this chapter.

Change is possible if we as a medical community choose to prioritize community health, health equity, and social justice outcomes. Community-based training removes barriers to care for patients and reduces barriers to practice for future physicians. In this chapter, we discuss models for curricular frameworks and funding for community-based GME training. We also discuss the need for policy-level changes to drive GME toward community-level accountability.

SECTION 2: PARTNERING COMMUNITIES AND GRADUATE MEDICAL EDUCATION PROGRAMS

Forms of Training in the Community

Many GME programs recognize the contributions of community to health and have attempted to integrate community resources into training over the years.[25] A 2023 monograph from State Health and Values Strategies, a Robert Wood Johnson Foundation grantee, describes a framework for community engagement of programs based on the degree of community involvement and the resulting impact of the program (Table 13.1). As community power increases, community impact also increases. Likewise, community integration into GME training exists along a spectrum, depending on the degree of community involvement in the training itself.

Until now, much of GME education involving communities has been at a community-informed or community-involved level, meaning the community has been considered, consulted, or involved at a superficial or transactional level. The community provides a service, such as teaching, and the residency provides a service, such as patient care. True integration does not exist, but residents gain exposure to community members, organizations, and community issues, while the community gains increased access to health care provided by the residency program (Fig. 13.1).

Community-informed or community-involved curricula take many forms, ranging from didactic to experiential to patient care.[26,27] Examples of existing community-informed or community-involved curricula maintain residents at the central teaching hospital training hub where they receive lectures about community engagement, population and community health, and social determinants of health. These lectures may involve community organizations and members coming to the training hub and speaking directly with learners. The curriculum may include learners taking field trips into the community. Several residencies have incorporated "windshield surveys" where learners drive through the community taking note of what they see regarding needs and assets within the community itself. The residents may use this information to design research or educational projects to help them take a deeper dive into what comprises a community and what challenges they could address.

Some medical schools and residencies engage in collaborations with community-based organizations.[28–30] These collaborations range from half-day field trips with brief community exposures to more committed involvements where students or residents spend multiple days providing a service, coordinating a project, or partnering with the community organization on a longitudinal plan for health care services, education, or other wellness-focused projects.[31,32]

Other existing residency curricula involve population health projects where residents review their own patient populations within a community and learn about

---

TABLE 13.1 **Transactional versus Transformational Engagement**
Transactional Engagement
• Checking a box
• Narrow engagement
• Seeking input on near-final product
• Results in superficial or technical change only
• Challenges: may lead to community fatigue, lack of trust
Transformational Engagement
• Sustainable relationships
• Transparency and "feedback loop"
• Results in cultural or structural change
• Challenges: resource intensive, requires institutional commitment and readiness

Adapted from State Health & Value Strategies. *Transformational Community Engagement to Advance Health Equity.* State Health & Value Strategies; 2023. https://www.rwjf.org/en/insights/our-research/2023/01/transformational-community-engagement-to-advance-health-equity.html.

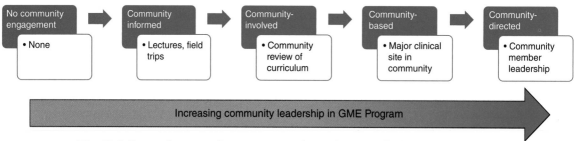

Fig. 13.1 Types of community engagement in graduate medical education (GME).

the epidemiology of the health of their own community.[33] These projects may include designing brief interventions that could impact the health of their own population.[34] Some include written or videos of reflections of their experiences, and others include residency-wide retreats focused on education and skill building within community-based care. Some residencies or medical schools may set up community rotation experiences that last from days to months, effectively resulting in longitudinal experiences.[35] Learners care for patients in the patients' community setting, rather than in the academic medical center setting.[33]

Community-informed and community-involved curricula are important steps on the pathway to fully engaging community members in medical education. They are defined by limited power-sharing with community members and limited impact on the community's health outcomes. Community-involved curricula have evidence of a relationship without community leadership. Many are precursors to other forms of community involvement. Once success is demonstrated with some community involvement, a program can develop deeper and more impactful ties.[36,37]

Some residencies provide community-based education, another step on the pathway. Community-based residencies have a major training site, such as a continuity clinic, located within the community itself, often within community health centers or federally qualified health centers (FQHCs). Starting in the 1990s, family medicine residencies began to explore how to accredit programs embedded in community health centers. In 1994 the Lawrence Family Medicine Residency Program in Massachusetts became the first community-accredited community health center-sponsored family medicine residency program. Community-based residents can use the experience of their continuity panel to learn more about social determinants of health, advocacy for their patients, or how their patients fit into the broader context of the community.[36,38–40]

Community-Directed Graduate Medical Education

Few existing curricula appear to fit the definition of **community-directed graduate medical education** (CDGME), also known as "community-driven" or "community-led," as defined by the 2023 Transformational Community Engagement to Advance Health Equity report from State Health and Value Strategies and Health Equity Solutions,[41] two policy institutes focused on achieving health equity. In these models, the community voice is present at a leadership level from inception to program assessment, and the GME program is accountable to community members. The goal of including the community in GME leadership is to create a residency where physicians are trained with community members directing key aspects of their curricula.[27]

This, in turn, may lead to improved health and equity outcomes, not only through patient care that builds upon the strengths of patients and communities, but also by creating a generation of physicians who have skills and experience with community-directed health care. These physicians will then be equipped to continue this work in their practice.

How this training looks will vary based on input from the stakeholders within the community as well as the residency training type and requirements from the ACGME. All specialties can be creative about partnering with community members in determining how to structure their experiences and provide the community with the care that it needs. The first step is for the subspecialties to identify the community or communities for whom they care. This conversation begins frequently with the medical system's historical shortcomings. Identifying, recognizing, and apologizing for historical and recent harms (even those not caused by the specific physicians involved) can be an important part of gaining trust and creating an effective partnership.

At that point, the community members can share their thoughts and ideas about what type of engagement they need from the specialists. In some cases, this may revolve around access and could include planning for subspecialty clinics to provide care in the community, through physical clinics, telemedicine options, and transportation provision for community members to facilitate access to needed specialty care. This must involve training in cultural humility so that the residents learn to build and maintain trusting partnerships with patients and providing patient-directed care. Community members may also prioritize training physicians who speak the language preferred by the community members themselves. Whatever the adaptations are to the training program, the most important part is that community members are engaged in planning processes, coupling their expertise with those of medical educators, voicing their priorities, and directing their ideas for solutions wherever possible.[26,27,42,43]

Example of a Community-Directed Graduate Medical Education Program

The Rush-Esperanza family medicine residency in Chicago is a THCGME-funded community-directed program with a community advisory board. The program is sponsored by an academic medical center, Rush University, and an FQHC, Esperanza Health Center. Residents see patients in the Brighton Park neighborhood of Chicago, a predominantly Latinx community on the southwest side of the city. Residents also rotate at a large academic medical center and community hospitals. The community advisory board is composed of members of the community and representatives of organizations rooted in the neighborhood.

As the program was being developed, Esperanza hosted a retreat to bring together the community advisory board and the future program academic leadership team. Community members were able to describe stories of ways their needs had not been met by the medical community in the past and their wishes for priorities in training future physicians in a system that better met their needs. They also described curricular priorities such as training in addiction medicine, cultural humility, and LGBTQ+ sensitivity. The advisory board set a priority that the residency program recruit residents who shared an ethnic identity and language fluency with the members of the community or who had a strong cultural understanding and mission orientation. This resulted in specific curricular development around these areas along with a recruitment effort that led by prioritizing bicultural and bilingual residents who now comprise the first two classes.

Today, the advisory board members continue to have an active role in program leadership, for which they are paid a stipend. They have an active and detailed role in some aspects of the program, a more advisory role in other aspects, and they have declined input into facets of the program where they feel they do not have expertise or interest. As an example, members of the advisory board were very interested in being involved in resident recruitment. Community members interview all residency applicants and provide input and perspective as future patients. At the advisory level, the board has participated in semiannual retreats and quarterly meetings with the program director on the program's mission, general direction, and specific strategic goals.

As the residency has matured, the advisory board has also evolved, with both predicted and unplanned member turnover and new directions and goals for the residency. For example, initially shared culture was highly prioritized in recruiting new residents. After 2 years, the advisory board recommended prioritizing mission fit alongside language skills, with shared culture being valuable, but not a top priority. The advisory board has also taken a substantial role in leading community engagement activities with the residents.

Community-Directed Participatory Education

In considering the core elements of the CDGME, the model of **Community-Based Participatory Research (CBPR)** provides a useful framework[44,45] (Table 13.2). Just as the Flexnerian model of medical education privileged specialized knowledge over the needs of people, the biomedical research conducted in elite institutions privileged testing of narrow hypotheses over the concerns of research participants. In response, beginning in the 1960s, movements in psychology, public health, education, nursing, and other fields pushed back on the question of ownership of knowledge and focused on the engagement of communities and

those most impacted by the conditions being studied.[46,47] The methods developed by these movements in turn informed the development of CBPR. The CBPR approach explicitly altered the balance of power such that research participants and community stakeholders were no longer subjects to be studied and thus required protection. Instead, they were autonomous agents in the research process, helping determine research questions, methods, and the interpretation of data. In this section, we propose a framework for developing and implementing CDGME programs that parallel principles that were developed for engaging in CBPR.[48]

In this walkover, the first principle of CDGME is the recognition of the community as the unit of identity. As noted in the introduction, community is not unidimensional; it may encompass history, race/ethnicity, faith, language, socioeconomic class, and other domains. The process of identifying the health priorities of the community and the goals of the residency program must begin with the voices of diverse members of the geographic area served by the residency program and its clinic. The second principle of community-directed GME is to build on strengths and resources within the community. How do community residents identify the strengths of their community? What are the mutual aid societies, non-profit agencies, businesses, and other resources that are the bedrock of their community? Programs should ask community members about local organizations that build community resilience and add to the infrastructure of the community as a way of seeking to understand the community where they provide care. [49]

The third principle involves a power-sharing process that attends to social inequalities through a collaborative, equitable partnership in all phases of the community-directed GME program. The community advisory board provides one method of creating collaborative partnerships for GME program leadership. The community advisory board and program faculty collaboratively choose outcome measures for the residency and determine the methods to ensure that those outcomes are achieved.

The fourth principle in the walkover from CPBR is that community-directed GME programs foster mutual colearning among all partners. Faculty and community come to the GME enterprise with different knowledge, experience, and beliefs. Partners must share their background and experience with each other for mutual benefit and to create new approaches to GME. One aspect of building shared understanding for residency oversight is to ensure that community partners are as familiar with the regulatory constraints of GME as the faculty. Unless such knowledge is explicitly shared, community members will remain disadvantaged in directing the program and risk being told by faculty members, the program director, or

TABLE 13.2   Applying Community-Based Participatory Research Elements to the Community-Directed Graduate Medical Education Concept: A Walkover.

Community-Based Participatory Research Elements	Community-Directed Graduate Medical Education Elements
Recognizes community as the unit of identity	Engage with diverse community members to identify the health priorities of the population served by the residency
Builds on strengths and resources in the community	Expand understanding of social determinants of health beyond factors which adversely impact the community Discover the social capital of the community: individual leaders, organizations, businesses, and the networks by which they interact
Facilitates collaborative, equitable partnership in all research phases and involves a power-sharing process that attends to social inequalities	Community members lead and facilitate Community Advisory Board Community members and faculty collaborate to develop the mission and methods used by the residency program
Promotes colearning and capacity building among all partners	Residency faculty ensure that community members understand the GME process Community members support faculty in learning history, culture, and resources of the community
Integrates and achieves a balance between research and action for the mutual benefit of all partners	Acknowledge imbalances of power between program faculty and community members Establish clear guidelines for communication and engagement
Emphasizes public health problems of local relevance and ecologic perspectives that recognize and attend to multiple determinants of disease	Integrate qualitative and quantitative data in approaching health problems Include public health and environmental data where available Center the lived experience of community members
Involves systems development through a cyclical and iterative process	Engage in continuous cycle of improvement by assessing progress toward goals and redesign program as needed Recognize that communities change over time: resources, built environment, etc.
Disseminates findings and knowledge gained to all partners and involves all partners in the dissemination process	Involve Community Advisory Board members as coauthors in preparing reports and dissemination of information
Plans for a long-term process and commitment to sustainability	Ensure that plans are made for sustainability; anticipate changes in federal funding, academic partnerships

Adapted from Israel BA, Schulz AJ, Parker EA, Becker AB. Review of community-based research: assessing partnership approaches to improve public health. *Ann Rev Pub Health*. 1998;19(1):173–202.

the designated institutional officer (rightly or wrongly) that certain proposed initiatives cannot be implemented due to ACGME rules. True sharing of power, as called out in the next principle, requires sharing of knowledge and understanding. As a corollary, program faculty must actively seek out knowledge of the community, including its history, culture, and resources, by entering communities as listeners and learners. These are not static processes but require

continued colearning for the mutual benefit of all partners and the community itself.

The fifth principle requires a balance between education and community action to the benefit of both partners. The program-community leadership may choose outcomes that directly impact the community at large (e.g., an expectation that medical trainees will participate in three community health outreach events per year), or they may choose to set other goals that do not lead to direct benefit to the community (choosing instead to focus on goals such as trainee recruitment). All partners in the program hold the expectation that the program will benefit the community and the trainees.

The sixth principle focuses on the local relevance of public health problems and ecological perspectives that recognize and attend to the multiple determinants of health and disease, both protective and harmful. Community-directed GME programs integrate epidemiologic data and the experience of community members in setting priority areas for programs. For example, in attending a community meeting, program faculty or residents hear that school absences due to childhood asthma were identified as a concern. Understanding the scope of the problem should involve review of diverse sources of information: public health reports, air quality data, school attendance records, and quality improvement data within the clinic or hospital. Program faculty and residents also need to identify resources within the community and seek the perspectives of community groups that want to ameliorate the problem.

The seventh principle requires that CDGME residencies engage in a continuous cycle of reassessment and redesign. For all the planning and collaborative development of the residency identified in the first six principles, conditions will inevitably change over time. The faculty-community leadership team should examine program clinical and academic outputs to assess if the goals of the program are being achieved. Program partners should be candid in examining their success in addressing structural barriers to equitable care. In the asthma example of the previous paragraph, the resident clinic could regularly analyze and share rates of avoidable pediatric asthma hospitalizations or prescribing rates of asthma controller medications. In addition, programs must also define a process to regularly examine changes the community is facing (economic, cultural, environmental) as well as challenges the program encounters (such as resident recruitment, academic challenges, accreditation).

The eighth principle involves the importance of disseminating outcomes and knowledge of CDGME programs to all partners and involve them in the dissemination process. The advisory board and other participating community partners should serve as coauthors on presentations, manuscripts, community forums, and other dissemination activities as a way of sharing information about the process and outcome of CDGME programs. Community members should be asked about preferred methods of dissemination, which may involve social media and community meetings as well as the use of less traditional forms of dissemination such as radio programs and short hard-copy newsletters.

The final principle involves a long-term process and commitment to sustainability. Ideally, partners would agree that the collaboration would continue, but a realistic plan for sustainability should be discussed. How to sustain the program, in the absence of funding or at reduced funding levels and with possible changes in accreditation standards, should be openly discussed. Overall, this principle emphasizes the importance of the relationship that has developed throughout the community-directed GME process.[50]

Implementation of the Advisory Board as a Core Feature of Community-Directed Graduate Medical Education Programs

Each of the principles described above can result in conflicts with community residents and patients of a clinical training site. Consider the following scenario:

Dr. Smith is the chair of the Department of Family Medicine at a large state university. After several years, he convinced university leadership to establish a family medicine residency with its Family Health Center located in a medically underserved community with a majority living at or below the federal poverty level near the main teaching hospital. His long-term goal is to attract top candidates. He envisions having those individuals complete inpatient rotations in specialty services at the teaching hospital where they can learn foundational medicine skills for family medicine practice. To build his program's reputation, residents will be required to complete and publish independent research that investigates health equity concerns they have observed in the local community. Dr. Smith has told colleagues that a key metric of success would be to place residency graduates in competitive fellowships across the country where they can continue leadership and research on health inequities. His colleagues at the medical school have been impressed with his progressive vision, and he looks forward to sharing that vision with patients and residents of the community where the Family Health Center will be located.

In this vignette, Dr. Smith's goals for the residency are informed by his experiences and hopes, and they may not be those of the community members. Some community members will reject the value of the residency, fearing that they will be cared for by "students" instead of the top-notch specialists that they see the medical center advertising all over the city. Some will conclude that the university is dropping into the neighborhood for its own self-interest and reject the program outright.

When implemented according to the CBPR principles discussed earlier, a community advisory board is an effective way of addressing many of these concerns. Such a board must include patients of the health center or clinic, as well as individuals representing key constituencies or stakeholders in the community and a diversity of ages and backgrounds. Skeptics or those who question the value of the residency represent invaluable sources of input. Individuals who represent interest in the health of the community include:

- Long-time neighborhood residents, block club leaders
- Members of community-based organizations
- Elected officials
- Youth organizers
- Religious leaders
- Business professionals
- Tribal officials or appointed leaders
- Community health board members
- Social service professionals

The Center for Health Care Strategies, a policy and health care innovation institute focusing on improving care for people with Medicaid, provides useful guidance on structuring a board.[51] The advisory board should be large enough to include a spectrum of the community but not so large that individuals cannot raise their concerns. We suggest 8–12 members. It is essential that advisory board members are treated as true leaders in the GME program. As such, just as residency faculty are paid, advisory board members should be offered a reasonable stipend for their participation in meetings.

Establishing ground rules for communication and collaboration is an early task for the advisory board. What are the residency decisions for which the advisory board will have input? Likewise, participants should be clear if there are decisions for which the advisory board will not be consulted. For example, faculty policy or labor laws may preclude the advisory board having authority for hiring or firing faculty or residents. Although this may lead to tense conversations, clarity is essential for the long-term impact of the advisory board.

The advisory board should be cochaired by a community member and program faculty. The agenda should be set by the community, but may include items such as the following:

- What qualities are important for residents of the program?
- How will residents learn about factors leading to health inequities? How can the advisory board support this training?
- How can residents, some of whom are likely to come from other areas, best engage with the community and learn about community strengths?
- What are the health challenges facing community members that residents should learn about and seek to address?

- What community resources should residents know about to refer their patients?
- How will the advisory board participate in medical resident interviewing and selection?
- What nonclinical skills are important for medical residents?

Perhaps the most important question for the advisory board to address is to define success for this community-directed residency program. A well-conceived community advisory board will serve as an expert panel for consultation, feedback, and troubleshooting for all programmatic considerations throughout the lifespan of a program, from conception to sunsetting. In the prior scenario, Dr. Smith defined success as academic publications and residents leaving the community when they graduated to attend fellowships. By contrast, the advisory board's definition of success may include residents who have a shared cultural understanding of the community, residents who are effective in connecting their patients to social care and resources, or graduates of the residency remaining in the community to improve access to health services. Collaboration between the advisory board and faculty of the residency should ideally result in a common understanding of desired outcomes. These outcomes should be specific and measurable and should be communicated with the wider community.

Integrating community into GME and GME into community is a fundamental step to effectively address health equity injustices in care delivery and outcomes.[52] Here, we have discussed GME programs directed by community members through a community advisory board and provided an example of a program already doing this. Using community-based participatory research as a framework, we have demonstrated a walkover to community-directed GME. In the next section, we discuss new models of GME funding and GME innovation required to achieve CDGME and to produce a more equitably distributed workforce.

SECTION 3: GRADUATE MEDICAL EDUCATION AND SOCIAL ACCOUNTABILITY

Improving Accountability With Current Funding Models

One of the barriers to wide implementation of community-directed GME is funding.[53,54] Of the $17 billion in total GME funding in 2019, Centers for Medicare and Medicaid Services (CMS) contributed $11 billion, making it the overwhelming driver of GME dollars.[21,55] CMS funding models assume a hospital-based training program.[56] The geographic clustering and inequitable distribution of physicians will remain the status quo without changes to significant GME funding that allow for funding to break away from the traditional CMS-driven, academic medical center-centered model.[57,58]

The goal of any innovative funding opportunity using public money should be to improve the health of the US population in a manner that reduces health inequities and increases access to care.[59-61] New funding often includes the expansion of primary care as a specific target because the per-capita number of primary care physicians in a population has been shown to correlate with lower population mortality and improved outcomes in a range of health conditions.[56,60] Prior to the passage of the Patient Protection and Affordable Care Act (the ACA) in 2010, efforts to create new primary care and rural training pathways succeeded at *decreasing* the per-capita supply of these clinicians between 2005 and 2015.[23,62] Expansion of community-focused programs should not be limited to primary care, however. Many communities lack access to specialty care, and these training programs should also be targeted for growth.[63]

Successful Models of Graduate Medical Education Funding to Reduce Disparities, Improve Health Equity, and Address Social Justice in Graduate Medical Education

Existing examples demonstrate how innovative funding in GME has moved beyond CMS and the academic medical center model to stimulate the growth of high-need specialties in high-need areas. Introduced earlier in the chapter, HRSA-funded THCGME supports community-based training in primary care specialties. THCGME funding began with the passage of the ACA in 2010, with periodic Congressional reallocation since then.[14,64] As with programs with CMS funding, the impact of clinical care from THCGME programs has not been studied. However, as described above, THCGME programs have intermediary outcomes that indicate a greater focus on community than previously seen, such as graduates practicing in medically underserved or rural areas. The focus on primary care programs also increases the impact on population health outcomes compared with residency graduates from specialty programs.[65-67]

HRSA also funds GME expansion in rural areas. In addition to primary care specialties, rural training grants support high-need specialties such as obstetrics/gynecology, general surgery, and psychiatry. More than 500 residents have trained in rural communities since the funding began in 2018.[68] The long-term clinical and geographic impact of these expansions is still to be determined. THCGME and rural funding both demonstrate ways of matching new funding streams to areas of highest need.

In 2014 Congress authorized funds to expand GME training through the Veterans Affairs (VA) system, with a goal of expanding access to care in underserved areas, particularly rural communities.[69] This funding allocation provided about 1500 new VA training slots, an increase of about 15%. The VA prioritized mental health services and primary care, while retaining flexibility to allocate the training spots to high-need programs in specialties other than primary care. As a result, by 2022, new VA GME sites were awarded in nearly every US state. Approximately 40% of the new GME positions were in primary care with nearly 25% more in addiction medicine or psychiatry. The remaining one-third of the new slots were allocated to high-priority specialties. These specialties were identified by the local VA health systems applying for the slots, allowing them to target areas of need. The VA expansion provides one model for future policies that equitably distribute physicians based on specialty and geography.[69]

Future Metrics to Promote Health Equity and Social Justice

Regardless of funding, GME's social accountability does not end with graduation.[70] A program's true impact is determined by the clinical outcomes its residents and graduates produce. Adding community health-focused metrics to currently reported GME metrics would center community outcomes as a priority in training. There is currently no requirement to demonstrate clinical or equity outcomes of any kind, but all GME programs in every specialty should be responsible for the clinical care they provide.[71-73]

Programs should be able to demonstrate their own clinical health outcomes in a range of measures relevant to the program and the community. Even for programs that are not yet community integrated, the GME system and funders should begin requesting reasonable data demonstrating positive contributions to the health of their patients.[74] Along with currently collected patient demographics, GME programs can be held accountable for demonstrating equity-specific outcomes, such as the distribution of patient ZIP code and income levels of people cared for by program trainees. Programs can demonstrate that these mirror local community needs. This kind of reporting would require collaboration among sponsoring institutions and accrediting bodies and could use existing infrastructure, such as accreditation data systems.

At a system level, GME can hold itself accountable for showing that GME programs are caring for patients across broad swaths of the US, reducing the geographic clustering of training that leads to future practice clustering. As noted, achieving this outcome will require leveraging existing funding sources outside of CMS as well as creative and innovative approaches to CMS-funded programs.

Programs can also be accountable for tracking where their graduates practice and accurately reporting rates of graduates practicing in medically underserved areas, rural areas, and community settings. Each new graduate will have individual preferences about their future practice, but without exposure to a robust, integrated, and healthy community training setting, few residents will understand the potential and rewards of community-driven medical practice. When experienced during training, physicians are better prepared for community-based practice and more likely to choose such a setting as a career.

CONCLUSION

In this chapter, we have discussed how GME became entrenched in hospitals and how training has been decentralized as a result. All modern GME has arisen in an era where patient care skills have been learned outside of the environment where patients live and work, with little exposure to community and social determinants of health. This contributes to inequity and injustice through an unequal distribution of physicians in the US and inadequate physician training in community health. It also denies patients and communities the opportunity to participate in the training of new physicians. GME, as an institution, has recognized the benefit of community training, and this chapter has reviewed various models of community-based GME. Over time, these models have shown varying degrees of community engagement, with earlier iterations tending toward peripheral or transactional community involvement. We have also discussed a new model of community-directed GME, in which the community has a role in setting the direction for the training program on the metrics that matter most to community members. Finally, this chapter has provided recommendations for increasing equity and social accountability within GME. All programs should report community health metrics and post-graduation outcome metrics to demonstrate the return to the public from the investment of public money into GME.

TAKE-HOME POINTS

1. Underserved communities have remained medically underserved through actions and choices on the part of the institution of medicine, including graduate medical education. This means that different actions and choices will be necessary to establish justice, reduce disparities, and improve health equity.
2. New physicians must train, in whole or in part, in the communities that most need care.
3. Community-directed graduate medical education communities and community members must have an equal role in the design and implementation of residency training that prepares future physicians to address the outcomes that most matter to patients.

4. Outcomes that would support true growth in social justice and health equity include accurate reporting of primary care graduates, graduates practicing in medically underserved areas, impact on health equity, and other clinical health outcomes in the communities the GME programs care for.

QUESTIONS FOR FURTHER THOUGHT

1. What institutional changes and resources will be required to implement the changes recommended in this chapter?
2. What policy changes may be required to implement the changes recommended in this chapter?

REFERENCES

1. MacQueen KM, McLellan E, Metzger DS, et al. What is community? an evidence-based definition for participatory public health. *Am J Public Health*. 2001;91(12):1929–1938. https://doi.org/10.2105/ajph.91.12.1929.
2. US Department of Health and Human Services. *Healthy People 2030: Social Determinants of Health*. https://health.gov/healthypeople/priority-areas/social-determinants-health.
3. Braveman P, Gottlieb L. The social determinants of health: it's time to consider the causes of the causes. *Public Health Rep*. 2014;129(Suppl 2):19–31. https://www.ncbi.nlm.nih.gov/pmc/articles/PMC3863696/.
4. Cassetti V, Powell K, Barnes A, Sanders T. A systematic scoping review of asset-based approaches to promote health in communities: development of a framework. *Glob Health Promot*. 2020;27(3):15–23. https://doi.org/10.1177/1757975919848925.
5. Institute of medicine Committee on Assuring the Health of the Public in the 21st Centure. *The Future of the Public's Health in the 21st Century*. National Academies Press (US); 2002. http://www.ncbi.nlm.nih.gov/books/NBK221239/.
6. Stern AM, Markel H. A historical perspective on the changing contours of medical residency programs. *J Pediatr*. 2004;144(1):1–2. https://doi.org/10.1016/j.jpeds.2003.11.005.
7. Duffy TP. The flexner report-100 years later. *Yale J Biol Med*. 2011;84(3):269–276.
8. Laws T. How should we respond to racist legacies in health professions education originating in the flexner report? *AMA J Ethics*. 2021;23(3):271. https://doi.org/10.1001/amajethics.2021.271.
9. Hunt S. The flexner report and black academic medicine: An assignment of place. *J Natl Med Assoc*. 1993;85(2):151–155. https://www.ncbi.nlm.nih.gov/pmc/articles/PMC2571842/.
10. Rosenblatt RA, Hart LG. Physicians and rural america. *West J Med*. 2000;173(5):348–351. https://www.ncbi.nlm.nih.gov/pmc/articles/PMC1071163/.
11. Gutierrez C, Scheid P. The history of family medicine and its impact in US health care delivery. *AAFPF*. 2002

12. American Board of Medical Specialties. https://www.abms.org/about-abms/our-story/.

13. Accreditation Council for Graduate Medical Education. *ACGME Data Resource Book 2021–22*. https://www.acgme.org/globalassets/pfassets/publicationsbooks/2021-2022_acgme__databook_document.pdf

14. HRSA, Health Workforce. *Teaching Health Center Graduate Medical Education Program*. https://bhw.hrsa.gov/sites/default/files/bureau-health-workforce/data-research/teaching-health-center-graduate-medical-education-annual-report-2021-2022.pdf

15. IHS Markit for the AAMC. *The Complexities of Physician Supply and Demand: Projections from 2019-2034*. AAMC; 2021. https://www.aamc.org/media/54681/download?attachment.

16. Agency for Healthcare Research and Quality. *Primary Care Workforce Facts and Stats No. 3*. 2018. https://www.ahrq.gov/research/findings/factsheets/primary/pcwork3/index.html.

17. Office USGA. *Physician Workforce: Locations and Types of Graduate Training Were Largely Unchanged, and Federal Efforts May Not be Sufficient to Meet Needs*. U.S. GAO. https://www.gao.gov/products/gao-17-411

18. Willis J, Antono B, Bazemore A, et al. *The State of Primary Care in the United States: A Chartbook of Facts and Statistics*. 2021. https://www.graham-center.org/content/dam/rgc/documents/publications-reports/reports/PrimaryCareChartbook2021.pdf

19. Starfield B, Shi L, Macinko J. Contribution of primary care to health systems and health. *Milbank Q*. 2005;83(3):457–502. https://doi.org/10.1111/j.1468-0009.2005.00409.x. https://www.ncbi.nlm.nih.gov/pmc/articles/PMC2690145/.

20. Teaching Health Center Planning and Development. *Teaching Health Center Planning and Development Technical Assistance*. https://www.hrsa.gov/sites/default/files/hrsa/advisory-committees/graduate-medical-edu/meetings/rural-residency-planning-development-technical-assistance-center.pdf

21. Phillips RL, George BC, Holmboe ES, Bazemore AW, Westfall JM, Bitton A. Measuring graduate medical education outcomes to honor the social contract. *Acad Med*. 2022;97(5):643–648. https://doi.org/10.1097/ACM.0000000000004592. https://www.ncbi.nlm.nih.gov/pmc/articles/PMC9028305/.

22. Davis CS, Roy T, Peterson LE, Bazemore AW. Evaluating the teaching health center graduate medical education model at 10 years: practice-based outcomes and opportunities. *J Grad Med Educ*. 2022;14(5):599–605. https://doi.org/10.4300/JGME-D-22-00187.1. https://www.ncbi.nlm.nih.gov/pmc/articles/PMC9580311/.

23. Chen C, Xierali I, Piwnica-Worms K, Phillips R. The redistribution of graduate medical education positions in 2005 failed to boost primary care or rural training. *Health Aff (Millwood)*. 2013;32(1):102–110. https://doi.org/10.1377/hlthaff.2012.0032.

24. Philips AP, Adashi EY. The teaching health center graduate medical education program: a permanent funding imperative. *J Grad Med Educ*. 2023;15(4):419–423. https://doi.org/10.4300/JGME-D-22-00879.1. https://www.ncbi.nlm.nih.gov/pmc/articles/PMC10449335/.

25. Prislin MD, Morohashi D, Dinh T, Sandoval J, Shimazu H. The community health center and family practice residency training. *Fam Med*. 1996;28(9):624–628.

26. Strasser RP. Community engagement: a key to successful rural clinical education. *Rural Remote Health*. 2010;10(3):1543. doi: 1543 [pii].

27. Strasser R, Worley P, Cristobal F, et al. Putting communities in the driver's seat: the realities of community-engaged medical education. *Acad Med*. 2015;90(11):1466–1470. https://doi.org/10.1097/ACM.0000000000000765.

28. Dobbie A, Kelly P, Sylvia E, Freeman J. Evaluating family medicine residency COPC programs: meeting the challenge. *Fam Med*. 2006;38(6):399–407.

29. Brill JR, Jackson TC, Stearns MA. Community medicine in action: an integrated, fourth-year urban continuity preceptorship. *Acad Med*. 2002;77(7):739. https://doi.org/10.1097/00001888-200207000-00025.

30. Brill JR, Ohly S, Stearns MA. Training community-responsive physicians. *Acad Med*. 2002;77(7):747. https://doi.org/10.1097/00001888-200207000-00036.

31. Fiore DC. A homeless shelter medical clinic organized and staffed by family practice residents. *West J Med*. 1995;163(6):537–540.

32. Gimpel N. Family medicine resident education: an innovative model of community medicine training. *J Commu Med Health Educ*. 2013;3(1). https://doi.org/10.4172/2161-0711.1000197.

33. Lochner J, Lankton R, Rindfleish K, Arndt B, Edgoose J. Transforming a family medicine residency into a community-oriented learning environment. *Fam Med*. 2018;50(7):518–525. https://doi.org/10.22454/FamMed.2018.118276. https://www.ncbi.nlm.nih.gov/pubmed/30005114.

34. Moushey E, Shomo A, Elder N, O'Dea C, Rahner D. Community partnered projects: Residents engaging with community health centers to improve care. *Fam Med*. 2014;46(9):718–723.

35. Summerlin HHJ, Landis SE, Olson PR. A community-oriented primary care experience for medical students and family practice residents. *Fam Med*. 1993;25(2):95–99.

36. Longlett SK, Kruse JE, Wesley RM. Community-oriented primary care: critical assessment and implications for resident education. *J Am Board Fam Pract*. 2001;14(2):141–147. Accessed Jul 18, 2023.

37. Knox KE, Lehmann W, Vogelgesang J, Simpson D. Community health, advocacy, and managing populations (CHAMP) longitudinal residency education and evaluation. *J Patient Cent Res Rev*. 2018;5(1):45–54. https://doi.org/10.17294/2330-0698.1580.

38. Longlett SK, Kruse JE, Wesley RM. Community-oriented primary care: Historical perspective. *J Am Board Fam Pract*. 2001;14(1):54–63.

39. Nutting P. *Community Oriented Primary Care: A Practical Assessment: Volume I: The Committee Report*. National Academies Press (US); 1984. http://www.ncbi.nlm.nih.gov/books/NBK217633/.

40. Takamura A, Misaki H, Takemura Y. Community and interns' perspectives on community-participatory medical education: from passive to active participation. *Fam Med.* 2017;49(7):507–513.

41. Health Equity Solutions. *Transformational Community Engagement to Advance Health Equity.* State Health and Value Strategies. https://www.rwjf.org/en/insights/our-research/2023/01/transformational-community-engagement-to-advance-health-equity.html.

42. Lehmann C, Liao W. The patient voice: Participation and engagement in family medicine practice and residency education. *Fam Med.* 2021;53(7):578–579. https://doi.org/10.22454/FamMed.2021.327569.

43. Ohta R, Ryu Y, Sano C. The contribution of citizens to community-based medical education in Japan: a systematic review. *Int J Environ Res Public Health.* 2021;18(4):1575. https://doi.org/10.3390/ijerph18041575. https://www.ncbi.nlm.nih.gov/pmc/articles/PMC7915629/.

44. Israel BA, Schulz AJ, Parker EA, et al. *Critical Issues in Developing and Following CBPR Principles.* Jossey-Bass and Pfeiffer Imprints, Wiley; 2018. https://iro.uiowa.edu/esploro/outputs/bookChapter/Critical-Issues-in-Developing-and-Following/9984214835102771.

45. Israel B, Schulz A, Parker E, et al. *Critical Issues in Developing and Following Community Based Participatory Research Principles.* 2008. https://www.semanticscholar.org/paper/Critical-issues-in-developing-and-following-based-Israel-Schulz/c4a57d13ba7f20f94a9c3c44bc343ea98cc2e6b6.

46. (OHRP) OfHRP. *The Belmont Report.* HHS.gov Web site. https://www.hhs.gov/ohrp/regulations-and-policy/belmont-report/index.html.

47. Minkler M, Wallerstein N. *Community-Based Participatory Research for Health: From Process to Outcomes.* 2 ed. Jossey-Bass; 2008:2.

48. Schlaudecker JD, Goodnow K, Goroncy A, et al. Meaningful partnerships: Stages of development of a patient and family advisory council at a family medicine residency clinic. *J Particip Med.* 2019;11(1):e12105. https://doi.org/10.2196/12105.

49. Jackson A, Blaxter L, Lewando-Hundt G. Participating in medical education: Views of patients and carers living in deprived communities. *Med Educ.* 2003;37(6):532–538. doi: 1535 [pii].

50. Crump C, Arniella G, Calman NS. Enhancing community health by improving physician participation. *J Community Med Health Educ.* 2016;6(5): 0711.1000470. Epub 2016 Oct 17. doi: 470 [pii].

51. Center for Health Care Strategies. *Design Recommendations for the Medical Member Advisory Committee.* Center for Health Care Strategies. https://www.chcs.org/resource/design-recommendations-for-the-medi-cal-member-advisory-committee/

52. Ford-Gilboe M, Wathen CN, Varcoe C, et al. How equity-oriented health care affects health: Key mechanisms and implications for primary health care practice and policy. *Milbank Q.* 2018;96(4):635–671. https://doi.org/10.1111/1468-0009.12349.

53. Yerramilli P, May FP, Kerry VB. Reducing health disparities requires financing people-centered primary care. *JAMA Health Forum.* 2021;2(2):e201573. https://doi.org/10.1001/jamahealthforum.2020.1573.

54. Schleiter K, Johnson L. Federal bills raise cap on medicare-funded residency positions and modify graduate medical education policies. *J Grad Med Educ.* 2021;13(4):602–606. https://doi.org/10.4300/JGME-D-21-00642.1. https://www.ncbi.nlm.nih.gov/pmc/articles/PMC8370355/.

55. Congressional Research Service. *Medicare Graduate Medical Education Payments: An Overview.* Congressional Research Service in Focus. 2022. https://crsreports.congress.gov/product/pdf/IF/IF10960

56. USC-Brookings Schaeffer Initiative. *Medicare Graduate Medical Education Funding Is Not Addressing the Primary Care Shortage: We Need a Radically Different Approach.* Brookings. https://www.brookings.edu/articles/medicare-graduate-medical-education-funding-is-not-addressing-the-primary-care-shortage-we-need-a-radically-different-approach/

57. Phillips RL, Bitton A. Tectonic shifts are needed in graduate medical education to ensure today's trainees are prepared to practice as tomorrow's physicians. *Acad Med.* 2014;89(11):1444–1445. https://doi.org/10.1097/ACM.0000000000000477.

58. Petterson SM, Robert L, Phillips J, Bazemore@@@ AW, Koinis GT. Unequal distribution of the U.S. primary care workforce. *afp.* 2013;87(11):online-online. https://www.aafp.org/pubs/afp/issues/2013/0601/od1.html

59. Weinstein DF. Optimizing GME by measuring its outcomes. *N Engl J Med.* 2017;377(21):2007–2009. https://doi.org/10.1056/NEJMp1711483.

60. Phillips KE, Haft H, Rauner B. *The key to Improving Population Health and Reducing Disparities: Primary Care Investment.* Health Affairs Forefront. https://www.healthaffairs.org/do/10.1377/forefront.20220725.733955/full/ doi: 10.1377/forefront.20220725.733955.

61. Chen C, Petterson S, Phillips RL, Mullan F, Bazemore A, O'Donnell SD. Toward graduate medical education (GME) accountability: measuring the outcomes of GME institutions. *Acad Med.* 2013;88(9):1267–1280. https://doi.org/10.1097/ACM.0b013e31829a3ce9.

62. Basu S, Berkowitz SA, Phillips RL, Bitton A, Landon BE, Phillips RS. Association of primary care physician supply with population mortality in the united states, 2005-2015. *JAMA Intern Med.* 2019;179(4):506–514. https://doi.org/10.1001/jamainternmed.2018.7624.

63. Fraher EKA, Holmes M. *A Methodology for Using Workforce Data to Decide Which Specialties and States to Target for GME Expansion.* https://www.shepscenter.unc.edu/wp-content/uploads/2016/12/y2_FraherKnaptonHolmes_ExecSumm_final.pdf

64. Chen C, Chen F, Mullan F. Teaching health centers: a new paradigm in graduate medical education. *Acad Med.* 2012;87(12):1752–1756. https://doi.org/10.1097/ACM.0b013e3182720f4d. https://www.ncbi.nlm.nih.gov/pmc/articles/PMC3761371/.

65. Green L, Miller W, Frey J, et al. The time is now: a plan to redesign family medicine residency education. *Fam Med*. 2022;54(1):7–15. https://doi.org/10.22454/FamMed.2022.197486. https://familymedicine/2022/january/gotler-2021-0315/.

66. Grumbach K. Forging a social movement to dismantle entrenched power and liberate primary care as a common good. *Ann Fam Med*. 2023;21(2):180–184. https://doi.org/10.1370/afm.2950. https://www.annfammed.org/content/21/2/180.

67. Parsons A, Unaka NI, Stewart C, et al. Seven practices for pursuing equity through learning health systems: notes from the field. *Learn Health Syst*. 2021;5(3):e10279. https://doi.org/10.1002/lrh2.10279. https://www.ncbi.nlm.nih.gov/pmc/articles/PMC8278437/.

68. Health Resources and Services Administration. *Rural Residency Planning and Development (RRPD) Program*. HRSA. https://www.hrsa.gov/rural-health/grants/rural-health-research-policy/rrpd.

69. Klink KA, Albanese AP, Bope ET, Sanders KM. Veterans affairs graduate medical education expansion addresses U.S. physician workforce needs. *Acad Med*. 2022;97(8):1144–1150. https://doi.org/10.1097/ACM.0000000000004545. https://www.ncbi.nlm.nih.gov/pmc/articles/PMC9311468/.

70. Kaufman A, Scott M, Andazola J, Fitzsimmons-Pattison D, Parajón L. Social accountability and graduate medical education. *Fam Med*. 2021;53(7):632–637. https://doi.org/10.22454/FamMed.2021.160888. https://familymedicine/2021/july-august/scott-2020-0565/.

71. Burke L, Khullar D, Orav EJ, Zheng J, Frakt A, Jha AK. Do academic medical centers disproportionately benefit the sickest patients? *Health Aff (Millwood)*. 2018;37(6):864–872. https://doi.org/10.1377/hlthaff.2017.1250.

72. Burke LG, Burke RC, Orav EJ, Duggan CE, Figueroa JF, Jha AK. Association of academic medical center presence with clinical outcomes at neighboring community hospitals among medicare beneficiaries. *JAMA Netw Open*. 2023;6(2):e2254559. https://doi.org/10.1001/jamanetworkopen.2022.54559. https://www.ncbi.nlm.nih.gov/pmc/articles/PMC9892959/.

73. Burke LG, Frakt AB, Khullar D, Orav EJ, Jha AK. Association between teaching status and mortality in US hospitals. *JAMA*. 2017;317(20):2105–2113. https://doi.org/10.1001/jama.2017.5702.

74. Gourevitch MN. Population health and the academic medical center: the time is right. *Acad Med*. 2014;89(4):544–549. https://doi.org/10.1097/ACM.0000000000000171. https://www.ncbi.nlm.nih.gov/pmc/articles/PMC4024242/.

ANNOTATED BIBLIOGRAPHY

Chen C, Petterson S, Phillips RL, Mullan F, Bazemore A, O'Donnell MS. Towards graduate medical education (GME) accountability: measuring the outcomes of GME institutions. *Acad Med*. 2013;88(9):1267.
A description of current workforce-related outcomes from GME funding and how these outcomes likely contribute to health and health equity.

Nutting PA, Connor E. *Community Oriented Primary Care: A Practical Assessment*. National Academies; 1984.
A foundational textbook of the concept of community-oriented primary care, this chapter describes a framework for assessing the effectiveness of the integration.

Israel BA, Schulz AJ, Parker EA, Becker AB. *Critical issues in developing and following community-based participatory research principles. Community-Based Participatory Research for Health*. Jossey-Bass; 2008:47–62.
This chapter lays the foundation for community-based participatory research, critical in this case for understanding the walkover between the community-directed aspects of CBPR and community-directed GME.

Phillips Jr RL, George BC, Holmboe ES, Bazemore AW, Westfall JM, Bitton A. Measuring graduate medical education outcomes to honor the social contract. *Acad Med*. 2022;97(5):643.
This paper describes the need and framework for GME accountability at the individual and system level to nudge the institution toward more just and equitable outcomes.

14

Social Responsibility as the North Star to Transform Medical Education

Miriam Hoffman, Ofelia Martinez, Kimberly M. Birdsall, Ora Batash, and Carmela Rocchetti

SUMMARY

Medical education is an extension and a core component of medicine and health care. It therefore has a fundamental responsibility to address the needs and problems of the society and communities it serves. While many medical schools articulate some aspect of this social responsibility in their aspirational missions, it is imperative and possible for a medical school's social responsibility to be the driving force behind the comprehensive development of the educational program. This should drive the content, methods, and structures of the school. Additionally, each institution should take a systematic approach to effectively translate lofty goals into specific activities, programs, and structures, enabling program evaluation and outcome assessment.

This chapter describes a transferable model that uses a philosophy and principles-driven framework that guided the comprehensive development of a new school of medicine. As a school tasked with building an educational program that addresses societal needs, we utilized a systematic, mission-driven approach to guide the development of the curriculum, pedagogical methods, and the structure of the educational program itself. This expands the context of medical education and the parties involved in the process of training health care professionals and involves partnering and integrating with entities from three realms: education/academic, health care delivery, and the community. These mutually beneficial partnerships strengthen the training students receive and can leverage medical education and trainees as drivers of change. This can be a challenging process as it amplifies voices not historically prioritized in medicine and medical education and requires institutional change and culture change.

We challenge medical schools to meet their obligation to address societal problems, redefine the context and partners involved in medical education, and provide a framework and guidance to move this work forward.

INTRODUCTION

Medical education, an extension and core component of medicine and health care, aims to address the needs and problems of the society and communities it serves. While many medical schools aspire to express some aspect of social responsibility in their mission statements, it is both imperative and possible for a medical school to actively pursue the development of a socially responsible and comprehensive educational program.

Social responsibility must drive the school's content, methods, and structures. Moreover, the school must take a systematic approach to ensure the effective translation of lofty goals into specific activities, programs, and structures within each institution, enabling program evaluation and outcome assessment. This chapter presents a transferable model using a philosophy and principles-driven framework that guided the comprehensive development of a new school of medicine and can serve as an example of how to enable medical education to meet its societal responsibility.[1-4]

This approach expands the context of medical education to include partners from three realms: educational/academic, health care delivery, and the community in the process of training health care professionals. Incorporating these partners can be challenging as it brings in voices not historically prioritized in medicine and medical education, demanding institutional and cultural change. We urge medical schools to fulfill their obligation to address societal problems, redefine the context and partners involved in medical education, and provide a framework and guidance to advance this work forward.

THE IMPERATIVE FOR CHANGE

The past century has seen remarkable advancements in medical science and technology. Our understanding of disease, bolstered by groundbreaking research and innovation, has transformed the landscape of health care, leading to a substantial increase in life expectancy globally. However, this progress has not been a universal experience; stark discrepancies persist, evidenced by an ongoing decline in life expectancy paired with exorbitantly rising health care costs particularly in the United States, as seen in Fig. 14.1.

Medical education represents a potent and necessary catalyst for meaningful change. Given its foundational role in shaping future health care providers, medical education has a unique capacity to embed new understandings, practices, and values deeply and durably, thereby making it a key driver for systematic change.[5-8]

Unfortunately, the historic design and execution of medical education predominantly focused on the **biological determinants of health**.[9,10] This approach, while indispensable, does not holistically encompass the complex, intersecting factors that contribute significantly to patient outcomes. Reflecting on the case in Box 14.1, a robust knowledge base on the pathophysiology and treatments

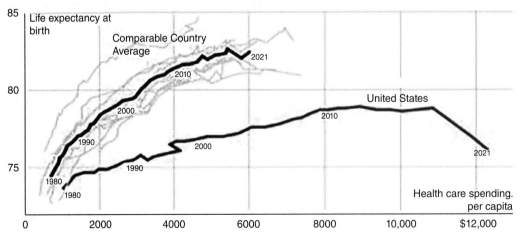

Fig. 14.1 Widening of life expectancy and health care spending discrepancies between the United States and comparable countries. (From Kurani N, Wager E. *How Does the Quality of the U.S. Health System Compare to Other Countries?* Peterson-KFF Health System Tracker; 2022. https://www.healthsystemtracker.org/chart-collection/quality-u-s-healthcare-system-compare-countries/.)

BOX 14.1 Case Example

Mr. S often visited the emergency department for asthma-related issues. He was well known to the doctors and staff at his local urban community hospital. After one recent emergency department visit, he was offered the opportunity to enroll in a direct **community health worker (CHW)** care coordination program.

Upon meeting with Mr. S, understanding his needs, and trying to conduct a home visit, the CHW learned that although he had insurance through Medicaid, he did not have regular primary care provider because no local providers were accepting new Medicaid patients. When he tried to see a doctor at the **federally qualified health center (FQHC)**, the care was good, but it took all day—even with an appointment. Mr. S shared that he prefers to go to the emergency department because it is closer to his home, it takes less time, and in his opinion, he receives better care.

Over the past 6 months, he has sought care in the emergency department ten times, resulting in multiple courses of steroids, antibiotics, admissions to the hospital, and many long days waiting to feel well enough to be discharged to home.

Aside from his challenge of finding a regular source of primary care, his main concern is his housing. When his landlord died a year ago, the building was sold to a developer, and he was evicted. Formerly a chef, he has been unemployed for 3 years and receives public food assistance plus $1000.00 per month from disability. The lowest cost housing he can find is $1200 per month, and no one will approve his application. He is on the subsidized housing waitlist, but it generally takes 5 years to obtain a subsidized housing voucher and find an apartment in his community.

To avoid staying in a shelter, Mr. S sleeps on a couch in a relative's basement. Mr. S expresses concerns about disrupted sleep due to frequent coughing and needing to wake up at night to use his albuterol inhaler. He feels the mold, dust, and cold temperature in the basement makes his asthma worse, but he frequently does not have the resources to purchase his over-the-counter allergy medications.

Mr. S expresses frustration about constantly feeling unwell and the frequent disruptions to his life due to his poor asthma control. He is knowledgeable about what triggers his asthma but is not able to control the triggers.

Upon further questioning, he shares that in exchange for his current housing, Mr. S gives his monthly food benefit to the family he is staying with; however, the food is regularly and quickly consumed by the four children in the household. This leaves him no choice but to walk across town for his one meal a day at the soup kitchen.

for asthma would be insufficient to care for Mr. S. His care requires a holistic and integrated approach to the factors that impact his health but are beyond his biology or genetics, such as his physical environment, lack of finances, and lack of access to care and medications. This may require a team of professionals, beyond just the physician.

The structural challenges which are often overlooked are the **social determinants of health (SDoH)**. SDoH refers to the variety of societal structures and influences that shape the conditions in which people are born, grow, live, work, and age.[11] These include, but are not limited to, socioeconomic status, education, neighborhood and physical environment, employment, race, social support networks, and access to health care. The collective impact of these determinants on an individual's health can be profound and far-reaching, influencing a wide range of health, functioning, and quality-of-life outcomes as well as risks as exemplified by Mr. S.

The traditional medical curriculum has been insufficient in equipping trainees with the knowledge, tools, and skills needed to adequately understand and respond to these social determinants. This critical educational gap has contributed to a multifaceted health care system that often fails to address the social context of disease, resulting in ongoing inequities in health care access, quality, and outcomes. Traditional medical education has also inadvertently failed its trainees by releasing them into a complex health care landscape without sufficient understanding of social determinants. This deficiency can lead to a sense of inadequacy, exacerbating provider burnout, and contributing to higher physician mortality rates.[12,13] It is imperative that we improve our educational approaches to better prepare and support our trainees, ensuring they are equipped not only to survive but to thrive in their vital roles.

The issues elucidated in the previous paragraph provide a glimpse into the profound challenges currently overshadowing health care in the United States.[14,15] These challenges underscore the urgent need for a paradigm shift in medical education. Our call to action is therefore that medical education must be reshaped and systematically driven by its responsibility to understand and address societal problems. While numerous medical schools incorporate elements of social accountability into their mission statements, often this commitment fails to go beyond words in a mission statement or it remains siloed in limited curricular offerings or extracurricular community service. It is not sufficient for societal needs to merely *inform* the work of medical education. Instead, social needs should become the primary driving force in the comprehensive development of the medical education program.[16–19]

This shift involves a reorientation, moving beyond a sole focus on biological determinants, to integrate the complex web of multiple interacting determinants of health (DoH)

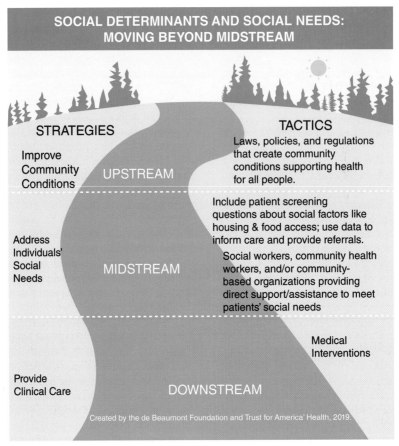

Fig. 14.2 Visual representation of the expanded lens needed to address root causes of poor health outcomes. (From Castrucci B, Auerbach J. *Meeting Individual Social Needs Falls Short of Addressing Social Determinants of Health.* Health Affairs Forefront; 2019. https://debeaumont.org/news/2019/meeting-individual-social-needs-falls-short-of-addressing-social-determinants-of-health/.)

into the heart of the curriculum. As illustrated by Fig. 14.2, social responsibility necessitates moving even earlier in the causal chain, to the upstream structural determinants that create the conditions, social policies, and other factors that drive health outcomes.

DRIVING CHANGE THROUGH EDUCATION

Comprehensive change in medical education represents a foundational step toward repairing and rebuilding an equitable and effective health care delivery system in the United States and lays the groundwork for meaningful progress in policy, practice, and patient engagement. Our approach to this transformation hinges on nurturing a culture rooted in relationship building, trust, and collaboration. To achieve this, we employ a systematic, mission-driven approach to

inform the development of our curriculum, instructional methods, and the overall structure of the educational program. This transformation seeks to prepare future health care leaders with the necessary competencies to comprehend and navigate the social context of health and disease. Our ultimate goal is to bridge gaps in care, form lasting partnerships, rebuild trust, and improve patient outcomes, creating a more equitable, responsive, and resilient health care system.

The Hackensack Meridian School of Medicine: A Case Study

Context

The Hackensack Meridian School of Medicine (HMSOM) in New Jersey illustrates how a socially accountable mission guided the development and structure of the school, incorporating regional as well as national societal needs. The school matriculated its charter class in the fall of 2018 and is a private medical school, housed within Hackensack Meridian Health, a large integrated health system.

New Jersey contains a unique context and a population with a set of demographic characteristics that mirrors the United States as a whole. New Jersey is recognized as one of the most socioeconomically and racially diverse states in the nation and has inequities in outcomes similar to what is seen nationally. Therefore this local context can provide a lens to view and consider the broader national landscape, as much of the health outcomes data mirror the national data available. One example in maternal mortality is shown in Figs. 14.3 and 14.4. These figures demonstrate

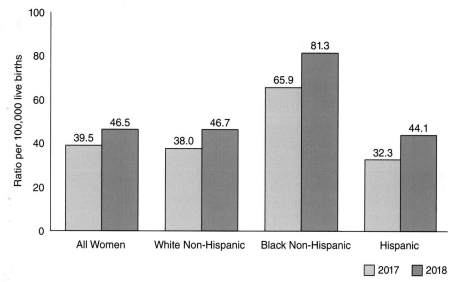

Fig. 14.3 NJ pregnancy-associated deaths by race/ethnicity. (New Jersey State Health Assessment Data. https://www-doh.state.nj.us/doh-shad/topic/Births.html.)

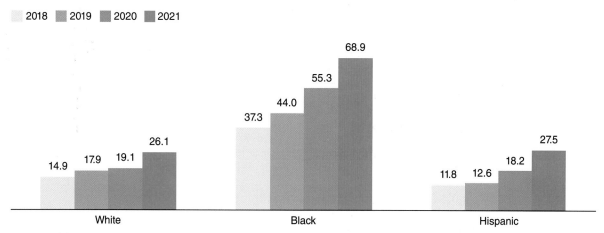

Fig. 14.4 Maternal mortality by race/ethnicity in the United States. (From Hill L, Artiga S, Ranji U. *Racial Equity and Health Policy Issue Brief.* KFF; 2022. https://www.kff.org/racial-equity-and-health-policy/issue-brief/racial-disparities-in-maternal-and-infant-health-current-status-and-efforts-to-address-them/.)

that maternal mortality is higher for Black women and that this inequity has worsened over time. Fig. 14.3 shows this trend in the context of New Jersey, while Fig. 14.4 shows this parallel trend in the United States broadly. The graphs illustrate differences in outcomes based on race and ethnicity. Although the terms "race" and "ethnicity" were historically understood as biologic, they are in fact social constructs. This concerning trend is but one example of the health inequities our school and our graduates are committed to addressing.

Additionally, the Hackensack Meridian Health network is the largest integrated health network in the state and spans north, central, and southern New Jersey, providing connection and insight to a wide variety of communities and needs. HMSOM utilizes the breadth of communities and clinical sites across the health system, including a wide range of types of municipalities and socioeconomic settings. As a result, the school is well positioned to serve as a case study of how to develop a systematic educational framework that is rooted in its social responsibility, both locally aware and responsive, and nationally relevant. Since the school's inception, HMSOM has been designed with a purpose: to address the health needs of its regional communities and beyond.

Systematic Mission-Driven Framework

When the original developers and partners convened to build a new medical school in New Jersey, the first focus was on developing the vision for the school. The vision developed by these collaborators' states: *Each person in New Jersey, and in the United States, regardless of race or socioeconomic status, will enjoy the highest levels of wellness in an economically and behaviorally sustainable fashion.* Once articulated, this gave clear direction to the goals and purpose of the school and led to the creation of the foundational philosophy upon which further development would rest. This philosophy asserts that a medical education program should fundamentally be designed to meet the needs and challenges that are facing the communities and society it is intended to serve.

We realize that this vision is broad and aspirational, as most vision statements are. In fact, our favorite definition of the word "vision" is *how is the world going to be different because of the work we are doing together?* We challenge all medical schools to create vision statements that are aspirational, driven by society's needs, and challenge the institution to meet their responsibility to society. The reality is that we have and will encounter challenges related to buy-in, engagement, and prioritization. Anticipating resistance and challenges is critical to enable success. Having a systematic approach to implementing a mission is an effective tool when faced with challenges. Additionally, areas

prioritized by the philosophy and its linked principles are beyond the historic focus of medical education. We do not intend to suggest that our team of medical educators and administrators will directly overhaul public policy, financial systems, or the social safety net. Rather, the foundational embedding of our vision into all aspects of the school is designed to develop the next generation of physicians who will incorporate this responsibility and their skills to implement changes in whatever career paths they choose—from individual patient care, population health, public policy, systems change, and more.

At the HMSOM, this informs all aspects of the educational program. Embracing our "blank slate," we worked deeply and intentionally to ensure that our mission informed every facet of the educational program—from curricular content to pedagogical methods and structural design. In this section we delve deeper into how the school's mission has been the driver of the content of the curriculum, the methods used, and the structure of the school itself.[20]

Philosophy

The foundational philosophy of the HMSOM includes three interconnected parts:

Part 1: A medical education program should be intentionally designed to meet society's health needs and to address relevant societal challenges head-on. In the context of the United States health care system currently, this includes poor quality of health outcomes, unacceptable health inequities, and poor value (i.e., high cost, poor quality) in the health care system.

Part 2: The pedagogical methods, curricular structure, and school programs and systems should be implemented to address the societal problems identified. This ensures that not only the content, but the methods and systems contribute meaningfully to mitigating the identified challenges.

Part 3: Responsible stewardship of resources is imperative. The structure and content of the educational program should be designed to ensure responsible stewardship of resources—belonging to the student, the institution, and society—with the goal of achieving the most value and effectiveness for the time and resources invested.

Once this three-part foundational philosophy was clearly defined, the team leading the development of the medical school created guiding principles that mapped directly to this three-part philosophy.

Guiding Principles

Six principles were derived from the foundational philosophy. These principles bridge from the higher-level philosophy to their application in the techniques. Table 14.1

TABLE 14.1 Six Principles Derived From the Foundational Philosophy

Principle A: Because the US health care system is fragmented, siloed, and dis-integrated from community and social systems and services, the determinants of health (i.e., a broad and integrated framework that includes all drivers of health outcomes), should inform the design and implementation of the curriculum.

It should drive both curricular content and curricular structure. Focus should be placed on integrating across traditional institutional and professional silos to guide the design and creation of all academic structures. Efforts should also be made to prevent silos from developing.

Principle B: Because community and context have a significant impact on health outcomes, a longitudinal community-engaged medical education program for learners should be implemented as a core aspect of the curriculum. This program should expose learners to the determinants of health and hone their skills in addressing them. This part of the curriculum should focus on individuals and populations and use a service-learning structure.

Principle C: Because the cognitive decisions that physicians make directly impact the quality, equity, and value of the health outcomes achieved, medical education training should address and target: (1) the ever-growing body of medical knowledge; (2) the development of higher order cognitive skills with learning that is deep, meaningful, and long-lasting, well beyond short-term test-taking hurdles; and (3) individual responsibility to use cognitive abilities to be part of the solution to societal problems.

Therefore, the curriculum should: (1) develop the students' ability to critically reason with a focus on patient-oriented and outcomes-focused clinical reasoning; (2) prioritize higher order cognitive goals, including active application of knowledge; (3) build competence in lifelong self-directed learning and adaptive expertise; and (4) set a competency expectation of a high level of clinical reasoning and diagnostic thinking that integrates basic science, clinical science, and health systems science early in the trajectory of medical training.[a]

Principle D: Physicians have a responsibility to advocate for and lead improvements to the structural determinants that diminish health outcomes and equity. Therefore, the curriculum should train students to understand and be skilled in addressing all determinants of health (DoH) on individual patient, population, and structural levels (i.e., micro-, meso-, and macro-system levels). Further, a professional identity formation curriculum should be leveraged to incorporate physician responsibility in areas related to all DoH.

Principle E: Because the identities and backgrounds of the physician workforce impact patient care, school programs and systems should promote the development of a diverse physician workforce that is optimized to produce high-quality, high-value, equitable health care.

Principle F: Because medical students have a range of developmental trajectories and time required to achieve competency, the educational program should be individualized to achieve: (1) the development of advanced skills, degrees, and certifications in each student related to their professional and educational goals; (2) flexibility of the educational program to support the development of core competencies, based on individual student developmental needs and time required; and (3) financial responsibility maximizing efficiency and minimizing educational debt.

These principles bridge from the higher level philosophy to their application in the techniques.

For example, our focus in evidence-based medicine goes beyond classroom-based epidemiology and critical appraisal and builds information mastery skills. This includes prioritizing patient-oriented evidence (e.g., mortality) rather than disease-oriented evidence (e.g., proxy markers such as blood test results). This is to counteract the reality that much medical decision-making is driven by expert opinion, assumptions about the impact of interventions on patient-oriented outcomes, and evidence that is lower on the hierarchy of evidence.

[a]We realize that a lot of medical schools will have articulated goals and curricula that sound similar to this principle. However, the crux of this principle is that the cognitive skills developed by the medical school curriculum should be singularly driven by the physician's responsibility to make clinical decisions that improve health outcomes and equity.

contains an explanation of each principle and demonstrates how each links to the foundational philosophy.

Techniques

Each principle above is linked to specific techniques that are the realization of the principles in the context of our school. These include curricular content, as well as methods and structure.

We provide three examples of our techniques and demonstrate how they are the application of a specific principle in our school's setting.

Example 1: Patient Presentation Problem-Based Learning Curriculum. The longitudinal **Patient Presentation Problem-Based Learning Curriculum (PPPC)** ensures a patient is at the center of student learning every week across phase 1 (16-month preclerkship curriculum). Students are presented with a case at the beginning of each week, which is analyzed in a stepwise manner. Students work in teams to determine the key clinical data, inclusive of determinants of health, to arrive at a reasonable differential diagnosis, diagnostic work-up, and plan. Students are expected to explain the relevance of the clinical data as they learn more content in each of the sessions during the week. All content that the students learn during the week—from the basic, clinical, and health systems science—links to the weekly case in some fashion. Cases integrate content from all determinants of health which we organized as biological, genetic, social, environmental, behavioral, and access to care. As a consolidating exercise, students generate a **concept map** each week integrating content from all the sciences and "tag" their concept map with the relevant determinants. The creation of weekly concept maps enables students to actively connect all scientific content to the determinants of health. In fact, it makes the determinants of health the lens through which students learn the entire curriculum. Cases are synthesized in small groups at the end of the week, so that students are able to validate their knowledge and apply it in a clinical context.

Each concept map shows how all content (basic, clinical, and health systems science) is framed using the weekly patient case and how students think about and link factors from all the determinants of health to the material they are learning. They then synthesize this to come to a holistic and integrated understanding of the factors at play in the patient's illness and clinical presentation.

This core component of our curriculum is an application of *Principle A*, which aims to harness the broad and integrated framework of the determinants of health in the design and implementation of the entire curriculum. It provides students with a broad lens into which they integrate what they are learning throughout medical school, enabling them to incorporate all the determinants into their clinical reasoning, diagnostic thinking, and patient management.

Example 2: Health Systems Science and the Human Dimension. The **health systems science** (HSS) longitudinal curriculum is a core thread of the curriculum alongside the clinical and basic sciences. HSS includes the principles, methods, and practice of improving quality, outcomes, and costs of health care delivery for patients and populations within a system of medical care. It includes the factors that impact health outcomes beyond the basic and clinical sciences. Students learn:

1. How health care systems and systems that affect health are structured, how they work, and what the drivers in a system are. This includes policy, financing, health law, medical ethics, health care inequities, and the determinants of health.
2. How to understand, use, and generate information and data via training in epidemiology, biostatistics, evidence-based medicine, information mastery, and research methods and
3. How to integrate 1 and 2 in order to think about medicine and the promotion of health (or disease) as occurring within a system. This includes public health, population health, quality improvement, and technology in medicine.

This core component of our curriculum is the application of a number of our principles, including *Principle D*, which focuses on training students to understand and be skilled in addressing all DoH on individual patient, population, and structural levels (i.e., micro-, meso-, and macro-system levels) in order to effect change. HSS content is critical in training students to be physicians who can shape the health care system to be one that addresses the three-part problem articulated in our foundational philosophy: (1) poor quality of health care outcomes, (2) poor value in the health care system, and (3) unacceptable health care inequities. To be effective physicians and leaders in the current and future landscape, students need competency in these areas to effect meaningful change at the level of the individual patient as well as at the level of populations and communities.

Our curriculum takes this further and integrates HSS with the Human Dimension curriculum which is a **community-engaged medical education** program (Box 14.2) that includes a focus on advocacy and systems. Knowledge and skills learned in the HSS thread are applied in the experiential service learning of the Human Dimension, which lasts the entire core curriculum. **Cultural humility** and professional identity formation are important synergistic aspects of this curriculum supporting achievement of these goals and competencies. Components of the Human Dimension include:

1. *Human Dimension Voices Program*, where students are matched with families from underserved areas for 3 years. Students become involved in all aspects of the family's life to understand the drivers of health, provide education, and navigate community resources to help the family to address goals they identify related to their health and well-being.
2. *Community Assessment and Community Health Projects*, where small groups of students are longitudinally immersed in a local community to complete a systematic community assessment identifying assets and challenges

BOX 14.2   Community-Engaged Medical Education—A Student's Experience

During Andy's first week of medical school, he and his small group were immersed in a nearby historically under-resourced community through a series of structured activities including a windshield tour, service learning, and meeting with community partners. On his first visit, Andy was struck by the traffic congestion in the community and considered the need to take mass transit on his subsequent visits to the area. A few weeks later, he returned to interview a community stakeholder, the director of a local food bank. Remembering the traffic, he considered taking mass transit but wasn't able to easily map out a quick route from his apartment, so he drove again. During the interview, the director of the food bank shared the many assets and challenges the organization and its clients face. Transportation to and from the facility was often a problem and limited not only the type of food clients could receive but also the quantities.

A few weeks later, Andy and a fellow student were paired with a family from the same community. This student dyad was assigned to develop a longitudinal relationship with this family over 3 years and work with that family to connect them to resources, help them access and navigate the medical system, and provide them with health education. Early on, it became clear the family needed to establish care with a primary care doctor. The diligent students eagerly researched local physicians to find that there was not a primary care provider or medical facility nearby nor easily accessible by bus, which was the family's main mode of transportation. When the students returned to discuss this with the family, they learned this gap in mass transit coverage was not only limiting the family's access to health care but to other important resources including employment opportunities. Andy and his partner continued to work with this family through their preclerkship and clerkship time.

As these students approached the end of the clerkship rotations, they actively took on the task of developing individual capstone advocacy projects. Each student identified a specific challenge and crafted a proposal to address it. Andy, determined to tackle the transportation limitation in the area where his matched family lived, set out to find a practical solution, even though he was initially unsure of the exact approach. Over the course of the year, he followed a capstone curriculum and was mentored by faculty and community leaders. Ultimately, Andy was able to create awareness about the lack of bus routes in the community, meet with the transit bus company, collect the data they requested, and propose a new bus route. Wanting to see his proposal get implemented, Andy continued this capstone initiative as a Phase 3 fourth-year student community elective, where he dedicated time to work on this advocacy project. At the time of Andy's graduation, the transit company added a bus route to the area, increasing the community's access to an abundance of resources.

Through this process the determinants of health came to life for Andy. He was able to learn the skills necessary to identify a problem, develop partnerships, and work collaboratively to build effective solutions while providing a tremendous service to the family and community he worked with.

---

of the community. This leads to a community health project, addressing an identified challenge that the student group implements with their community partners.

3. *Human Dimension Capstone,* where each student completes a scholarly project focusing on one DoH, including a literature-grounded analysis and proposed systems-level solution.

Example 3: 3+1 Curriculum Model. The overall structure of our curriculum is a 3+1 model. This means that all students complete the same generally 3-year core curriculum followed by an individualized Phase 3. Students work with their advisers and mentors to build a program that meets their professional and educational goals as well as their developmental needs. It enables them to meet their academic requirements in the amount of time they need, addresses their personal and financial needs, and sets them up for success in their identified areas of interest and growth. Combined with the individualized final 5 months of the core curriculum, this affords students 17 months of individualization of their educational program. This approach provides flexibility, allowing students to focus on areas of interest and enhancing knowledge and skills when needed, without incurring additional financial debt. Students choose from a wide variety of offerings, including obtaining a master's degree or certificate, clinical immersions, research experiences, community-based projects, and electives, all designed to meet educational competencies. The Phase 3 Residency (P3R) program allows students to graduate after the 3-year core curriculum and enter residency within Hackensack Meridian Health.

This not only supports diversity in the student body and clinician workforce, but also removes obstacles for learners to fully explore aspects of medicine and other fields related to their interests.

There are multiple ways in which this structure provides financial and economic value, as targeted in *Part 3 of our*

Foundational Philosophy. This is an important goal given the impact of debt and finances on student career choice, practice patterns, and overall societal educational debt burden. Students can graduate in 3 years after completing their core requirements, entering the workforce 1 year earlier and with 1 year less of educational debt. They can also obtain a graduate degree or certificate, graduating in 4 years with two degrees. The robust advising process leading to each student's individualized program also provides experiences that are goal-oriented and higher impact than what is typically seen in fourth-year medical school curricula.

This structural aspect of our curriculum is the application of *Principle F*, which recognizes that each medical student comes to their education from a unique position and that programs should be individualized to support their success both within and beyond medical school. In addition, for students who need more time to achieve their foundational competencies than given in the 3-year core curriculum, part of their individualized time can be used to accommodate the longer time needed in the core curriculum. It is important to highlight that one fixed structure and length for a medical school curriculum will not support the needs of all students. Some can accelerate their program and goals (e.g., graduating in 3 years or obtaining two degrees in 4 years), and some will need more time to achieve success in the core curriculum. This individualized approach also supports students from various backgrounds, including those who are historically underrepresented in medicine. This structural intervention allows students the flexibility they may need and plays a crucial role in diversifying the health care workforce, supporting the achievement of *Principle E*.

Toward Achieving Our Mission

The school has graduated three classes, with physicians who are thriving in their residency training. Students and graduates are having great success in their clinical performance and on all national licensing examinations. For example, the most recent Association of American Medical Colleges (AAMC) Resident Readiness Survey assessing our graduates' residency performance, residency program directors reported 100% of graduates met or exceeded overall performance expectations; in addition, 28% of our first graduating class have been appointed as chief residents. This suggests that a school can achieve both clinical and academic success while building social accountability robustly into the educational program and its expectations of students. The success of the school's ability to realize its philosophy and goals has been recognized by regional accreditors. Likewise, the school recently received full accreditation from the Liaison Committee on Medical Education, another marker of the success and execution of this mission-driven program.

MAKING CHANGE AND TRANSFERRING TO YOUR CONTEXT

The utilization of our systematic mission-driven approach to guide the development of curriculum, pedagogical methods, and the structure of the educational program can be applied to new schools or existing schools that are undergoing curricular reform. This can be done in part or in whole but in order to advance this social responsibility mission-driven work across the medical educational system, all schools must be challenged to incorporate some actionable pieces of the approach. Institutions may be resistant to full adoption, which is why the approach enables—and encourages—the incorporation of at least some fundamentals without necessarily changing everything. Although the foundational philosophy and principles are held constant, every school exists in a unique context with specific mission, maturity level, resources, strengths, and challenges. As such, the implementation techniques and timeframe will be unique to each school or program.

Understanding and Analyzing Your Context

When social responsibility is the comprehensive driving force behind an educational program, it is necessary to have a deep understanding of many aspects of the local context in which the program will operate. It is an iterative process with leaders from the medical school, the community, and the health care delivery system which involves face-to-face meetings, ongoing discussions, and work sessions. It involves asking and answering questions, identifying priorities, strengths, and challenges, and takes dedicated time, focus, and a skilled team. It is, however, worth the investment as this is the critical first step to a successful integration of your mission-driven approach.

Three components of your context should be analyzed in order to solidify partnerships, understand motives, establish priorities, obtain buy-in, and ultimately implement your mission-driven approach. These components are: (1) the local community, (2) the health care delivery system, and (3) the educational landscape.

The information and questions below are not exhaustive, but examples of the types of issues and considerations you should engage with. Identifying the right stakeholders and constituencies to find the answers to these questions will vary by setting. Sometimes the information you are seeking will be explicit and even part of published reports, and sometimes it will be more complex and take more time to learn.

Understanding Your Community

There are many ways that societies assess and understand the nature, priorities, and needs of their communities. Currently, in the United States, the health status and

---

BOX 14.3 Understanding Your Local Community—Questions to Ask

- How do you define your community?
- What are the cultural norms of your community?
- What are the demographics and social determinants of health specific to the community?
- What are the key health care inequities?
- What are the assets in the community?
- What are the main challenges facing community members?
- Who are the people/organizations community members go to when they are in need?
- Who are the official and unofficial leaders of the community?
- What is the role of the local health department?
- What is the relationship of the local health department to the state?
- How does the health department function within the community?
- Are political priorities and the needs of the people in your community aligned?

BOX 14.4 Understanding Local Health Care Delivery Systems—Questions to Ask

- Are you working with one or multiple health care delivery providers in your location?
- What is the relationship between the community and local health care providers? What is the level of trust?
- Are there existing community-based programs that deliver services such as community health centers?
- What is the landscape of health care payors? How are payor networks structured and how does this impact the delivery of care?
- What are the financial drivers in the health care landscape? For example, are health insurance programs incentivizing care management and population health?
- What are the motivations of physicians and other health care providers?
- Are there adequate physical and financial resources for providers to deliver care?
- What is the relationship between the health care delivery institution(s) and the academic institution (ownership, financial, affiliation, etc.)?
- Where are there areas for mission-driven collaboration and partnership between the health care delivery partners?
- What impact would the incorporation of a mission-driven approach have financially on the health care delivery system?

---

priorities of a community can be identified through review of the publicly available community health needs assessments (CHNA) and community health improvement plan (CHIP) documents. These documents are updated every 3 to 5 years and will provide foundational information about the demographics, socio-economics, health status, key health inequities, and main challenges facing the community as well as the long-term plan to address these issues.

This is important information but not enough to fully understand the community. To ensure a comprehensive understanding of the community, we must take a combined qualitative and quantitative approach as well as the time necessary to learn the community's unwritten cultural norms, priorities, anchor institutions, assets, trusted local leaders/organizations, and political landscape. This is an ongoing process of understanding and must be updated periodically because as communities change—through political leadership, demographics, etc.—the community context will likely change (Box 14.3).

Understanding Your Health Care Delivery System

The health care delivery system where medical students will learn and practice clinically is a critical component of their training and professional identity formation. As such, it is important to integrate your mission, philosophy, and approach into the health care delivery system, as much as possible. This will take time, patience, and perseverance, and begins with analyzing the nuances of the system including its

network, funding structure, mission, and the motivation of health care providers. Understanding your health care system, however it is structured, enables you to identify avenues for collaboration to support the integration of your mission-driven approach. It is important to note that educational institutions will have varying types of relationships and degrees of influence on health care delivery, so building allies and partners is critical, as described in the "Building Institutional Support and Making Change" section (Box 14.4).

Understanding Your Academic Landscape

Another key contextual factor to understand is the educational landscape of your medical school or training program. There are many shapes and forms of academic partnerships and alliances which can create opportunities as well as challenges for your mission-driven agenda. Assessing the institutional landscape is a similar process to assessing the community or health care landscape, in that you need to understand the priorities, mission, resources, and leaders.

Developing an understanding of the landscape will take time and attention as academic relationships take many

BOX 14.5   Understanding Your Educational Landscape—Questions to Ask

- What is the history, mission, and foundational principles of the organizations that are part of your educational landscape?
- What is the organizational and financial structure of the institution?
- What is the relationship between the community and the academic institutions? What is the level of trust?
- Are there other programs that can be integrated into your approach such as nursing, public health, social work, law, political science?
- What are the power structures and dynamics within the institution and between the institution and the community?
- What are research and scholarship opportunities?
- Are there advocates/champions of your model within the institution including at the leadership level?
- Does the health care system train other learners and trainees? How does this impact capacity for your learners and opportunities for collaboration?
- What impact would the incorporation of a mission-driven approach have financially for the institution?

forms across undergraduate and graduate higher education institutions. Medical students are often integrated with students from other health professions, graduate medical education residents, and medical students from other schools. In many cases, medical schools are part of larger universities, but this is not always the case. In academic medical affiliations, one institution usually has primary financial responsibility and therefore greater influence. Understanding the flow of funds between institutions as well as power dynamics is an important component to take into consideration. A particularly important and dynamic shift currently taking place in the academic medicine landscape is the increasing affiliation and/or ownership of medical schools by health systems.

Another academic area to understand is the interprofessional training programs in your local context. Interdisciplinary academic partnerships integrated into health professions education is essential for preparing future physicians to work successfully in complex systems and interprofessional teams. Identifying and providing opportunities for interdisciplinary initiatives builds capacity and trust at the student, institutional, and professional levels, and across professional disciplines (Box 14.5).

Understanding and analyzing your context is the first step in building strategic partnerships within the community, health care delivery, and educational systems. Thoughtful evaluation makes barriers and resources easier to identify, illuminating areas that enable partnership and the development of an effective implementation plan. The timing of this work is an important consideration as it is best to form partnerships when system conditions are favorable for the adoption of your approach.

As partnerships develop, trust is established resulting in the emergence of new insights, approaches, and collaboration across all components. This is where your skilled team will support integration of continual learning and growth, because as your understanding evolves, and as needs, priorities, and leaders change, partnerships will also change. This fluid and cyclical process is necessary because strategic, dynamic partnerships are critical to transform medical education to be based on societal needs. Transformation cannot be successful if the integration of philosophy and principles takes place only within the walls of a medical school. Success requires true collaborative partnerships in the community, medical, and educational systems to ensure transformative real-life learning for students.

BUILDING INSTITUTIONAL SUPPORT AND MAKING CHANGE

Health systems should have a unique interest in incorporating a mission-driven framework because results of multiple pilot projects indicate addressing social determinants of health can help improve patient outcomes and experience, reduce readmissions, and have the potential for significant cost savings. Building upon this knowledge and successes, the creation of a medical education system driven by social responsibility, where physicians gain a true understanding and experience of the social determinants of health, will not only produce a new kind of physician and result in positive changes in communities but also has the potential to result in tremendous cost savings for health systems.

Developing support from institutional leaders is critical for sustained efforts in this work. While this may be a tall order, it can be built over time. Medical educators should not wait for broad and robust support before attempting to make these changes in their curricula and institutions. Rather, they should work creatively to find partners and collaborators with shared and/or synergistic goals. These can be found in many places—from patient safety and quality within health care delivery systems to other health professions schools to community-based entities such as community health centers or community-based nonprofit organizations. Pilot programs can be used to demonstrate proof of concept, to gain support, and to develop faculty, staff, and systems.

Working to build support and achieve these goals requires perseverance and strategy. You must look for people in your institution who can be advocates and champions and build relationships with them. This takes effort and time and is an ongoing process; but culture can change over time. Be mindful of how you sustain the motivation, enthusiasm, trust, and partnership of your team, allies, and partners. The ultimate goal is to achieve sustainable executive-level support, while building culture change which can begin at the foundation of an institution.

Working to achieve these goals will involve people and entities not historically involved in medical education. Medical educators will have to think outside the historic box (of medicine), to look for partnerships and key players who they can learn from and who can be part of the process of medical education.

Additionally, building medical education based on societal needs means that you are impacted by and vulnerable to complex societal factors, more than you would have historically needed to attend to. This can include societal values, public policy, and legal proceedings, and will vary based on local and federal factors. Therefore you need to maintain a clear focus on your mission so that you are not distracted or deterred from it, while being able to respond to and collaborate with societal entities, such as policymakers, community groups, and municipalities.

An example of this dynamic situation can be seen in the 2023 rulings from the US Supreme Court that impact the role of diversity, equity, and inclusion (DEI) initiatives in higher education. This ruling has a wide range of potential impacts, and a first reaction may be that DEI goals will not be achieved. However, using a systematic and comprehensive approach linking a school's mission to all aspects of the educational program means that aspects like DEI demographics within admissions are only one component of a health care workforce mission. As described in Example 3, the health care workforce mission drove multiple aspects of our school, such as the creation of the school's 3+1 model. Likewise, the integration of community-engaged medical education is another way to expand the range of persons who apply to the health professions and the nature of the training they receive, both also impacting health care workforce outcomes.

CONCLUSION

In this chapter we challenge medical educators to develop and change their programs to be comprehensively and directly driven by their responsibility to address societal problems. This is also an opportunity for medical education to drive change in medicine and health care delivery. While we more commonly think of health care delivery impacting medical education, educational endeavors can be leveraged to develop faculty, prioritize integrated approaches to

care, and build a health care workforce with an approach to medicine that integrates all the factors that impact health outcomes. While we are focused on undergraduate medical education in the example in this chapter, this approach can and does apply to graduate medical education, continuing professional development, and other health professions education. Indeed, integration and collaboration between health professions education, health care delivery, and community-based entities is needed to ultimately improve health outcomes and health equity within a society, as illustrated in Fig. 14.5.

Using societal needs as the driving force behind educational program development can be a shift for physicians and medical educators. It creates a broader context for medical education and expands who is included in that process.

As we reflect on the many advances we have made as a society in the diminishment of disease and suffering and the extension of life expectancy, we know that significant problems remain that we must address. We cannot ignore the inequities in outcomes within our society, as well as the reality of overall worsening outcomes and poor value in the United States due to the fragmented nature and narrow view of interventions to improve health.

As medical educators we are forging the next generation of physicians. This brings with it great responsibility, as well as great opportunity. We have the opportunity to create physicians who understand and integrate *all* the factors that drive health outcomes into their care of patients, who are skilled change agents and who have a deep sense of their responsibility to the communities and society they serve. It is only with a medical education system that has a systematic and clear focus on our fundamental responsibility to society that we will be able to improve the health outcomes and health equity within our society.

TAKE-HOME POINTS

1. Medical education, an extension of and core component of medicine, fundamentally has a responsibility to address the needs and problems of the society and communities it serves.
2. This should inform the content the school focuses on as well as the methods chosen and the structures of the school and its programs.
3. A systematic approach should be taken to link from a vision to specific principles that are then applied in each institution's local context. This will prevent lofty goals from being no more than well intentioned words in a mission statement.
4. The example shared in this chapter can be transferred, in part or in whole, to other schools and contexts by

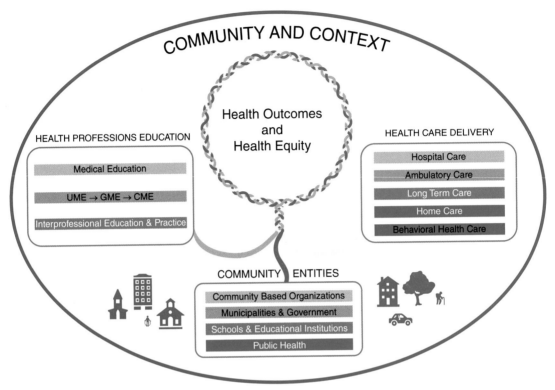

Fig. 14.5 Integration and partnership to improve health outcomes and health equity.

holding the foundational philosophy and principles constant and applying them in other contexts.

5. Given current challenges and structures within health care in the United States, collaboration and integration with community entities is needed. To implement this, institutions should follow the tenets of Community-Engaged Medical Education.

6. Understanding and analyzing the context of your community, health care delivery, and academic systems is a critical and ongoing process.

7. Institutional support is important and can be built over time. Medical educators need to work creatively to find partners and collaborators with shared and/or synergistic goals.

8. Working to achieve these goals is hard and will involve people and entities not historically involved in medical education. Medical educators should look for partnerships and key players who we can learn from and who can be part of the process of medical education.

REFERENCES

1. Ko M, Heslin KC, Edelstein RA, Grumbach K. The role of medical education in reducing health care disparities: the first ten years of the UCLA/Drew Medical Education Program. *J Gen Intern Med.* 2007;22(5):625–631.

2. Murray RB, Larkins S, Russell H, Ewen S, Prideaux D. Medical schools as agents of change: socially accountable medical education. *Med J Aust.* 2012;196(10):653. https://doi.org/10.5694/mja11.11473.

3. Reeve C, Woolley T, Ross SJ, et al. The impact of socially-accountable health professional education: A systematic review of the literature. *Med Teach.* 2017;39(1):67–73. https://doi.org/10.1080/0142159X.2016.1231914.

4. Rourke J. Social accountability: a framework for medical schools to improve the health of the populations they serve. *Acad Med.* 2018;93(8):1120–1124. https://doi.org/10.1097/ACM.0000000000002239.

5. Schroeder SA. We Can Do Better - Improving the Health of the American People. *NEJM.* 2007;357:221–1228. https://doi.org/10.1056/NEJMsa073350.

6. Strasser R, Worley P, Cristobal F, et al. Putting communities in the driver's seat: the realities of community-engaged medical education. *Acad Med.* 2015;90(11):1466–1470.

7. Weiner S. *Medical Schools Overhaul Curricula to Fight Inequities.* Association of American Medical Colleges; 2021. https://www.aamc.org/news-insights/medical-schools-overhaul-curricula-fight-inequities.

8. Woollard B, Boelen C. Seeking impact of medical schools on health: meeting the challenges of social accountability. *Med Educ.* 2012;46(1):21–27. https://doi.org/10.1111/j.1365-2923.2011.04081.x.

9. Hood CM, Gennuso KP, Swain GR, Catlin BB. County health rankings: relationships between determinant factors and health outcomes. *Am J Prevent Med.* 2016;50(2):129–135. https://doi.org/10.1016/j.amepre.2015.08.024.

10. Hunt JB, Bonham C, Jones L. Understanding the goals of service learning and community-based medical education: a systematic review. *Acad Med.* 2011;86(2):246–251.

11. CDC. *Social Determinants of Health.* Centers for Disease Control and Prevention; 2022. https://www.cdc.gov/about/sdoh/index.html

12. Kung A, Cheung T, Knox M, et al. Capacity to address social needs affects primary care clinician burnout. *Ann Fam Med.* 2019;17(6):487–494. https://doi.org/10.1370/afm.2470.

13. Duarte D, El-Hagrassy MM, Couto TCE, Gurgel W, Fregni F, Correa H. Male and female physician suicidality: a systematic review and meta-analysis. *JAMA Psychiatry.* 2020;77(6):587–597. https://doi.org/10.1001/jamapsychiatry.2020.0011.

14. Cianciolo AT, Regehr G. Learning theory and educational intervention: producing meaningful evidence of impact through layered analysis. *Acad Med.* 2019;94(6):789–794. https://doi.org/10.1097/ACM.0000000000002591.

15. Committee on Educating Health Professionals to Address the Social Determinants of Health. Board on Global Health. Institute of Medicine. National Academies of Sciences. Engineering, and Medicine. *A Framework for Educating Health Professionals to Address the Social Determinants of Health.* National Academies Press (US); 2016.

16. Preston R, Larkins S, Taylor J, Judd J. Building blocks for social accountability: a conceptual framework to guide medical schools. *BMC Med Educ.* 2016;16(1):227. https://doi.org/10.1186/s12909-016-0741-y.

17. Arebalos MR, Botor FL, Simanton E, Young J. Required longitudinal service-learning and its effects on medical students' attitudes toward the underserved. *Med Sci Educ.* 2021;31(5):1639–1643.

18. Barber C, van der Vleuten C, Leppink J, Chahine S. Social accountability frameworks and their implications for medical education and program evaluation: a narrative review. *Acad Med.* 2020;95(12):1945–1954. https://doi.org/10.1097/ACM.0000000000003731.

19. Boelen C, Woollard R. Social accountability: the extra leap to excellence for educational institutions. *Med Teach.* 2011;33(8):614–619. https://doi.org/10.3109/0142159X.2011.590248.

20. Ellaway RH, Van Roy K, Preston R, et al. Translating medical school social missions to student experiences. *Med Educ.* 2018;52(2):171–181. https://doi.org/10.1111/medu.13417.

PART VI

Case Studies: Leadership, Culture, and Climate Change

15

Leveraging the Underrepresented in Medicine Minority Faculty Experience
A Platform for Addressing Health Equity and Racial Justice in Medical Education

Janet H. Southerland, Kendall M. Campbell, and Charles P. Mouton

OUTLINE

SUMMARY

The lack of a diverse cohort of faculty has garnered more attention over the past four decades as it relates to health inequities. There have been some gains, but significant concerns remain. Underrepresented in medicine (URM) faculty play a pivotal role in training the next generation of health care providers in research and discovery and in direct clinical care, thus contributing to closing the gap in the significant health inequities experienced nationally and worldwide. Although this group continues to be underrepresented in the health care professions, URM faculty provide mentorship opportunities for learners, especially those who are from marginalized and underrepresented groups, as well as provide new perspectives on health inequities research and community care. Understanding and communicating the value of URM faculty as conduits for information sharing among peers, learners, and others in academic environments, coupled with the diversity of educational opportunities and richness of academic environments needs further emphasis. Because of the lived experiences of URM faculty and the diversity of cultures and backgrounds they bring to the learning environment, these faculty are perfect models to teach issues of culture, racial justice, and health equity to learners across the education continuum. A better understanding of faculty backgrounds and experiences as part of the recruitment, retention, and progression of historically marginalized faculty will be essential to increasing faculty numbers and longevity in health professions education. This chapter provides a historical perspective and culminates with a platform to maximize the contributions of URM faculty. This platform emphasizes the value of the URM faculty experience across the missions of education, research, and clinical care and highlights their lived experience and cultural diversity as additional domains they bring to the work role. It also highlights the impacts of inequitable environments in academic institutions and historical injustice as constrictors to the contributions of this group and demonstrates the platform needed for URM faculty talent to be realized in addressing health equity and racial justice.

INTRODUCTION

Dismantling racism, promoting health equity, and creating platforms for addressing racial justice are necessary and have become needed and important work of academic health systems.[1,2] Work in the area is mired in a history of racial injustice that has permeated our medical establishment, from institutional racism to the minority tax and gate blocking of those groups that have been historically marginalized and often don't receive support to promote career success.[3,4] Faculty who are underrepresented in the health professions come from marginalized communities including people who identify as Black or African American, Latinx (Hispanic or Latino), or American Indian and Alaska Native (AIAN), Native Hawaiian, and other Pacific Islander.[5,6] Underrepresented in medicine (URM) along with others are crucial to the missions of academic health centers. The lack of a diverse cohort of faculty has garnered more attention over the past four decades as it relates to health inequities. There have been some gains, but significant concerns remain.[7] URM faculty play a pivotal role in training the next generation of health care providers in research and discovery and in direct clinical care, thus contributing to closing the gap in the significant health inequities experienced nationally and worldwide. Although this group continues to be underrepresented in the health care professions, URM faculty provide mentorship opportunities for learners, especially those who are from marginalized and underrepresented groups, as well as provide new perspectives on health inequities research and community populations.[8,9]

Academic health centers have created initiatives to increase the presence of URM faculty, and the Association of American Medical Colleges (AAMC) has also dedicated resources and provided data to better inform academic institutions on how to promote the recruitment, retention, and advancement of those who are URM. Also, the AAMC has clarified and broadened their definition of "underrepresented" in medicine (also URM) based on the representation of marginalized groups in the general population.[10] Additionally, other notable organizations developed programs to address the needs of those underrepresented in medicine and other health professions, including the Harold Amos (medicine, dentistry, nursing) Medical Faculty Development Program at the Robert Wood Johnson Foundation. Other organizations that have contributed programs are the Society of Teachers for Family Medicine, National Institutes of Health (NIH), National Science Foundation, and W.K. Kellogg Foundation along with a multitude of university-sponsored and university-supported programs. Understanding and communicating the value of URM faculty as conduits for information sharing among peers, learners, and others in academic environments, coupled with the diversity of educational opportunities and richness of academic environments, needs further emphasis.

Because of the lived experiences of URM faculty and the diversity of cultures and backgrounds they bring to the learning environment, these faculty are perfect models to teach issues of culture, racial justice, and health equity to learners across the education continuum. Development of diverse leaders in academia ensures that role models are available to demonstrate compassionate care to all communities. URM faculty leaders often possess specialized experience in community engagement, the public health exposome, population health and health systems, health policy, and the development of new technologies including personalized medicine and genomics. A better understanding of faculty backgrounds and experiences as part of the recruitment, retention, and progression of historically marginalized faculty will be essential to increasing faculty numbers and longevity in health professions education. This chapter provides a historical perspective and culminates with a platform to maximize the contributions of URM faculty. This platform emphasizes the value of the URM faculty experience across the missions of education, research, and clinical care, and highlights their lived experience and cultural diversity as additional domains they bring to the work role. It also highlights the impacts of inequitable environments in academic institutions and historical injustice as constrictors to the contributions of this group and demonstrates the platform needed for URM faculty talent to be realized in addressing health equity and racial justice.

BACKGROUND

Understanding the History of the Underrepresented in Medicine Faculty Experience in Academic Medicine

To know where we need to go, we should first explore how we got here. The **19th through early 20th centuries** presented challenges and exclusions. Early in US history, academic medicine was dominated by White males, and minoritized individuals faced significant barriers to entry into medicine as well as other health professions.[11] Eventually, women and other racial and ethnic groups were able to gain admission, leading a category of "first to lead" efforts. There have been many URM individuals who served as firsts and paved the way for faculty from marginalized backgrounds to participate in advancing medical education opportunities. Howard University College of Medicine opened in 1868, and the faculty included the first African American to serve on a medical school faculty. Dr. Alexander T. Augusta, who received his medical degree from the University of Toronto, served as a professor of surgery. In 1953 Dr. Grace Marilyn James became the first African American female to serve as medical school faculty when she was appointed to the faculty at her alma mater, the University of Louisville. Dr. Susan LaFlesche Picotte was the first Native American female to serve as a faculty member at her alma mater, the Women's Medical College of Pennsylvania. Dr. Jeanne Sinkford served as the first

African American and first female dean of a dental school in the United States in 1975. Since the time of these URM pioneers in health professions education, conversations around racial justice, diversity, and equity have gained momentum in society at large and have led to increased attention to race and equity within academic medicine. The tripartite approach to medical education through teaching, clinical care, and research is foundational to training physicians and other health professionals. While discriminatory practices and systemic racism limited opportunities to pursue medical education and faculty positions, it has become apparent in the current landscape that the role of diverse faculty members is required to adequately prepare a workforce that is competent, skilled, and ready to meet the needs of a variety of communities nationally and internationally. The exclusion of URM faculty persisted well into the 21st century. The year **1910**, with the publication of the Flexner report by the Carnegie Foundation, marked a radical transformation in the nature and process of medical education, with a resulting elimination of proprietary schools and the establishment of the biomedical model as the gold standard of medical training.[12] After the release of the report, only two of the nation's seven Black medical schools survived. It is projected that if the schools had not been closed, that some 30,000 to 35,000 Black physicians over the past century would have been trained.[13]

Barriers to Professional Equity

The civil rights movement that followed decades later from the **1950s to 1960s** sparked broader discussions about racial equality and prompted some academic institutions to start addressing racial disparities in medical education and faculty representation. Academic medicine through its URM faculty played an important role in the struggle. Many URM health professionals were denied membership in the majority of professional organizations and thus founded similar organizations to meet their professional needs. Through organizations like the National Medical Association and its journal editor Dr. W. Montague Cobb, URM physicians continued the push for equality and justice. However, progress for equality of URM faculty continued to be slow, and URM individuals continued to face challenges in accessing leadership roles and meaningful participation in research and education. In the **1970s through the 1980s**, implementation of affirmative action policies aimed to increase diversity in academic institutions, including medical schools and other health professions schools. Programs established to increase URM applicants and matriculants such as the Health Resources and Services Administration (HRSA) Centers of Excellence Programs in Minority Health began to make a rapid change in admission patterns across medical schools. These programs as well as other affirmative action initiatives led to a gradual increase in URM representation among medical students and some movement in increasing URM faculty. Affirmative action faced legal challenges and retrenchment from the federal government, which affected its continued implementation and led to debates about its effectiveness. Due to continuous efforts to eliminate the small gains made during this period and efforts which continue until today, affirmative action is no longer a viable mechanism for helping achieve racial equity.

Pathway Programs

Pipeline and mentorship programs emerged from **1990 to 2000**. The AAMC 3000 by 2000 program to increase URM medical students, the AAMC Health Services Research Institute, and numerous NIH-sponsored minority summer research institutes began to train URM faculty for academic careers. During this period of time, other national organizations, medical schools, and academic medical centers began establishing pipeline programs and mentorship initiatives to support URM individuals at various stages of their academic careers. These efforts aimed to increase the number of URM students, residents, and faculty members, with a focus on providing resources and guidance.[14-16] In 2003 the Institute of Medicine (IOM) issued a report on health disparities titled "Unequal Treatment" that made recommendations to increase diversity in the workforce, integrate cultural competency in education, and increase research focused on health disparities.[15] Over 20 years later, we have fallen woefully short. After 2010, diversity, equity, and inclusion initiatives led to growing recognition of the need to create inclusive environments that supported the success of URM faculty members as well as other groups, such as individuals with disabilities, established by the Equality Act of 2010.[17] Further, many medical schools and academic institutions launched comprehensive diversity and inclusion activities aimed at addressing structural inequalities, promoting cultural competence, and fostering a sense of belonging for URM individuals. Unfortunately, these programs met the headwinds of the Bakke and Hopwood Supreme Court decisions along with the Reagan and Bush Administrations' dismantling of federal support and funding for professional education. Currently, we continue to battle newer initiatives aimed at dismantling diversity and inclusion efforts. Various states have passed legislation banning diversity and inclusion efforts in higher education and the Supreme Court of the United States ruling in the Students for Fair Admissions, Inc. v. President & Fellows of Harvard College in 2022 eliminated the consideration of race in college admissions.[18] Throughout, URM faculty have continued to make progress in helping academic institutions meet their missions. Despite the progress made, URM faculty members continue to face

challenges that include microaggressions, implicit bias, lack of diverse leadership representation, challenges with promotion and tenure, and inequities in obtaining research funding. A recent *New England Journal of Medicine* special report authored by Kamran et al.[19] indicates that there still exists "sluggishness" in increasing URM diversity in the US medical student body. This sluggishness also persists in both academic medical school faculty and leadership, with little improvement being observed over time.[19]

CHALLENGES TO UNDERREPRESENTED IN MEDICINE FACULTY IN ACADEMIA

Barriers Impacting Underrepresented in Medicine Faculty Progress

Present-day threats to the issues of academic freedom and existential threats to the academy are sure to cause indirectly and/or directly even greater barriers/challenges for URM faculty. Efforts toward achieving social justice and health equity are being undermined by educational censorship (banning teaching of critical race theory), political and university leadership intervention in faculty recruitment and promotion, the paucity of Black males in medicine, and the banning of the use of race in admissions decisions. URM faculty feel these threats both internally and externally. In some states, academic medical centers can no longer support URM faculty with Diversity, Equity, and Inclusion offices and institutional resources focused on diversity. These attacks also provide a not-so-subtle reinforcement of an institutional culture that states URM faculty do not belong in our academic medical centers. If academic medicine still plans to live up to the challenge of addressing health inequities, these threats and challenges to URM faculty must be overcome. While individuals from underrepresented backgrounds make up about 37.6% of the US population based on the 2020 US census, only 9.8% of faculty in medical education are from underrepresented backgrounds. In addition, underrepresented minority nurses make up 19.2% of full-time nursing faculty,[20] while underrepresented minority dentists made up about 11% of full-time faculty[21,22] compared to those from majority backgrounds. These statistics speak to the urgent need of academic medicine to recruit and develop URM faculty who can contribute to improving health equity. Traditional faculty career success is predicated on the ability of faculty to be productive in the areas of education, research, and clinical care—the proverbial three-legged stool. Thus, clinical and research training is an essential component of any faculty's preparation. The history of URM faculty in clinical care and research is framed by the thought that these faculty were not able to do research or be scientists. The plan was for URM individuals to provide clinical care as sanitation doctors to keep "Black" disease from passing to "White" people.[19,23] The tradition of creating barriers and isolation continues but has taken a different form of systematic biases to maintain the status quo. For example, primary care is the most diverse specialty in medicine, and other specialty areas struggle with having diversity in terms of gender and/or race and ethnicity.[24] While there is still emphasis placed on making progress in increasing the representation of faculty underrepresented in medicine, this move is in keeping with the thinking that URM doctors are best suited for clinical work and population-based care.[25] Beyond the challenges faced by minorities to receive a clinical education, URM faculty face barriers in one of academic medicine's key mission areas—research. Of the over 300,000 currently funded scientists, only 1.8% are Black and only 6% Hispanic. The award rate for NIH R01s is 10.2% for the Black principal investigators compared to 18.5% for the White principal investigators, and Whites are almost twice as likely to get funded compared to Blacks.[26–28] This racial bias persists even after controlling for a variety of factors predicting funding success as well as cultivating a successful career in the academic setting.[29] Given this bias in funding opportunities, many URM scientists face a lack of adequate research resources including equipment, supplies, space, and mentorship. They also do not receive the support of having post-doctoral training and graduate students or opportunities to participate as part of their research teams. These challenges have a direct effect on the ability of URM faculty to achieve promotion and tenure. Many promotion and tenure rules focus on the demonstration of scholarly productivity as well as a broad recognition of excellence and national/international reputation by a faculty's peer group. These goals become difficult to achieve without sustained funding to support a research career that extends past the institution. Also, URM faculty frequently apply to and receive funding for programs and projects with a community engagement, social sciences focus.[30] While recognizing the need for substantive work in both areas, URM faculty may be at a disadvantage compared to more foundational science researchers. While the NIH has encouraged more community engagement and is focused on health promotion and disease prevention, 51% of extramural funding goes to basic, foundational, or clinical research.[31,32] If URM faculty lack the support to be successful at attracting external (namely NIH) funding, they have difficulty demonstrating the value of their research and the institution. Added to these concerns are the limited number of URM faculty available for peer review and service on editorial boards.[33] Because URM faculty do more health inequities research than well-represented counterparts, it can be challenging to get a peer review based on merit of the research apart from bias against the content. This is especially problematic when URM faculty write about issues of racism and discrimination when

there are those who feel that racism does not exist. It could be argued that this is the case in those states that have decided to ban diversity, equity, and inclusion work. The message is that the focus should be on equality and not equity, and the national conversation around anti-Blackness along with other forms of discrimination such as institutional racism that is alive and well is no longer needed.[34,35]

UNDUE BURDENS ON UNDERREPRESENTED IN MEDICINE FACULTY

Access Denied

The history of education for URM faculty, and in particular Black faculty, has been a troubled one. From the need to educate themselves to having to fight against school boards and school districts for adequate textbooks, classrooms, and teachers. Inequitable educational environments have also historically placed enormous burdens that hinder the success of URM faculty.[36] The narrative of URMs in the United States includes small, inadequate facilities, one-room schoolhouses, multiage classrooms, and secondhand books. URM faculty experienced separate but unequal educational environments with attempts on every front to keep them from learning, excelling, and achieving. While integration helped Black and other minoritized people move forward, it came with racism, discrimination, and bias. Racist structures, institutionalized racism, and systems that benefit some and disadvantage others still exist. Even now these systems exist, propagated by advances in technology where some form group chats and exclude certain employees.[37] Even though minoritized individuals have had a challenging time in education, they have shown resilience and courage and have advanced the field. Historically, Black colleges and universities (HBCUs) contribute some of the best and brightest talent to our health care workforce and beyond. To leaders in health professions, dentistry, nursing, and medicine, the impact of HBCUs, though fewer, has in many cases outpaced the contributions of predominantly White institutions in producing URM medical professional health care workforce.[38] Not to mention, that in many of our academic institutions, it is those URM faculty who often lead diversity, equity, and inclusion initiatives, who are the ones adversely impacted the most by racist, inequitable, and noninclusive environments.

Challenges to Leadership and Promotion

As previously mentioned, URM faculty often face barriers in accessing research funding, mentorship, and academic opportunities for leadership, limiting their ability to progress in their careers. Mentorship, sponsorship, and advocacy have not traditionally been offered to URM faculty in navigating the promotion and tenure process as part of institutional decorum. The lack of diverse representation horizontally and vertically on some campuses reinforces the negative views held by the majority peers regarding URM faculty and students. The few URM faculty are often overwhelmed with the number of students they need to help, their service obligations to help their institution become more inclusive, and the community needs for better, more engaged health care. This lack of URM presence in medical education institutions has perpetuated the cycle of exclusion. Limited representation has further led to a lack of diverse perspectives in shaping the various components of medical education, research agendas, and health care policies.[39] Recognition awards, funding, and senior leadership roles remain pervasive. A study by Dickins et al. showed that faculty diversity was imperative in decreasing the threat and burden of stereotyping among other things.[40] To begin to adequately recover, effectively address, and remove the many barriers URM faculty continue to face in medical education, it is important to acknowledge past wrongs, actively work to dismantle systemic barriers, promote diversity, equity, inclusion, and belonging, and foster environments that value and respect individuals from all backgrounds. Institutions also must commit to ongoing efforts to rectify these historical injustices and create a more equitable and inclusive medical education system.

Challenges in Clinical Care and Modeling for Teaching Health Equity and Racial Justice

The report "Unequal Treatment: Confronting Racial and Ethnic Disparities in Health Care" released by the IOM in 2003 recommended an increase of underrepresented minority groups in the health care workforce along with integration of cross-cultural education as part of health care training and advancement in research efforts to identify sources of disparities and promising interventions.[41] It is well documented that a workforce that mirrors marginalized populations and communities leads to improved health outcomes. There is also evidence that URM students and junior faculty also benefit from faculty who look like them and can serve as role models.[42] Additionally, recent data indicate marginalized communities where Black doctors serve experience increased life expectancy.[38] Patients prefer physicians who look like them and that they can relate to and often the mere presence of Black faculty increases trust, enhancing the physician-patient relationship.[43] Low URM faculty numbers often result in missing out on advances in research, education, and clinical care. Physician-patient racial concordance has been shown to have a significant impact on a variety of health outcomes. Patient-provider racial and ethnic concordance (seeing a minority physician who is of the same race or ethnicity of

the patient) results in improvements in time spent together (between patient and provider), medication adherence, shared decision-making, wait times for treatment, cholesterol screening, patient comprehension of cancer risk, patient perception of treatment decisions, and increased consent for preventive services.

IMPROVING THE UNDERREPRESENTED IN MEDICINE FACULTY PRESENCE AND EXPERIENCE IN ACADEMIA

A Concordant Future

The "only one" phenomenon is a common theme for URM faculty at majority institutions. Due to low URM faculty numbers, faculty in these groups experience feelings of isolation and exclusion that are not uncommon even today. The need for URM faculty to train an adequate URM health care workforce is reinforced by data on the positive effects of racial concordance between health providers and their patients. Racial concordance between the health care professional and patient correlates with improved patient health outcomes, patient satisfaction, and communication. Patient-provider racial and ethnic concordance (seeing a minority physician that is of the same race and ethnicity of the patient) results in improvements in (1) time spent together (between patient and provider),[44] (2) medication adherence,[45] (3) shared decision-making,[46] (4) wait times for treatment,[47] (5) cholesterol screening,[48] (6) patient comprehension of cancer risk,[49] (7) patient perception of treatment decisions,[50,51] (8) reduced implicit bias (by provider),[52] (9) patient engagement is higher,[53] and (10) increased consent for preventive services.[54] The importance of patient-provider racial concordance may loom even larger as the health care environment begins to have a greater focus on value-based care and population health management. Racial concordance may be one of the overlooked and underutilized tools to help advance health equity and improve health outcomes. If these benefits are to be realized, URM faculty will be needed to help educate the next generation of URM clinicians and give them the tools to fight for racial justice in health care.

Underrepresented in Medicine Faculty: The Lived Experience

Underrepresented minoritized faculty play a crucial role in promoting health equity and racial and social justice in a variety of ways. Their presence, contributions, and lived experiences bring unique perspectives, experiences, and insights that are essential for creating more inclusive and equitable health care systems. URM faculty serve as role models for URM students and trainees. Seeing individuals who look like them in leadership, in the classroom, and in clinics can inspire students to pursue careers in medicine and provide evidence that success is attainable despite the legacy of exclusion of URM individuals. The presence of URM faculty helps address feelings of isolation and inadequacy that URM students may experience. URM faculty members often bring firsthand knowledge of the cultural, social, and economic factors that can impact health care outcomes in marginalized communities. URM faculty can contribute to the development of curricula that incorporate culturally competent components for care, help address health inequities, and emphasize patient-centered approaches. Medical education is enriched by URM faculty by contributing diverse perspectives to scholarship and research. Their experiences can shed light on root causes of disparate health outcomes, social determinants of health, and other issues that might not receive adequate attention with their insights and feedback.

As URM faculty they can challenge and dispel biased assumptions and stereotypes about racial and ethnic minorities. They can bring attention to issues such as implicit biases and help trainees from all backgrounds develop the skills needed to provide equitable care to patients. These faculty can also influence teaching practices by advocating for inclusive pedagogical content that respects the diversity of backgrounds and learning styles among students. Further, integration of diverse case studies and scenarios into education materials can help with removing stereotypes and address biases. URM faculty help in promoting institutional changes by advocating for and promoting development of an inclusive environment. They have historically been instrumental in shaping policies related to admissions, recruitment, retention, mentorship, fostering a more welcoming and supportive educational environment. Additionally, URM faculty expertise is critical in addressing health inequities through guiding learning experiences in the classroom through patient care and advanced training opportunities. Their research and clinical work provide guidance in understanding and mitigating root causes of health inequities. Historically, URM **faculty** have had strong ties to underserved communities, placing them in a position of trust that allows them to engage in community outreach, education, and advocacy more easily.

This level of engagement has helped to bridge the gaps that exist between academic institutions and schools of medicine and the communities they serve. Also, URM faculty are given or assume leadership roles responsible for diversity, equity, and inclusion initiatives that often include advocating for policy changes and requiring them to drive the transformation of the medical and academic institutions. Typically, these positions are underresourced and underfunded, leaving those individuals to shoulder the burden of shifting the campus culture to be more equitable and inclusive. Also, this work has not been recognized in the promotion and tenure process, leaving many minoritized faculty in these roles to be viewed as unproductive. Recent changes in policy by state legislatures across the country targeting and banning diversity, equity, and inclusion activities will only create more barriers to URM faculty who have made this part of the scholarly and academic pathway.

URM faculty have a multifaceted impact on clinical care and medical education contributing to more innovative care models to support patient care and students/trainees. Personal experiences and narratives can foster empathy helping others understand challenges faced by marginalized populations while motivating others to advocate for system changes. Their insights and efforts are essential for dismantling systemic barriers, addressing health inequities, and broadly promoting a more just and inclusive health care system.

Growth and Development

To effectively promote faculty retention and development, we must move from the deficit model of looking at URM faculty that posits that something is inherently wrong with them and their approach to the work of academic medicine. Included in this approach is the misunderstanding by White or well-represented faculty as to why URM faculty make certain decisions or act in certain ways.[55] We believe this thinking is based in racism and stereotyping in that URM or Black people were thought to be mentally inferior, slow, and hard to learn.[56] We have to transition from using stereotypes and stigmatizing URM faculty to a more progressive and equitable approach that seeks to address inequities by considering the broader context and systemic factors that contribute to them. This approach acknowledges that individuals from underrepresented minority groups may face unique challenges but emphasizes the importance of providing equitable opportunities, reducing biases, and dismantling discriminatory systems to achieve more equitable outcomes. Efforts to promote diversity, equity, and inclusion involve addressing structural inequalities and creating a more inclusive and supportive environment for underrepresented minorities. This approach extends beyond a skills-based approach and considers how culture, the lived experience of more senior URM faculty, and how we interact with White faculty impact our faculty experience.

Representation in Leadership Positions and Decision-Making Bodies

Key to leadership in academic medicine for URM faculty is mentorship, opportunities, and expansion of networks that evolve these relationships. The study by Coe et al.

proposed a mentoring model that describes potential pathways to leadership positions and intentional use of multidimensional mentoring teams as critically important for successfully navigating the path to leadership in academic medicine. Developing URM faculty leaders is critical to the diversity, equity, and inclusion needs of academic health centers, as these leaders may be more attuned to the needs of communities and have direct access to people, budgets, and resources needed to change policy and enact equitable change. Careful attention needs to be paid to not create pseudoleaders, URM faculty leaders placed in leadership positions because of the diversity they bring when they have not received the appropriate training.[33,57]

Establishing Underrepresented in Medicine Faculty Networks and Support Systems

Establishing URM faculty networks and support systems is crucial for creating a supportive and inclusive environment within medical institutions. These networks and systems can provide a platform for URM faculty to connect, share experiences, seek mentorship, and advocate for change. This can be accomplished through national and local organizations that are the majority minority. These organizations cater to unique needs and can address the various challenges faculty face in majority schools. Having URM faculty champions within schools is also important. Individuals who are willing to take the lead in initiating and organizing efforts foster a sense of community and belonging among URM faculty by consistently providing meaningful engagement opportunities. Creating a welcoming environment for all while advocating for systemic changes that will prompt belonging and includes open lines of communication is essential. Components of sustainable support systems and networks involve clear development goals and objectives, regular development activities, adequate resources and funding, personal and professional growth opportunities, advocacy and collaborations, and leadership training. Establishing URM faculty networks and support systems requires dedication, ongoing effort, and collaboration within health sciences institutions. When done effectively, these networks can contribute to the retention, advancement, and success of URM faculty within medical institutions while promoting diversity and equity in medicine and health care.

FRAMEWORK FOR INSTITUTIONAL SUPPORT AND CAREER SUCCESS

An effective framework for promoting URM faculty development and retention in medical education requires a comprehensive and holistic approach that addresses various aspects of faculty recruitment, support, and advancement.

The potential framework requires diverse recruitment strategies that are targeted and actively seek those candidates who have been marginalized in medicine. There is a requirement for collaboration with external networks and organizations that support these groups as well as duplicating successful programs at schools across the country. Efforts must be inclusive and will require recruitment practices that incorporate bias awareness training and have diverse search committee members.

Recruitment and Retention

Once onboarded, URM faculty require mentorship and sponsorship. Mentorship is important to support career development. Programs that provide a mentoring team that is individualized and provide opportunities for sponsorship have been shown to be effective in expanding networks and helping with advancement.[58-60] For URM faculty, sponsorship may be more important than mentorship, especially in the setting of cross-cultural professional relationships and especially involving White male leaders. Sponsors open the door for URM faculty by providing opportunities like lead authorship on a manuscript, introductions to a colleague at a prestigious university, or resources like an extra staff member or more lab space. Along with instrumental mentoring and mentoring on specific projects, sponsorship has the potential to propel the URM faculty member's career forward toward greater achievement. Professional development helps URM faculty obtain resources for skill-building, leadership development, and research collaboration. URM faculty also need opportunities to share experiences and strategies for navigating culturally sensitive and complex health equity scenarios. Institutions must address inequity in workload distribution and types of work assignments. URM faculty are often disproportionately burdened with increased teaching loads, diversity-related activities, and committee assignments that interfere with career progression through the promotion and tenure process. Above all, long-term institutional commitment must be realized through creating safe and inclusive spaces, providing equitable compensation, recognition in the form of advancement and promotion, and fair and transparent evaluations. By implementing a comprehensive framework that encompasses recruitment, support, development, and advancement, medical institutions can create an environment that fosters the growth and retention of URM faculty, leading to a more diverse, inclusive, and equitable medical education landscape.

Model for Change, Progress, and Success

Understanding the wide domain of contributions that URM faculty bring to academic medicine is key to understanding how to support those contributions and faculty

Supporting the Contributions of URM Faculty

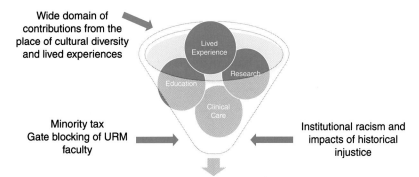

Fig. 15.1 Phase one: supporting the contributions of underrepresented in medicine (URM) faculty.

advancement. That wide domain not only encompasses talent brought to the traditional missions of education, clinical care, and research, but also includes contributions from cultural diversity and the URM lived experience that can impact the perspectives of learners, fellow faculty, senior leaders, and beyond. To depict a platform from which to share those contributions and how institutions can work to promote the contributions of URM faculty, we have defined three distinct phases to accentuate needed areas of focus. Phase one (Fig. 15.1) depicts the impacts of the minority tax, gate blocking of URM faculty, institutional racism, and historical injustice on URM faculty members, to essentially narrow the domains of contributions this group makes to the academic environment and institution at large.[3,4] This narrowing is a narrowing in scope as well as a narrowing in volume and is essentially a stifling of URM faculty talent to the detriment of the institution.

The narrowing of the domain of contributions of URM faculty has consequences for both the faculty member as well as the institution, and this narrowing has to be appreciated and dismantled to promote URM faculty success. Consequences to the faculty member include feelings of imposterism, reverse imposterism, and being made a pseudoleader by the institution.[53] These feelings that result from experiences at the institution cause URM faculty to leave academic medicine many times only after 5 years of service.[61] The impact of their departure hinders mentoring opportunities for learners and the climate of the academic environment for those URM faculty who are left behind. Being left behind has the potential to increase the diversity efforts disparity for those faculty as well as increase their likelihood of being isolated or overlooked by the institution.[62,63] Because of constricted contributions of URM faculty, impacts to the institution include missed

opportunities at innovation across the missions of education, care, and research and the disadvantage of having a homogeneous work environment filled with group think and limited diversity of viewpoints and ideas. Recognizing the narrowing of the domain of contributions by URM faculty is a must for senior leaders of academic health centers. Clues can include the absence of the URM voice on important issues in the institution, as well as a lack of interest, mission discordance, and at its extreme, a disdain for the institution. Arriving at the place where the domain of contributions of URM faculty is supported is where our academic institutions need to focus.

Even though we have shared much that impacts the presence of URM faculty in academic medicine, there are two foundational issues to be addressed by academic institutions to support the contributions of URM faculty. They include creating pillars of psychological safety and institutional equity. We depict them as pillars because they have to not only be foundational, but supportive for the entire organization. Phase two (Fig. 15.2) follows Phase one and depicts what psychological safety and institutional equity can do for the URM faculty member. Psychological safety is the larger, immediately important pillar of the two as that pillar needs to be created first. It's from a safe environment that strides can be made to promote institutional equity as all faculty will feel comfortable making recommendations to improve the environment. A psychologically safe environment for URM faculty can be described as one in which this group can share openly their opinions without the fear of retribution, loss of opportunities, or mistreatment.[64] In a psychologically safe environment, institutional equity can be approached because the voices of URM faculty can be heard and appreciated. These two pillars set the stage for contributions of URM faculty that can not only lead to

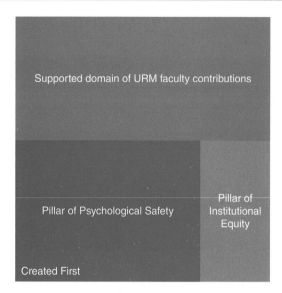

Narrowed domain of
contributions

Pillars created by the academic institution
to support URM faculty contributions

Fig. 15.2 Phase two: pillars created by the academic institution to support underrepresented in medicine (URM) faculty contributions.

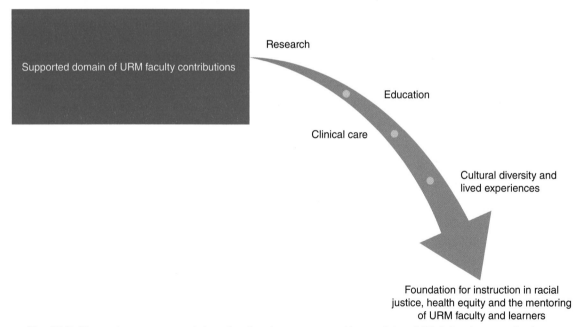

Fig. 15.3 Phase three: supported domain of underrepresented in medicine (URM) faculty contributions.

advances across the traditional missions of education, care, and research but can lead to larger innovations and break-throughs because of the maximization of support for the diversity voice of the organization.

When URM faculty feel and recognize that they are sup-ported and their contributions valued, it is important to cre-ate retention and advancement plans and help their growth into their role as academic faculty. Faculty development opportunities across the domains of education, research, and clinical care are a must and should only be undertaken after Phase two has been addressed. In addition to traditional faculty development, this group benefits from academic environments that promote their individual learning and cultivate their career interests, similar to the precision medicine approach in clinical care.[65] Not only do they benefit from approaches that promote individual learning in the setting of psychological safety, but they also thrive in "for us, by us" academic and faculty development environments.[66] Similar to clinical environments where patients prefer racially concordant clinicians and where health outcomes and mortality rates can be improved in those settings, faculty development for URM faculty provided by URM faculty has the potential to demonstrate higher levels of success. The impacts of the shared URM faculty experience cannot be minimized when it comes to faculty development for this group.

Faculty development for any faculty member is never declared a completed process. We all continue to grow in our roles, learning new things and gaining new experiences to help provide better care to our patients, education to our learners, and innovations that change health care. There does, however, need to be a platform from which we teach racial justice and health equity and from which we mentor new URM faculty and learners. This platform is created in Phase three (Fig. 15.3) and comes from an environment where the domain of URM faculty contributions is supported. In addition to research, education, and clinical care experiences, URM faculty can draw from their cultural diversity and lived experience to provide educational support across the domains of racial justice and health equity. Academic institutions must be careful to recognize this talent and not overburden it, creating a diversity pressure for these faculty. Considerations need to be given to using URM faculty talent and expertise to train well-represented and other faculty to help address these issues in academic medicine.

Phases one, two, and three, in that order of succession, are needed to bring URM faculty to the place of equitable and meaningful contributions to our academic health centers.

STRATEGIES FOR INTEGRATING HEALTH EQUITY AND RACIAL JUSTICE FOR UNDERREPRESENTED IN MEDICINE FACULTY IN MEDICAL EDUCATION

Integrating health equity and racial justice into medical education is essential to ensure that future health care professionals are equipped to address the inequities and biases that exist within health care systems. Here are some strategies that have been and should continue to be effectively integrated into medical education: (1) curriculum reform, (2) case-based learning, (3) interprofessional education,

(4) community engagement, (5) cultural competence, (6) unconscious and implicit bias, (7) patient and caregiver narratives and perspectives, (8) reflection, and (9) research opportunities. Qualitative studies support implicit biases in evaluation of URM students, especially more objective evaluations; some URM students feel they have to be exceptional to achieve average standing.[67] URM faculty representation on curriculum committees can serve to assist with identifying and eliminating bias, explicit and implicit, that has traditionally marred medical education and the selection process for faculty and students. It is understood that biases are part of human nature, and the understanding is grounded in social and behavioral sciences that focus on decision theories. Issues of fairness, self-control, emotional satisfaction, social pressure, and cultural norms are directly incorporated into how we make choices[68] that probably play a central role in maintaining the status quo related to improving URM representation. Dedicated modules or coursework on health equity, structural racism, and bias integrated throughout the curriculum can potentially help those in medical education to combat the propensity to follow our nature while we lean more into the best approaches to nurturing to improve URM faculty presence. Additionally, URM faculty can enhance case-based learning by providing content that highlights equity and disparity concerns along with social and cultural factors that impact health outcomes for underrepresented patients. Interprofessional educational options within the curriculum can also introduce options for collaboration providing support for URM faculty that can help with communication, academic success, and elimination of isolation. Multidisciplinary teams have been shown to be effective in caring for patients who are present for care with complex medical issues and problems. Training in this manner also improves continuity and quality of health care.[69]

URM faculty are also essential in establishing partnerships with organizations that represent or support marginalized people to provide students with firsthand experiences of the social determinants of health and health inequities impacting communities of color. Meaningful service-learning opportunities that connect students with underserved populations help garner trust. Implicit bias within health education settings has been shown to contribute to challenges in recruiting and retaining future health professionals from racial and ethnic minorities and hampers diversification efforts.[70] Ensuring proper training for non-URM faculty around unconscious bias and cultural competence that focuses on better understanding of cultural differences, overcoming biases, and delivering culturally sensitive care will help with reducing the burden and minority tax borne by URM educators and clinicians in academia.[71] Changing demographics across the US has produced diverse cultures and languages that now require health care providers to target the care they provide to be individualized and patient centered.[3] To achieve this type of result, a sufficient cohort of medical providers and educators reflective of the changes in demographics is necessary to better understand patient perspectives and experiences with health care to achieve better health and outcomes. Sharing patient narratives and experiences related to health inequities also can be invaluable additions to educating and training future generations. Integrating health equity and racial justice into medical education requires a multifaceted approach that involves curriculum design, faculty development, experiential learning, and ongoing evaluation. By incorporating these strategies, medical institutions can help shape a new generation of health care professionals who are committed to addressing disparities and promoting equity in health care.

LEVERAGING HEALTH EQUITY AND RACIAL JUSTICE EDUCATION IN THE CLINICAL ENVIRONMENT

Leveraging health equity and racial justice education in the clinical environment is crucial for ensuring that health care providers deliver equitable care to all patients. One effective model involves the recruitment and retention of URM faculty members as part of the plan of integrating tenets of cultural competence and equitable care into the clinical setting systematically. The clinical environment is often an extension of what is taught in the classroom. Preclinical education that introduces health equity and social justice concepts early in the curriculum will provide a foundational understanding as learners progress to the clinic setting. Leveraging simulation and technology has become a viable option to integrate concepts for training related to social justice and health equity in preparation for clinical practice. Virtual reality, natural language processing, artificial intelligence, machine learning, and patient simulators are currently being used to provide inpatient and outpatient care experiences involving diverse patient groups. Feedback is received in real time, and students are able to practice and learn in low- and high-risk scenarios. These tools can be used to identify specific challenges, fill knowledge gaps, and improve skill acquisition. In addition, training can be conducted to simulate team-based care and interprofessional education to build high-quality and high-functioning teams. Attention to designing clinical experiences that specifically expose trainees to best practices in addressing health inequities and providing equitable care is part of medical education, but there seems to be little to no calibration in the provision of training for clinical faculty located in the institution or at rotation sites in understanding social justice and health equity issues surrounding care. Offering ongoing training and workshops for health care

providers to stay updated on best practices for promoting health equity and racial justice is essential. Further, assessment of knowledge, attitudes, and skills related to health equity and racial justice through feedback from peers and self-assessment can be helpful to guiding continuous improvement. By including these steps, medical institutions can ensure that health equity and racial justice education become an integral part of the clinical environment, preparing future health care providers to deliver care that is culturally sensitive, equitable, and responsive to the needs of diverse patient populations.

FUTURE DIRECTIONS: ADVANCING HEALTH EQUITY AND RACIAL JUSTICE IN MEDICAL EDUCATION

In today's rapidly evolving health care landscape, considerations for the future in promoting social justice and health equity in medical education remain a critical endeavor. Several future directions and trends are emerging to advance these goals and ensure that medical education addresses the complexities of diverse populations, social determinants of health, and the impact of systemic racism. The most proximal and most obvious future direction is strengthening and advancing the pathways to produce more minoritized faculty that will fulfill a multipronged approach to educating a competent and confident workforce. This work stretches across multiple domains and requires a team lift of senior leaders in academic health systems, training programs, medical societies, funding agencies, and policymakers. Not only do we need programs that extend back to grade school to expose learners to careers in the health professions, but we need these programs to also provide academic strengthening, address educational inequities in marginalized communities, and dismantle practices that infuse racism into different facets of health. These needed changes are not novel or innovative and have been discussed before, but change has been slow in increasing the numbers of minoritized faculty in academic medicine and in particular Black men. There are many factors that contribute to the problem, but enduring bias, unconscious or conscious, is a reasonable target for meaningful change and improvement.

There are other approaches to be considered to increase the presence of faculty in this cohort. They not only include paying off student loans to make education more accessible, but also paying mortgages, paying home down payments, buying office practices, and building more medical and health professions schools targeting learners from underrepresented and rural backgrounds. Other areas of promise that should be considered are those marginalized resident physicians, many of whom are already motivated to pursue additional educational growth and development as academicians. Strengthening existing programs and creating new ones that facilitate entry of a resident physician into an academic career are a must to increase numbers of URM faculty. Designing programs from a place of psychological safety and institutional equity and structuring them to provide faculty development and training to care for diverse populations can be helpful in preparation for an early career faculty member. Additionally, promoting career advancement and longevity would be the desired outcome as the faculty shortage continues to increase. Key directions/take aways to promote improvement in URM faculty representation as guidance for leadership involve:

- Integration of a culturally competent curriculum (with continuous evaluation and adaptation)
- Understanding of implicit bias and antiracism and how it impacts health outcomes
- Ethics and social responsibility
- Consideration of global health equity models
- Advocacy and policy engagement
- Health inequities research and education
- Interprofessional education and team-based care
- Community engagement and partnerships
- Culturally aware patient-centered clinical care
- Technology and innovation
- Longitudinal training
- Resilience training

Ongoing challenges and areas that have need for improvement:

- Promoting research and scholarship on health equity and social justice
- National and international collaborations in advancing the health equity agenda
- Creating content using technology and innovation to address health equity and access issues

The future of social justice and health equity in medical and health education requires a multidimensional approach that spans curricula, faculty development, research, community engagement, policy, and advocacy. By embracing these directions and greater faculty representation across the population, medical institutions and academic health centers can make valuable contributions to a more equitable and inclusive health care system that addresses the needs of all patients and communities.

REFERENCES

1. Raphael JL, Freed GL, Ampah SB, et al. Faculty perspectives on diversity, equity, and inclusion: building a foundation for pediatrics. *Pediatrics*. 2023;151(4).
2. Acosta DA, Skorton DJ. Making 'Good Trouble': time for organized medicine to call for racial justice in medical education and health care. *Am J Med*. 2021;134(10):1203–1209. https://doi.org/10.1016/j.amjmed.2021.04.034.
3. Rodríguez JE, Campbell KM, Pololi LH. Addressing disparities in academic medicine: what of the minority tax? *BMC Med Educ*. 2015;15(1):6. https://doi.org/10.1186/s12909-015-0290-9.
4. Amaechi O, Foster KE, Tumin D, Campbell KM. Addressing the gate blocking of minority faculty. *J Natl Med Assoc*. 2021;113(5):517–521. https://doi.org/10.1016/j.jnma.2021.04.002.
5. About the Topic of Race (census.gov); National Research Council (US) Panel on Race, Ethnicity, and Health in Later Life; Anderson NB, Bulatao RA, Cohen B editors. Washington (DC) National Academies Press (US); 2004.
6. Anderson NB, Bulatao RA, Cohen B, eds. *National Research Council (US) Panel on Race, Ethnicity, and Health in Later Life*. National Academies Press(US); 2004.
7. Filut A, Alvarez M, Carnes M. Discrimination toward physicians of color: a systematic review. *J Natl Med Assoc*. 2020;112(2):117–140. https://doi.org/10.1016/j.jnma.2020.02.008.
8. Fassiotto M, Flores B, Victor R, et al. Rank equity index: measuring parity in the advancement of underrepresented populations in academic medicine. *Acad Med*. 2020;95(12):1844–1852. https://doi.org/10.1097/ACM.0000000000003720.
9. Pololi LH, Evans AT, Gibbs BK, Krupat E, Brennan RT, Civian JT. The experience of minority faculty who are underrepresented in medicine, at 26 representative U.S. Medical Schools. *Acad Med*. 2013;88(9):1308–1314. https://doi.org/10.1097/ACM.0b013e31829eefff.
10. AAMC. *Underrepresented in Medicine Definition*. Association of American Medical Colleges. https://www.aamc.org/what-we-do/equity-diversity-inclusion/underrepresented-in-medicine.
11. Byrd WM, Clayton LA. Race, medicine, and health care in the United States: a historical survey. *J Natl Med Assoc*. 2001;93(3 Suppl):11S–34S.
12. Duffy TP. The Flexner report--100 years later. *Yale J Biol Med*. 2011;84(3):269–276. https://www.ncbi.nlm.nih.gov/pubmed/21966046.
13. St. Fleur N. *Listen: How One 1910 Report Curtailed Black Medical Education for Over a Century*. STAT; 2022. https://www.statnews.com/2022/04/04/color-code-flexner-report-curtailed-black-medical-education/.
14. Sullivan LW. *Missing Persons: Minorities in the Health Professions, A Report of the Sullivan Commission on Diversity in the Healthcare Workforce*. 2004. https://campaignforaction.org/wp-content/uploads/2016/04/SullivanReport-Diversity-in-Healthcare-Workforce1.pdf.
15. Smedley BD, Butler AS, Bristow LR, eds. *In the Nation's Compelling Interest*. The National Academies Press; 2004. http://doi.org/10.17226/10885.
16. Garcia G, Nation CL, Parker NH. *Commissioned Papers: Contribution A: Increasing Diversity in the Health Professions: A Look at Best Practices in Admissions. In the Nation's Compelling Interest*. National Academies Press; 2004:231–272.

17. Nivet MA. Minorities in academic medicine: review of the literature. *J Vasc Surg*. 2010;51(4):S53–S58. https://doi.org/10.1016/j.jvs.2009.09.064.

18. Students for Fair Admissions, Inc. v. President and Fellows of Harvard College. No. 20–1199. Argued October 31, 2022—Decided June 29, 2023. https://www.supremecourt.gov/opinions/22pdf/20-1199_hgdj.pdf.

19. Kamran SC, Winkfield KM, Reede JY, Vapiwala N. Intersectional analysis of U.S. Medical Faculty Diversity over four decades. *N Engl J Med*. 2022;386(14):1363–1371. https://doi.org/10.1056/NEJMsr2114909.

20. American Association of Colleges of Nurses. *Fact Sheet: Enhancing Diversity in the Nursing Workforce*. American Association of Colleges of Nurses; 2023. https://www.aacnnursing.org/Portals/0/PDFs/Fact-Sheets/Enhancing-Diversity-Factsheet.pdf.

21. Smith SG, Banks PB, Istrate EC, Davis AJ, Johnson KR, West KP. Anti-racism structures in academic dentistry: supporting underrepresented racially/ethnically diverse faculty. *J Public Health Dent*. 2022;82(Suppl 1(Suppl 1)):103–113.

22. Data USA. *Dentists Detailed Occupation*. https://datausa.io/profile/soc/dentists#.

23. Sullivan LW, Suez Mittman I. The state of diversity in the health professions a century after Flexner. *Acad Med*. 2010;85(2):246–253. https://doi.org/10.1097/ACM.0b013e3181c88145.

24. Asaad Babker. Impact of the Flexner's report on health professional education. *N.a. J Adv Res Rev*. 2023;19(3):939–941. https://doi.org/10.30574/wjarr.2023.19.3.1888.

25. Nguemeni Tiako MJ, Johnson S, Muhammad M, Osman NY, Solomon SR. Association between racial and ethnic diversity in medical specialties and residency application rates. *JAMA Netw Open*. 2022;5(11):e2240817. https://doi.org/10.1001/jamanetworkopen.2022.40817.

26. Xierali IM, Nivet MA, Rayburn WF. Diversity of department chairs in family medicine at US Medical Schools. *J Am Board Fam Med*. 2022;35(1):152–157. https://doi.org/10.3122/JABFM.2022.01.210298.

27. Ginther DK, Schaffer WT, Schnell J, et al. Race, ethnicity, and NIH research awards. *Science*. 2011;333(6045):1015–1019. https://doi.org/10.1126/science.1196783.

28. Wiley Z, Hanna J, Kobaidze K, Franks N. Team science: advancing women and black, indigenous, and other people of color on the pathway of conducting clinical research. *Ther Adv Infect Dis*. 2023;10. https://doi.org/10.1177/20499361231159501. 20499361231159501.

29. Erosheva EA, Grant S, Chen M, Lindner MD, Nakamura RK, Lee CJ. NIH peer review: criterion scores completely account for racial disparities in overall impact scores. *Sci Adv*. 2020;6(23):eaaz4868. https://doi.org/10.1126/sciadv.aaz4868.

30. Cruz TH, Borrego ME, Page-Reeves J. Increasing the Number of Underrepresented Minority Behavioral Health Researchers Partnering With Underresourced Communities: Lessons Learned From a Pilot Research Project Program. *Health Promot Practice*. 2020;21(6):865–871. https://doi.org/10.1177/1524839920907554.

31. National Institutes of Health. *Budget*. https://www.nih.gov/about-nih/what-we-do/budget.

32. Strauss D, Gran-Ruaz S, Osman M, Williams MT, Faber SC. Racism and censorship in the editorial and peer review process. *Front Psychol*. 2023;14:1120938. https://doi.org/10.3389/fpsyg.2023.1120938.

33. Rodríguez JE, Campbell KM, Washington JC. Dismantling anti-Black racism in medicine. *Am Fam Physician*. 2021;104(6):555–556.

34. Braveman PA, Arkin E, Proctor D, Kauh T, Holm N. Systemic and structural racism: definitions, examples, health damages, and approaches to dismantling. *Health Aff (Millwood)*. 2022;41(2):171–178. https://doi.org/10.1377/hlthaff.2021.01394.

35. Smedley BD, Stith AY, Colburn L, Evans CH. *The Right Thing to Do, The Smart Thing to Do*. National Academies Press; 2001. http://doi.org/10.17226/10186.

36. Tulshyan R. *Ask an Expert: My Team Members Keep Leaving Me Out*. Harvard Business Review, Ascend; 2021. https://hbr.org/2021/01/ask-an-expert-my-team-members-keep-leaving-me-out.

37. Noonan A, Lindong I, Jaitley VN. The role of historically Black colleges and universities in training the health care workforce. *Am J Public Health*. 2013;103(3):412–415. https://doi.org/10.2105/AJPH.2012.300726.

38. Shen MJ, Peterson EB, Costas-Muñiz R, et al. The effects of race and racial concordance on patient-physician communication. *J Racial Ethnic Health Disparities*. 2018;5(1):117–140. https://doi.org/10.1007/s40615-017-0350-4.

39. Dickins K, Levinson D, Smith SG, Humphrey HJ. The minority student voice at one medical school: lessons for all? *Acad Med*. 2013;88(1):73–79. https://doi.org/10.1097/ACM.0b013e3182769513.

40. Jackson CS, Gracia JN. Addressing health and health-care disparities: the role of a diverse workforce and the social determinants of health. *Public Health Rep*. 2014;129(1_suppl2):57–61. https://doi.org/10.1177/00333549141291S211.

41. Carethers JM. Facilitating minority medical education, research, and faculty. *Dig Dis Sci*. 2016;61(6):1436–1439. https://doi.org/10.1007/s10620-016-4057-x.

42. Snyder JE, Upton RD, Hassett TC, Lee H, Nouri Z, Dill M. Black representation in the primary care physician workforce and its association with population life expectancy and mortality rates in the US. *JAMA Netw Open*. 2023;6(4):e236687. https://doi.org/10.1001/jamanetworkopen.2023.6687.

43. Stevens GD, Shi L, Cooper LA. Patient-provider racial and ethnic concordance and parent reports of the primary care experiences of children. *Ann Fam Med*. 2003;1(2):105–112. https://doi.org/10.1370/afm.27.

44. Traylor AH, Schmittdiel JA, Uratsu CS, Mangione CM, Subramanian U. Adherence to cardiovascular disease medications: does patient-provider race/ethnicity and language concordance matter? *J Gen Intern Med*.

2010;25(11):1172–1177. https://doi.org/10.1007/s11606-010-1424-8.

45. Cooper-Patrick L, Gallo JJ, Gonzales JJ, et al. Race, gender, and partnership in the patient-physician relationship. *JAMA*. 1999;282(6):583–589. https://doi.org/10.1001/jama.282.6.583.

46. Harrison A, Appleby J. Reducing waiting times for hospital treatment: lessons from the English NHS. *J Health Serv Res Policy*. 2009;14(3):168–173. https://doi.org/10.1258/jhsrp.2008.008118.

47. Strumpf EC. Racial/ethnic disparities in primary care: the role of physician-patient concordance. *Med Care*. 2011;49(5):496–503. https://doi.org/10.1097/MLR.0b013e31820fbee4.

48. Persky S, Kaphingst KA, Allen VC, Senay I. Effects of patient-provider race concordance and smoking status on lung cancer risk perception accuracy among African Americans. *Ann Behav Med*. 2013;45(3):308–317. https://doi.org/10.1007/s12160-013-9475-9.

49. Saha S, Beach MC. Impact of physician race on patient decision-making and ratings of physicians: a randomized experiment using video vignettes. *J Gen Intern Med*. 2020;35(4):1084–1091. https://doi.org/10.1007/s11606-020-05646-z.

50. Penner LA, Dovidio JF, Gonzalez R, et al. The effects of oncologist implicit racial bias in racially discordant oncology interactions. *J Clin Oncol*. 2016;34(24):2874–2880. https://doi.org/10.1200/JCO.2015.66.3658.

51. Hagiwara N, Slatcher RB, Eggly S, Penner LA. Physician racial bias and word use during racially discordant medical interactions. *Health Commun*. 2017;32(4):401–408. https://doi.org/10.1080/10410236.2016.1138389.

52. Alsan M, Garrick O, Graziani G. Does diversity matter for health? Experimental evidence from Oakland. *Am Econ Rev*. 2019;109(12):4071–4111. https://doi.org/10.1257/aer.20181446.

53. Powell W, Richmond J, Mohottige D, Yen I, Joslyn A, Corbie-Smith G. Medical mistrust, racism, and delays in preventive health screening among African-American men. *Behav Med*. 2019;45(2):102–117. https://doi.org/10.1080/08964289.2019.1585327.

54. Hudson B, Campbell KM. Does criticism of minority faculty result from a lack of senior leadership training and accountability? *Acad Med*. 2020;95(12):1792. https://doi.org/10.1097/ACM.0000000000003735.

55. Reinhardt JM. The Negro: is he a biological inferior? *Am J Soc*. 1927;33(2):248–261. https://doi.org/10.1086/214384.

56. Santiago-Delgado Z, Rojas DP, Campbell KM. Pseudo leadership as a contributor to the URM faculty experience. *J Natl Med Assoc*. 2023;115(1):73–76. https://doi.org/10.1016/j.jnma.2022.11.003.

57. Rodriguez JE, Figueroa E, Campbell KM, et al. Towards a common lexicon for equity, diversity, and inclusion work in academic medicine. *BMC Med Educ*. 2022;22(1):703. https://doi.org/10.1186/s12909-022-03736-6.

58. Bonifacino E, Ufomata EO, Farkas AH, Turner R, Corbelli JA. Mentorship of underrepresented physicians and trainees in academic medicine: a systematic review. *J Gen Intern*

Med. 2021;36(4):1023–1034. https://doi.org/10.1007/s11606-020-06478-7.

59. South-Paul JE, Campbell KM, Poll-Hunter N, Murrell AJ. Mentoring as a buffer for the syndemic impact of racism and COVID-19 among diverse faculty within academic medicine. *Int J Environ Res Public Health*. 2021;18(9):4921. https://doi.org/10.3390/ijerph18094921.

60. Beech BM, Calles-Escandon J, Hairston KG, Langdon SE, Latham-Sadler BA, Bell RA. Mentoring programs for underrepresented minority faculty in academic medical centers: a systematic review of the literature. *Acad Med*. 2013;88(4):541–549. https://doi.org/10.1097/ACM.0b013e31828589e3.

61. Cropsey KL, Masho SW, Shiang R, Sikka V, Kornstein SG, Hampton CL. Why do faculty leave? Reasons for attrition of women and minority faculty from a medical school: four-year results. *J Womens Health (Larchmt)*. 2008;17(7):1111–1118. https://doi.org/10.1089/jwh.2007.0582.

62. Campbell KM. The diversity efforts disparity in academic medicine. *Int J Environ Res Public Health*. 2021;18(9):4529. https://doi.org/10.3390/ijerph18094529.

63. Campbell KM. Mitigating the isolation of minoritized faculty in academic medicine. *J Gen Intern Med*. 2023;38(7):1751–1755. https://doi.org/10.1007/s11606-022-07982-8.

64. Foster KE, Robles J, Anim T, et al. What do underrepresented in medicine junior family medicine faculty value from a faculty development experience? *Fam Med*. 2022;54(9):729–733. https://doi.org/10.22454/FamMed.2022.895447.

65. Gameiro GR, Sinkunas V, Liguori GR, Auler-Júnior JOC. Precision medicine: changing the way we think about healthcare. *Clinics (Sao Paulo)*. 2018;73:e723. https://doi.org/10.6061/clinics/2017/e723.

66. Robles J, Anim T, Wusu MH, et al. An approach to faculty development for underrepresented minorities in medicine. *South Med J*. 2021;114(9):579–582. https://doi.org/10.14423/SMJ.0000000000001290.

67. Joseph OR, Flint SW, Raymond-Williams R, Awadzi R, Johnson J. Understanding healthcare students' experiences of racial bias: a narrative review of the role of implicit bias and potential interventions in educational settings. *Int J Environ Res Public Health*. 2021;18(23):12771. https://doi.org/10.3390/ijerph182312771.

68. Mellers BA. Decision research: behavioral. In: Smelser NJ, Baltes PB, eds. *International Encyclopedia of Social and Behavioral Sciences*. 1st ed. Elsevier Science & Technology; 2001:3318–3323.

69. Taberna M, Gil Moncayo F, Jané-Salas E, et al. The multidisciplinary team (MDT) approach and quality of care. *Front Oncol*. 2020;10:85. https://doi.org/10.3389/fonc.2020.00085.

70. Marcelin JR, Siraj DS, Victor R, Kotadia S, Maldonado YA. The impact of unconscious bias in healthcare: how to recognize and mitigate it. *J Infect Dis*. 2019;220(Supplement_2):S62–S73. https://doi.org/10.1093/infdis/jiz214.

71. Williams DR, Cooper LA. Reducing racial inequities in health: using what we already know to take action. *Int J Environ Res Public Health*. 2019;16(4):606. https://doi.org/10.3390/ijerph16040606.

16

Dismantling the Complex Systems of Power and Privilege in Medical Education Through Change Management

Priya S. Garg, Abbas A. Hyderi, Eva M. Aagaard, and Stephanie E. Mann

SUMMARY

The road to social justice and health equity is contingent upon addressing and correcting the inequities in medicine and health care. The long-standing history of structural racism in the United States has contributed to ongoing health inequities stemming from policies and practices that influence medical practice and medical education. Eliminating these inequities will require addressing and dismantling the complex relationship between power and privilege perpetuating the structural barriers that impact health care and the educational programs that train the health care system's physicians and other health professionals. As we examine our own institutions and local context, medical educators have an opportunity and moral imperative to acknowledge and utilize our power and privilege to change the narrative and interrupt the status quo perpetuating the policies, practices, and processes that promote racism and racist practices. Breaking down these persistent barriers to racial equity requires an understanding of change management and the emotional elements (e.g., avoidance, rationalization, silence) that can hinder transformation. In this chapter, we provide a brief historical perspective describing the structures, processes, and practices that have led to the hierarchy of power and privilege that exists in the United States and how it impacts current-day medicine and our learners and faculty across the continuum of medical education. We present a practical eight-step approach integrating Kotter's well-known principles of change management with the Bridges' Transition Model to manage the human transitions that underlie change. We explore these frameworks through the lens of antiracism and provide concrete examples drawn from the literature and our experiences as physicians and educational leaders at our different institutions.

INTRODUCTION

Medical education is an upstream driver of change in health care and a key element required to address health inequities. In general, medical educators have failed to name racism as a key structural driver of health inequities and health care disparities. Medical education traditionally focuses on teaching students about health care disparities and the differences in disease prevalence that exist between racial groups rather than explaining the why (including racism) and how (social constructs) these differences have

come to be. Changing learner understanding of race-based disparities in medicine requires medical education leaders to evaluate their educational programs, policies, and practices for racism at every level.

In 2020, after the death of George Floyd, Breonna Taylor, and countless others, medical educators across the country were called to action by their students, many asking their medical schools to evaluate medical education and its historical practices. In examining the history of medicine, countless current-day racist practices in medicine and medical education revealed themselves. At this inflection point in history, medical education leaders must take necessary steps toward making lasting antiracist change in medical education. To do so, we must educate ourselves on the historical racist practices in medicine (Table 16.1) and develop strategies to dismantle power and privilege in medicine and medical education. Change management skills are critical to implementing antiracist policies and practices, and an understanding of the emotional impact of transition is important to support success. Learning from other organizations through case studies and examples can accelerate the change process and support the creation of a sustainable, antiracist learning environment throughout the continuum of medical education.

POWER AND PRIVILEGE

A significant step in mitigating and eliminating the public health crisis of racism is to address and eliminate two of the drivers that perpetuate racism—power and privilege. In

TABLE 16.1   Brief History of Racism in Medicine[1-6]

Year	Event	Description
1781	J. Marion Sims' Gynecological Experiments	Sims conducted unethical gynecological experiments on enslaved Black women without anesthesia
1932–72	Tuskegee Syphilis Study	African American men with syphilis were denied treatment to study the natural progression
1951	Henrietta Lacks and HeLa Cells	Cells taken without consent from Henrietta Lacks, an African American woman, were used for research without acknowledgment
1960s–70s	Forced Sterilization	Black and Native American women were disproportionately subjected to involuntary sterilization
1970s–80s	Lead Poisoning in Public Housing	Minority communities were disproportionately exposed to lead due to discriminatory housing policies
1990s	Racial Disparities in Pain Management	Studies revealed racial bias in the prescription and management of pain, with minorities receiving inadequate treatment
2020	COVID-19 Disparities	Minority communities experienced higher rates of COVID-19 infection and death due to systemic health care inequalities

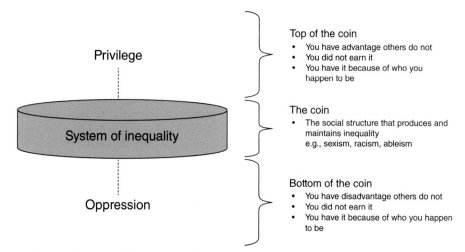

Fig. 16.1 The coin model. (From Nixon SA. The coin model of privilege and critical allyship: implications for health. *BMC Public Health*. 2019;19(1):1637.)

the next section, we explore power and privilege through a theoretical framework called the **Coin Model**[7] and discuss the opportunities to dismantle that power and privilege through medical education.

The Coin Model

Dismantling the complex interplay of power and privilege is the foundation of Nixon's Coin Model of Privilege and Allyship[7] (Fig. 16.1). This model describes a conceptual framework for health inequities as avoidable consequences of social structures resulting from privilege. Using the analogy of a coin representing a social structure, Nixon describes the two sides of the metaphorical coin representing those who are privileged on the top of the coin and those who are oppressed (i.e., marginalized, disadvantaged, vulnerable, high-risk populations) as being on the bottom of the coin. A critical element of this framework is that *both* positions are unjust. Creating equity is not about moving people from the bottom to the top but rather dismantling the systems (i.e., the coins) that cause these inequities. Although potential solutions must include interventions to improve the opportunities available to vulnerable groups (bottom of the coin), we must also focus on the system (the coin) and create solutions that will change the policies and mindset of those who have created or are part of the system. In addition, those at the top of the coin need to recognize that there are two sides to the coin, including the unearned advantages of the dominant group and ask and answer difficult questions such as "What benefits from privilege did I have?" and "How did my actions reinforce systemic inequities?"

HISTORICAL PERSPECTIVES AND CURRENT STATE IN MEDICINE

Ignoring the history and evolution of the impact of racism on the health and well-being of all patients has led us to the current state of health inequities (see Table 16.1). As Nixon describes in the Coin Model, health inequities are widespread and persistent with the root causes attributed to social, political, and economic disparities grounded in long-standing practices favoring and perpetuating White privilege and the failure to account for and address structural racism.[8,9] Racism and the racialization of Black, Indigenous, and people of color have been embedded in health care and medical education for centuries. Civil rights and social policies made over the last 300 years have resulted in structural racism that produces differential conditions between White Americans and racial and ethnic minorities in the five key areas of the social determinants of health (education, employment, health care, housing, and public health), leading to racial health inequities.

For example, **redlining**,[10] a legal discriminatory practice in which mortgage lenders denied loans often because of racial characteristics, resulted in Black Americans being excluded from certain neighborhoods and created segregation across many cities in the United States. This persistence of racial segregation resulted in Black Americans living in communities with a lack of access to many factors needed for optimal health (healthy food, employment, sanitation services, green space) which continues to influence health and lead to the health inequities we see today.[8,10]

Medicine and medical education itself have also perpetuated many false beliefs related to minoritized populations including failing to teach that race is a social construct. It is now well understood that any difference seen in health between races is predominantly due to social inequities like the ones we have discussed above. In addition, centuries of scientific experimentation and research on Black Americans without their consent has led to a mistrust of the health system.[11] Unfortunately, many providers lack the knowledge and awareness of the history of experimentation on Black Americans (see Table 16.1) and the understanding of the "why" behind the present-day mistrust. The two sides of the coin are strong in medicine, and medical education must be rigorously attentive to the depths of oppression and privilege that have led to health inequity. Learners must be taught the structural determinants, including racism, that have historically impacted health and continue to impact health and be inspired to action to ensure health equity for future generations.

Looking Forward

To move forward, we need to reframe the approach to addressing health inequities by focusing on the social structures that disadvantage nondominant groups. Leaders within the health system at the policy, health care delivery, and academic levels must consider and work to dismantle the practices that unintentionally reinforce inequities despite the time pressures in practice that exist. These practices derive from potentially biased assumptions and structures that inform, enable, and influence the care, education, and research provided to some and not to others. Useful questions include: Are there providers who have an awareness of the historical perspectives available to address questions and concerns and influence decision-making? Has the hospital, clinic, or health system partnered with the local community and government to think about employment policies, access to transportation, and resources in the community that have disadvantaged these groups? In health care, there are two sides to the coin and the future must focus on thinking about the advantages and privileges that exist in the system by learning from historically marginalized groups and health system leaders leveraging their privilege to create awareness and collective action.

A Call to Medical Educators

As academic health centers across the United States prioritize antiracist strategies, education leaders are seeking tools, frameworks, expertise, and programs that are best suited to support the ongoing evolution of antiracist practices. Antiracism is not an identity but a process in which we must all continually engage.[12] Further, to create an antiracist culture in medicine, we must consider how we can recognize structural racism not just in health care, but also in medical education and then advocate for change. Systemic structures within medical education have led to the current lack of racial diversity of students entering and graduating from medical school, entering and staying within certain specialties, the lack of diversity of physician leadership, and the framing of health care inequities as a problem with marginalized populations rather than an in-depth exploration of the societal injustices that explain why these health inequities exist.

Like health care, medical education is a large ecosystem of individuals and institutions with structures and policies in place that have systematically advantaged individuals from majority populations and disadvantaged those from non-majority populations. One perspective to consider in medicine is that privilege has impacted those who have been given the opportunity to enter the field and the opportunities available if allowed to enter. The majority of medical students are White Americans, and despite the fact that 13% of the US population are Black Americans, medicine has lagged behind with only 5.7% of US doctors being Black Americans. Finally, once entered into medical school and residency, recent studies have demonstrated consistent inequities in grading outcomes,[13] entrance into **Alpha Omega Alpha Honor Medical Society**,[14] increased rates of attrition from residency, and differential experiences of learning.[15] As medical education leaders, we have recognized that to change the advantages in our field, we have to begin with systems starting long before medical school. These include developing connections with the early education system, high school pathway programs, and shaping messages about science along with exposure to early mentorship and role models for Black American students. But it also involves changing our system of medical education to make it more equitable to enter, learn, and achieve within medicine. Changing the complex dynamics of power and privilege requires a multifaceted, longitudinal approach that will ensure individuals and organizations develop the skills and capacity within their own ecosystem to engage in a manner that fosters individual, community, and system change.

HOW TO MANAGE THE TRANSITION TO CHANGE—KOTTER AND BRIDGES

As our institutions strive to create an antiracist environment, we must appreciate that the implementation process is and will be complex. Implementation requires not only adept change management skills but also a parallel understanding of the emotional impact of the transition and associated steps necessary to create a sustainable, antiracist environment. In this section, we provide examples from our individual and institutional efforts to create an antiracist culture and how we applied two well-known change management strategies, Kotter's Organizational Change Model[16] and Bridges' Transition Model,[17] to support meaningful attenuation of both sides of the coin.

The three phases of Kotter's Eight-Step Organizational Change Model are: (1) create a climate for change, (2) engage and enable the whole organization, and (3) implement and sustain the change. Within each phase are essential steps as described in Table 16.2.

William Bridges' three-stage model (Fig. 16.2) focuses on the transitions (emotional reaction to acknowledging and letting go of power and privilege) that individuals within an organization will experience and must be managed if the change is to be successful. Changes are situational, whereas transitions are more psychological. Individuals recognize that whenever a change takes place, it means that something is ending. That ending can cause strong emotions, including anger, fear, denial, sadness, and surprise. As the realization that change is happening sets in, people move toward a neutral zone. This zone is characterized by emotions of confusion, frustration, skepticism, or apathy. Often in this phase, there are a large number of questions and a feeling that there is never enough clarity. It can be easy to lose momentum when in the neutral zone, backsliding to previous behaviors. Finally, as the change takes hold, most people move toward a place of new beginnings with excitement, energy, and a sense of commitment to the new way of thinking, doing, or being.

Specific to antiracism, White fragility insulates most White Americans from racial discomfort. Beginning a discussion of racism in any organization will result in behaviors of argumentation, silence, and denial.[18] This discomfort has to be acknowledged by those in the dominant, privileged group. In the neutral zone, members of marginalized groups may well express feelings of skepticism about whether change will ever occur or frustration at having to wait for change. As antiracism work continues, leaders must think about the underlying feelings of shame that are likely to arise from acknowledging the privilege that has existed as a member of the dominant group.

In both change models, to manage the transition, listening and communication are key. Assessing readiness for change is an important first step. This can be particularly complex in antiracism work where open communication

---

TABLE 16.2 Bridges' Transition Model and Kotter's Change Management Steps

- Create a climate for change
  - Create a sense of urgency and importance
  - Build guiding teams to support the work
  - Get the vision right
- Engage and enable the whole organization
  - Communicate for buy-in and alignment
  - Enable action and remove barriers
  - Create and celebrate short-term wins
- Implement and sustain the change
  - Do not let up and, rather, measure and build on what is working and adjust those things that are not
  - Make it stick by embedding it in the culture, structures, policies, and processes

---

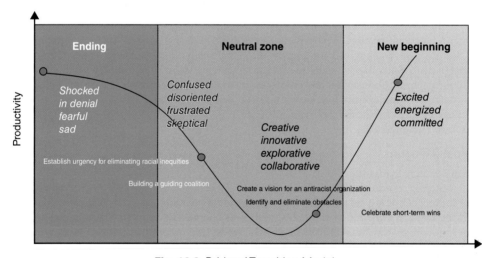

Fig. 16.2 Bridges' Transition Model.

about barriers to change and long-standing belief systems may be difficult to dislodge. A force field analysis can be a useful tool to understand drivers of and resistors to change.[19] Prior to embarking on a major change initiative, like specific elements of antiracism work we note next, this tool can support determining whether the time is right to move forward. For example, is there sufficient support from senior leadership and other individuals critical to the change you are trying to make? If there are state political headwinds, what barriers exist and in which areas? How can they be overcome or minimized? Are there other major change initiatives occurring at the same time and how does this deplete or reinforce your resources? With antiracism work, human resources are critical. What else are people occupied with and can they dedicate the time you need? What support and engagement do you have from learners, faculty, accrediting bodies, etc.?

Once a decision to move forward is made, clarity from leadership that change will happen and why it is needed is critical. Listening for underlying cares and concerns about the change that may have been missed or misunderstood helps to clarify and address issues along the way and allows leaders to provide the emotional support necessary to help people move through and embrace or at least accept the transition. This is especially critical in antiracism work because of the complex impact on people based on their own experiences, backgrounds, and belief systems. As a result, the change management process often requires training multiple leaders in the team on not just what to expect, but also how you believe change will impact their individual units (admissions, student affairs, curriculum, etc.) and the people working in them and how to address issues as they arise. Checking in regularly with leaders and individuals involved in the transition to understand what they are seeing and hearing to target communication and address backslides is vital. Finally, helping everyone see what the outcomes are that you hope for and how these support the broader mission of the institution (or unit), as well as how they can individually and collectively contribute to the change, is a key responsibility for all leaders.

Applying Kotter's Eight-Step Approach to Antiracism

As educational leaders, we have played a role in leading our organizations through Kotter's eight-step process to change organizational culture toward a more antiracist learning environment. We also engaged the Bridges' Transition Model to move our organizations through these stages. We have worked both locally and nationally and have learned many lessons through the process. Here we highlight the antiracist concepts and principles that apply to each step of the Kotter Model and provide practical examples that

can be used at other institutions. We also describe experiences with the Bridges' Transition Model in some of these examples.

Step 1: Inspire People to Act and Create a Sense of Urgency Around Antiracism Initiatives

The killing of George Floyd, Breonna Taylor, and the many other unnamed racial minorities by police officers served as a watershed moment that spurred activism and questioning of the systemic racism that continues in the United States. Across the country, our medical students spoke up and shared their concerns about racist perspectives and practices that were being perpetuated in current-day medicine. At two of our institutions, Boston University Chobanian and Avedisian School of Medicine and Washington University School of Medicine, the recognition of racism began before these horrible events as students were already questioning the practices that were apparent to them as new and early learners in the medical community.

Example 1: At Washington University School of Medicine, initial action toward antiracism was spurred by national attention to discrepancies in election to Alpha Omega Alpha (AOA) Medical Honor Society by race. Leadership decided to study our outcomes with regard to AOA selection. When we identified inequities based on race, it spurred a deeper investigation into our own grading data, and we demonstrated, as others have, that there were significant differences in clinical grades by race.[13] The Senior Associate Dean for Education and the Associate Dean for Program Evaluation and Continuous Quality Improvement presented those data to the department chairs and senior leadership. This spurred a desire for action and a willingness to look deeply at our grading processes and make immediate changes, including discontinuing AOA selection until we could eliminate inequities. As the announcement was made to faculty and students across the school, some voiced significant concerns about discontinuing AOA, including anger and fear. Some voiced concern that they felt the school was suggesting that if they had received AOA designation, that they were themselves being branded as racist. To address these concerns, multiple members of the leadership team including the Senior Associate Dean for Education and the Dean met with individuals and held meetings with groups to listen, correct misunderstandings, and explain the decision, while remaining steadfast that this was the decision and it was not going to be reversed.

Example 2: At Boston University Chobanian and Avedisian School of Medicine, several second-year medical students raised concerns about what they were hearing in the classroom. Specifically, students described faculty claims that certain diseases were more prevalent in Black

Americans and that while the reasons were unknown, they may be due to racial differences. This led to the development of an antiracism vertical integration group and an immediate analysis of the curriculum to identify how and where racism was manifesting. The findings of the curricular analysis were shared with the medical school community.[20]

In both examples, demonstrating racism through data was extremely powerful and an important way to create a sense of urgency. With racism, there is often an initial phase of denial as individuals begin to feel attacked or that they are being called racist rather than recognizing the systems of oppression that are everywhere. Analyzing institutional data in areas known to have vulnerabilities like admissions, awards/honors, and curricula can create the sense of urgency that is needed. In our experiences, data also moved our organizations from the neutral zone to new beginnings later in our journeys, spurring innovation and new energy.

To support leaders in identifying areas of potential focus, the Association of American Medical Colleges (AAMC) created the **Diversity, Inclusion, Culture, and Equity (DICE) Inventory** and supported the creation of the **Medical Education Senior Leaders (MESL) Antiracism Task Force Institutional Self-Assessment Toolkit**.[21] These can also be used to measure progress (steps 7 and 8).

Step 2: Build a Small but Empowered Coalition of Individuals Committed to Identifying and Systematically Addressing Policies and Practices That Support Antiracist Outcomes

After creating a sense of urgency, it is critical to create a knowledgeable and credible team. The guiding team must bring a sense of trust and believability that can motivate their peers to take action. With work related to antiracism, we have found that many institutions will ask students or minority faculty and staff alone to lead this work because of their passion for it. In our experience, it is vital that the guiding coalition include both students and faculty and majority and minority individuals. Faculty have the knowledge needed to understand the inner workings and are more aware of policies, processes, and the barriers that may exist and be brought up by peer faculty. Students are also essential to the team because they are strong motivators for change and can recognize and speak authentically to the impact of processes on students. Members of the dominant and minority group and experts from disciplines within and outside of medicine should also be included to ensure both lived experiences and political and social headwinds can be identified early in the process. Given that racism is a social construct, experts from areas outside of medicine can provide relevant knowledge and help to communicate the vision from a more knowledgeable viewpoint.

Example 1: At two of our institutions (Washington University School of Medicine and the University of Toledo College of Medicine and Life Sciences) a task force was developed and empowered by the governing body of the medical school to investigate underlying causes for and to make recommendations to eliminate grading disparities.[13,15] The task force engaged students, faculty, course leaders, equity, diversity, and inclusion leaders, and others to interrogate the extant literature and identify national and local system factors as well as local interpersonal and personal biases that may be at play. Based on these results, they brought forth recommendations for change. These were vetted by the governing body and resulted in additional work groups empowered with specific charges. These institutions worked on making changes to the curriculum and assessment structures, providing enhanced testing support for all learners, and developing required training for all faculty and housestaff.

Example 2: At Kaiser Permanente Bernard J. Tyson School of Medicine, members of the Office of Medical Education and the Office of Equity, Inclusion, and Diversity formed an Inclusive Curriculum Workgroup of faculty and staff. This workgroup is involved in curriculum review and support as well as faculty development including implementing a series of educational sessions titled "Unlearning Race-Based Medicine."

Step 3: Develop a Shared Vision of the Work and the Future Antiracist Learning Environment That It Will Bring

For all organizations moving toward an antiracist culture, communicating the vision in a clear and concise way is critical. Antiracism in medical education is about equitable health for all. The vision for dismantling racism in medical education must include the clear connection between systemic racism and health inequities. When the connection between health and systemic racism becomes clear through the vision, the buy-in becomes greater. Antiracism can become conflated with political views, so it is critical that the focus remain on health equity as the intended future state. With antiracism in medical education, this is important when articulating the vision to leaders and faculty across the many learning environments and health systems in which we work.

Example 1: To communicate a vision for the future and immediate next steps, all of our organizations developed and disseminated commitments to antiracism. Senior leaders communicated the commitments in emails, town halls, and other forums to ensure wide dissemination. We have learned that it is critical with antiracism for the leadership to repeatedly communicate their vision and commitment and to be prepared to deal with different constituents' reactions to antiracism-focused vision. As tragedies from racism continue to occur locally and nationally, many of our institutions use those moments to acknowledge our commitment to antiracism and reshare the vision. This communication can prevent backslide from the neutral zone and maintain momentum toward change.

Example 2: In 2021 the AAMC Medical Education Senior Leaders (MESL) group representing medical education deans from medical schools across the country endorsed a document created by their antiracism rapid action team. The document entitled *Creating Action to Eliminate Racism in Medical Education* included an antiracism vision statement for medical education. The document stated the following: *As members of AAMC MESL, we condemn the structures of racism that have allowed inequities in medicine and medical education to persist and are committed to combating racism in medical education by creating policies and changes that will support an antiracist learning environment and culture.* This shared vision generated by a geographically diverse group of medical education senior leaders provided a roadmap to support our efforts to move forward antiracism initiatives within our own organizations.

Step 4: Communicate to Help Ensure Buy-in for Antiracist Initiatives

Engaging and enabling the whole organization to move toward an antiracist learning environment and culture requires communication focusing on the emotions and fears that arise when change is about to take place. At this stage, leadership and the guiding team must think about the questions that are likely to come from the negative emotions many will feel when the new vision and direction is articulated. Racism in particular creates strong emotions, and many people focus on the individual and interpersonal level and believe the change is about them being racist rather than addressing the historical structures that embed racism throughout medicine and medical education.

As the examples given thus far illustrate, the iterative addition of more people with each step and each change helps to ensure that individuals can feel a part of the change and are able to contribute. Developing groups with specific goals can allow for this broader engagement but may require dedicated time or resources. These groups are often best led or supported by members of the initial guiding coalition to ensure alignment with the overall vision and coordination across change initiatives, while ensuring resources are allocated as needed. Including leaders from different areas, key constituents, and learners in the groups themselves generates new energy and creates additional voices to disseminate the message of change among peers in informal and formal ways.

Example 1: At Kaiser Permanente Bernard J. Tyson School of Medicine a position for a Faculty Director of Inclusive Curriculum was created with one support staff person. The Faculty Director provides oversight for the Inclusive Curriculum Workgroup comprised of faculty and staff from key offices and all departments (described previously in Step 3), the Equity, Inclusion, and Diversity curriculum thread, and related faculty development and facilitates communication about these initiatives.

Example 2: At Boston University Chobanian and Avedisian School of Medicine a website was created focused on antiracism and inclusive curriculum. The website included additional faculty and students as expert consultants who are available to faculty as their curriculum is revised and changes are tried. This enlisted a greater number of people and created more champions beyond the initial core coalition who could advance the vision and generate new ideas.

Step 5: Enable Action and Identify and Remove Barriers to Inaction for Antiracist Initiatives

At this stage, senior leaders may benefit from distancing themselves from the details of doing the work of making change to focus instead on managing and coordinating the work of others. This allows the senior leaders to anticipate and address barriers, enhance collaboration across groups, and ensure key constituents are kept abreast of impending changes. Barriers that commonly arise include those that are political, financial, and structural. The most common structural barrier to completing work in these areas is time. One mechanism to address this problem is to proactively carve out time for work groups to get things done during pre-existing time set aside for such work. Eliminating or reducing unnecessary meetings can also help. By thoughtfully considering the people involved and their other commitments, it is possible to create a working group that can effectively collaborate to get the job done. Political and financial barriers are also common and vary by school, program, and state.

Example 1: Political barriers to antiracism work are significant in many of our states and institutions. For example, several states have passed anti-DEI education legislation, and the 2023 US Supreme Court decision regarding race-conscious admission will have far-reaching impacts on medical school admissions. Senior leaders can collaborate with internal government affairs units, other schools, and lobbying organizations to fight against such measures locally. If such laws have already been passed, or in the case of the Supreme Court decision in race-conscious admissions, working with legal counsel to fully understand the laws and their interpretation will be critical. Identifying and working with other institutions in similar predicaments can help generate creative solutions to overcome barriers and work around racist policies. Even within very strict laws and regulations, senior leaders can work to address internal processes and procedures or drive support resources for those most impacted by such laws or policies.

Example 2: Financial prioritization is ever present within academic medical centers. The education mission and its initiatives are frequently threatened with loss of funding. Within education, the majority of our budget goes toward salary expenses and funding people's time. To address these barriers, buy-in from senior leaders including the dean and department chairs is crucial. Working directly with them to free up the time of the most knowledgeable, passionate, and successful leads should be a priority. If that is not possible, consider aligning work for individuals or groups or help them set priorities based on what is most likely to be immediately successful while not losing sight of long-term plans and strategies. Often giving permission to drop a prior commitment to something that is no longer as important is just as important as asking someone to take on something new.

Step 6: Create and Celebrate Short-Term Successes to Sustain Engagement in Antiracism and Health Equity

The work of antiracism is long term. The structural inequities and biases that plague our systems and processes took more than a century to develop. They will not be dismantled overnight. Clarity about this truth is important for everyone involved in change initiatives. To sustain the work, it is helpful to identify potential quick wins.

When launching a new initiative, celebrate it through announcements, acknowledge its leaders, and provide support for those individuals to present their work at conferences. Be sure to recognize quick and early accomplishments and positive outcomes.

Example 1: Across all four of our institutions early and ongoing wins have been celebrated through routine communication channels and processes thereby creating collective community enthusiasm and support for the changes. Examples of such wins have been changes in the grading process to de-emphasize the weight of standardized testing, creating an elective in health equity and justice, converting the admissions process to holistic review, and creating faculty development in bias mitigation in admissions, assessment, and letter writing. The celebrations help to move people from the neutral zone to the belief in the new beginning, changing the mood to one of acceptance or even excitement for what is possible.

Example 2: At the University of Toledo College of Medicine and Life Sciences, a health equity task force was created in response to a student-led mandate for greater focus on antiracism within the curriculum. Students were a critical element of communication and dissemination

of information to their classmates. Within 8 months, the school's commitment was further demonstrated as the task force led to the creation of a longitudinal health equity curricular thread that was directed by a well-respected faculty member known for her commitment to diversity, equity, and inclusion. The faculty appointment and curricular thread were communicated to students through medical education newsletters, email, and the Dean's monthly update. All communications emphasized the school's ongoing commitment to antiracism.

Step 7: Sustain Antiracist Change Through Monitoring Progress, Adjusting, and Progressive Implementation

For these initiatives to be sustainable, it is crucial that we measure impact. Clearly articulating the goals of each initiative and outlining expected outcomes allows us to measure whether or not they were achieved. This helps feed those short-term wins, generates excitement about what has been achieved, allows course correction when errors have been made, and supports dissemination of the work locally to key constituents and nationally. The latter further supports the development and promotion of the individual faculty who have worked so diligently. Many faculty do not have program evaluation skills. Consider collaborating with a local or regional program evaluation unit or bringing in a consultant, if possible, to support this work. Alternatively, identify colleagues in research domains who may be able to serve as mentors to faculty or students to support a scholarly approach to their work.

Example 1: All four of our institutions participated with several other medical school leaders on the AAMC Medical Education Senior Leaders (MESL) Antiracism Task Force and helped develop and pilot an Institutional Self-Assessment Toolkit.[21] The toolkit is intended for internal organizational use only, without any comparison to other schools or data shared externally, with measures in the areas of mission, governance and resources, educational programs, students/learners, and the learning environment. It asks schools to self-report on each measure using the three-item scale: has not yet begun, is in progress, or is done with ongoing continuous quality improvement. The intended output is an action plan that prioritizes one to three goals for the next year using the SMART (specific, measurable, attainable, realistic, and time-bound) framework[22] paying attention to context, resources, and support. Setting these goals and using robust evaluation methods to periodically track how an institution is doing in these areas as well as to identify additional areas of opportunity exemplifies this step. Ideally this progress and the key initiatives are communicated to internal constituents for both accountability and to sustain momentum.

Example 2: At Kaiser Permanente Bernard J. Tyson School of Medicine, we utilized an equity- and human-centered design framework to integrate the entirety of the educational program's interested parties (faculty, staff, and students) in the cocreation and implementation of a scorecard tool that evaluates the learner experience and curricular content in three core constructs (representation, critical conscientiousness, and inclusive environment). The tool is under ongoing refinement, including being integrated into the usual curriculum governance processes and being extended to the clinical learning environment.

Step 8: Institutionalize the Change Through New Antiracist Policies and Procedures and Ensure that Ongoing Evaluations of the Changes Are Being Made to Ensure Sustainability

Ultimately, to ensure that these change initiatives are sustained, they must be embedded in the policies, procedures, and culture of the institution. Without this, a backslide is inevitable. Policies and procedures that support holistic review in admissions or require bias training for admissions committee members or faculty and housestaff involved in assessment are examples of best practices. Building support programs for all students that include a holistic view of well-being and providing specific support for those students who show early signs of struggling can address some structural racism issues while staying within the bounds of more restrictive legal statutes.

Example 1: At Washington University School of Medicine, we created a subcommittee of our curriculum oversight body charged explicitly with reviewing policies, procedures, curricula, and outcomes through an antiracism lens. The subcommittee is comprised of educational leaders; equity, diversity, and inclusion champions; students; and housestaff to ensure broad representation, but it is nimble enough in size to complete the work. The subcommittee completed an evaluation of our programs using a variety of tools and made suggestions for important priority areas. It also created a scorecard to monitor progress. It regularly reviews curricular content including admissions rubrics; lectures or other pedagogical materials with a historically race-based approach; clinical cases used in the classroom or standardized patient suite; assessment questions; and educational program outcomes.

Example 2: At Boston University Chobanian and Avedisian School of Medicine, an established annual educational quality improvement process added a new question asking faculty to describe what changes they have made to their course or clerkship to create a more antiracist learning environment.[23] This new question within an existing institutional process requires faculty to annually evaluate their antiracist changes and promotes ongoing innovation

in antiracism and health equity in medical education. The changes are shared annually with the education committees to highlight the work that is being done and the areas of opportunity.

Throughout each of these steps in the Kotter framework, it is critical to attend to the emotional burden of transition as outlined previously. Communicating frequently, listening to fundamental cares and concerns, addressing issues as they arise, anticipating barriers, proactively addressing barriers, and working to secure a large cohort of people who understand why the work is important, what they can do to support it, and where it is eventually going is essential. As senior leaders, we also benefited from communicating about our work with each other and our regional and national medical education and DEI community.

CONCLUSION

The road to **social justice** and **health equity** is not a destination but a journey for all involved in medical education to identify and address how power and privilege operate within our institutions to perpetuate outcomes associated with historical patterns of inequities. It is incumbent on medical education institutions to commit to the process of becoming antiracist organizations. Change management endeavors will need to acknowledge the parallel emotional process that must be considered as changes are made that unravel and eliminate the complex interplay of power and privilege that impact the health of our patients. This work requires collaboration within the institution, across institutions, and among people. Intentional team building, networking, and collaboration aid in forward progress and help sustain momentum. Together, we can progressively chip away at both sides of the power and privilege coin.

REFERENCES

1. Price GN, Darity WA. The economics of race and eugenic sterilization in North Carolina: 1958-1968. *Econ Hum Biol.* 2010;8(2):261–272. https://doi.org/10.1016/j.ehb.2010.01.002.
2. Brandt AM. Racism and research: the case of the Tuskegee syphilis study. *Hastings Cent Rep.* 1978;8:21–29.
3. Skloot R. *The Immortal Life of Henrietta Lacks.* Crown Publishers; 2010.
4. Jacobs DJ. Lead poisoning in private and public housing: the legacy still before us. *Am J Public Health.* 2019;109(6):830–832.
5. Anderson KO, Green CR, Payne R. Racial and ethnic disparities in pain: causes and consequences of unequal care. *J Pain.* 2009;10(12):1187–1204.
6. Alcendor DJ. Racial disparities-associated COVID-19 mortality among minority populations in the US. *J Clin Med.* 2020;9(8):2442.

7. Nixon SA. The coin model of privilege and critical allyship: implications for health. *BMC Public Health*. 2019;19:1637.

8. Bailey ZD, Krieger N, Agénor M, Graves J, Linos N, Bassett MT. Structural racism and health inequities in the USA: evidence and interventions. *Lancet*. 2017;389(10077):1453–1463.

9. Yearby R, Clark B, Figueroa JF. Structural racism in historical and modern US health care policy: study examines structural racism in historical and modern US health care policy. *Health Aff (Millwood)*. 2022;41(2):187–194.

10. Egede LE, Walker RJ, Campbell JA, Linde S, Hawks LC, Burgess KM. Modern day consequences of historic redlining: finding a path forward. *J Gen Intern Med*. 2023;38(6):1534–1537. https://doi.org/10.1007/s11606-023-08051-4.

11. Wells L, Gowda A. A legacy of mistrust: African Americans and the US healthcare system. *Proceedings of UCLA health*. 2020;24:1–3.

12. Kendi IX. *How to be an antiracist*. One world; 2023.

13. Colson ER, Pérez M, Blaylock L, et al. Washington University School of Medicine in St. Louis case study: a process for understanding and addressing bias in clerkship grading. *Acad Med*. 2020;95(12S):S131–S135. doi: 10.1097/ACM.0000000000003702

14. Teherani A, Hauer KE, Fernandez A, King Jr TE, Lucey C. How small differences in assessed clinical performance amplify to large differences in grades and awards: a cascade with serious consequences for students underrepresented in medicine. *Acad Med*. 2018;93(9):1286–1292. https://doi.org/10.1097/ACM.0000000000002323.

15. Hanson JL, Pérez M, Mason HRC, et al. Racial/ethnic disparities in clerkship grading: perspectives of students and teachers. *Acad Med*. 2022;97(11S):S35–S45. https://doi.org/10.1097/ACM.0000000000004914.

16. Kotter JP. *Leading Change*. Harvard Business School Press; 1996.

17. Bridges W, Mitchell S. Leading transition: a new model for change. *Leader to Leader*. 2000;16(3):30–36.

18. DiAngelo R. *White Fragility: Why It's So Hard for White People to Talk about Racism*. Beacon Press; 2018.

19. Thomas J. Force field analysis: a new way to evaluate your strategy. *Long Range Plann*. 1985;18(6):54–59. https://doi.org/10.1016/0024-6301(85)90064-0.

20. Green KA, Wolinsky R, Parnell SJ, et al. Deconstructing racism, hierarchy, and power in medical education: guiding principles on inclusive curriculum design. *Acad Med*. 2022;97(6):804–811. https://doi.org/10.1097/ACM.0000000000004531.

21. Association of American Medical Colleges. *Creating Action to Eliminate Racism in Medical Education*. Association of American Medical Colleges. 2020. https://www.aamc.org/media/63351/download

22. Conzemius A, O'Neill J. *The Power of SMART Goals: Using Goals to Improve Student Learning*. Solution Tree Press; 2009.

23. Nathan AS, Del Campo D, Garg PS. Where are we now? Evaluating the one year impact of an anti-racism curriculum review. *Med Teach*. 2024. doi:10.1080/0142159X.2024.2316852

17

Reimagining Health Care Professional Education to Embrace Socioeconomically Diverse Learners

Stephen Maloney, Jonathan Foo, Michelle You You, Jennifer Cleland, and Kieran Walsh

OUTLINE

SUMMARY

Health care professions education is critical. The United States must have a system of health care professions education that supports the training and professional development of adequate numbers of professionals who can deliver the care the population requires. Yet health care professions education is expensive, with significant costs, including but not limited to curriculum design, assessment, and evaluation. A substantial amount of this cost falls upon the learner, in both explicit fees and hidden costs of participation. These can be barriers for prospective students from certain societal groups entering and thriving in health care education. There is a need to take active steps to embrace socioeconomically diverse learners.

This chapter develops the concepts of cost and value as applied to health professions education. It explores the tensions in considering cost alongside education excellence and the different perspectives and viewpoints from which issues of cost and value can be considered. The lens of cost and value is then applied to the choices faced by institutions around admissions processes and designing cost-effective curricula. The chapter provides practical solutions as well as research approaches to expand the evidence base for informing cost-effective education in the health professions.

SECTION 1: BACKGROUND

Health care professions education is critically important. The United States must have a system of health professions education that supports the training and professional development of adequate numbers of high-quality professionals who can deliver the care the population requires.

Health professions education is also expensive. It includes a myriad of significant costs—including, but not limited to, curriculum design, assessment, and evaluation. These costs add up. The mean cost of US medical education today is about $300,000 per student.[1] A substantial amount of this cost falls upon the learner, in both explicit fees and hidden costs of participation. This can be a barrier for prospective students from certain societal groups who wish to enter medical or other health professions education programs. At present, 75% of US medical students come from families in the top 20% of household incomes,[2] but without participation of all societal groups, there can be limited social justice and social mobility in health professions education. There is a need to take active steps to entice and embrace socioeconomically diverse learners. Barriers to full participation can relate to gender or race or a host of other factors. We have made progress by breaking down some of these barriers. But the significant barrier of cost remains. In this chapter, we discuss how health care professions education might be reimagined within the United States so that we can make more cost-conscious decisions around health professions education—embracing and supporting greater learner socioeconomic diversity in our programs and in our health workforce.

Tensions From an Emerging Field

The art and science of applying cost and value approaches to health professions education is an emerging field. It can provide us with a new lens through which to view the challenges ubiquitous to health professions educators and education institutions across the globe. One of these challenges is addressing equity and diversity in health professions education. Although economic data alone do not tell us which decision we should make, they offer fresh perspectives by which to reimagine solutions and to guide decision-making in pursuit of our goals. However, in exploring the field of cost and value and its application to medical education, you may have to overcome some tensions inherent in our health professions education upbringing: your identity as an educator and the culture of pursuing educational excellence no matter the cost.

It is readily accepted that health economic data have a significant role in guiding government and health service expenditure to optimize health outcomes. However, the field of health professions education is often reluctant to accept the same economic principles and reasoning when applied to optimizing health professions education outcomes. Insights into why this reluctance exists can be obtained from the international health professions education community through recent work led by Cleland et al. who conducted interviews of global thought leaders in health professions education from across the United States, Canada, the Netherlands, Denmark,

Australia, the Middle East, and China.[3] Aside from a lack of confidence in the knowledge and skills required, there was concern that obtaining evidence on the costs and benefits of our educational decision-making could result in unwanted accountability and subsequent loss of autonomy. It was therefore considered important, but risky. For example, what if the data did not support their current decision-making, showing that the option selected was more costly and less effective than an alternative? Would they then be forced to change direction? Perceptions of professional identity also played an influential role, with the viewpoint that analyzing costs and benefits is not the reason or purpose they went into educational research but rather their pursuit of educational excellence. However, if the challenges listed prevent us from making evidence-based decisions, then they are also barriers to reimagining the evolution of our profession.

SECTION 2: A COMMON LANGUAGE

Health professions training has not routinely equipped its learners with the economic literacy to interpret studies of educational costs and benefits. What one person understands by "cost" in health professions education is likely to be different from another person. Part of the solution for moving toward cost-effective education therefore requires orientating to some key economic terms and principles.

Health professions educators are likely conscious of the financial costs within education such as the fees typically paid by students or the outgoing expenses of educational institutions through staff and faculty wages, materials, and clinical placement payments. However, the true cost also includes all the tangible and intangible energy and effort that then cannot be put to another cause (i.e., the "opportunity cost"). Given that there are finite resources available to use for health professions education, those involved in the health professions education system must consider the opportunity cost if educators are to optimize outcomes from our educational effort. A simple cost analysis can assist in exploring educational inputs in monetary terms for two alternatives without consideration of the outputs. Better again, the assistance of an economic evaluation which looks at both the costs and the benefits of two feasible alternatives can be even more powerful. The specific types of educational questions with which these analyses can assist are discussed within the recommended solutions to these issues later in this chapter.

Perspective Matters

Although multiple definitions and formulas exist for the term "value," it should be considered as a judgment about the ratio of inputs (economic cost) to the outputs or educational benefits. When comparing two options, the one that provides the greater value is the one that yields the greatest ratio of benefits to the relative effort or cost. What makes the concept of value more nuanced is that it can vary depending on whose viewpoint it is being considered from. This point is illustrated by the example of a student-led clinic.

Student-led clinics are settings where students are engaged in delivering health services. Student clinics have a wide range of involved groups or interested parties, each with their own "costs of participation," their own outcomes of interest, and therefore their own viewpoint on value. Value from the viewpoint of the learner might focus on learning outcomes as well as exposure to various clinical specialities that they may otherwise not be able to experience. Value from the viewpoint of the educational institution may focus on the clinic enabling an increase in placement hours and student numbers, enabling greater enrollment and revenue from student enrolment. Value from the viewpoint of the health service may focus on additional services rendered. Value from the viewpoint of society may be concerned with reduced emergency department utilization or health outcomes provided to an otherwise underserved population.

No matter the viewpoint, making informed decisions about value requires a reference point—a feasible alternative by which to make a comparison. It is easier to make a choice when one knows both the cost and benefits of the next option. Unfortunately, health professions education falls short in this area. A systematic review led by Cook et al. mapping the research methods, costs, and economic benefits of physician continuing professional development, found that of their 111 included papers, only 22% provided a comparison against an alternative.[4] Naturally, when one party's costs are reduced, another's may have increased. This important relationship between parties is why many high-quality studies explore multiple partys' perspectives. Within the context of considering multiple perspectives, a study by Foo et al. showed a total additional cost of US$9371 per student failing in clinical education from the perspective of all parties considered. But students bear the majority of this burden, incurring 49% of costs, followed by the government (22%), the education institution (18%), the health service organization (10%), and the clinical educator (1%).[5] We believe their study also highlights the argument that we have an interdependent relationship of outcomes, with a shared interest and responsibility for the education of tomorrow's health workforce.

The Societal Viewpoint

A diverse health workforce can decrease health inequities. It is therefore unfortunate that representation by minority groups in US training is declining.[6] However, it is difficult to create impact from initiatives when health professions education is such a large and dynamic system. Training the US health professional workforce has become big business, as it is in many countries. Global expenditure now exceeds 100 billion USD annually. It has also become increasingly competitive, driving up entry scores and student fees and adding further pressure to the costs of participation. Society is not only served by having diverse socioeconomic groups enter medical programs, but by ensuring that all have the ability to support themselves to thrive throughout the entire program. The progression of students to being meaningfully employed and retained within our health workforce increases the return on our societies' educational investments. A learner who does not succeed within a program or who leaves their profession prematurely represents an economic loss to society. A public medical program without transparency or accountability for their health professions education spend, which cannot demonstrate the cost-effectiveness of its approaches, presents an unknown financial risk for society. For example, the 2023 US Department of Education Financial Value Transparency and Gainful Employment regulation requires postsecondary programs to provide increased transparency around expected costs, financial aid, and expected earnings for graduates.[7] The societal viewpoint is summarized well by the Prato Statement on cost and value in health care professional education, which states that one of the drivers of cost and value research in health professions education is to drive education that is sustainable, accessible, and able to meet future health care requirements.[8]

Section 3 will look at the return on investment from our course admission processes. Section 4 will look at some key touch points within health professions programs to help us imagine low-cost, transparent education practices. Section 5 will further explore the role of cost and value in reimagining research for global impact, bridging the research-to-practice divide, and expanding the evidence base for cost-effective medical education.

SECTION 3: ADMISSION TO MEDICAL PROGRAMS

Association for American Medical Colleges (AAMC) data show that those from lower socioeconomic status (SES) groups have lower acceptance rates into medical school, making up 24.2% of applicants but only 21.5% of acceptees.[9] This theme of low SES diversity among medical students is consistent with information from our international colleagues, with the medical profession consisting predominantly of individuals from affluent backgrounds. For example, 80% of UK medical school applicants come from only 20% of UK high schools, and half of UK schools have sent no applicants to medicine in recent years.[10] In fact, across the world, young people with the academic and personal attributes to successfully study medicine and become doctors experience disadvantages associated with sociodemographic factors such as ethnicity, minority group membership, or low income.[11] These disadvantages lead to underparticipation in medicine and higher education more generally. The reasons for this are often multifaceted, interconnected within a myriad of wider, complex structural and societal issues including ethnic minority inequalities, parental education,[12] personal aspirations,[13] educational attainment,[14] and family and peer influences and expectations.[15]

The lack of diversity in medicine has caused concern that medical schools may not be promoting social mobility nor creating the best possible workforces to care for the populations they serve.[16-18] Given this, governments have attempted to widen participation to education and medicine via macrolevel policies, the broad aim of which are to reduce discrepancies between the rates of participation of different demographic groups of students in higher education generally[19] and medical education specifically.[20] The focal groups for widening access are heavily determined by each country's historical and current social issues, from racial groups,[21,22] indigenous populations such as Aboriginal and Torres Strait Islanders in Australia,[22,23] rural communities,[24] and lower socioeconomic groups.

These widening participation policies are then enacted by universities and medical schools via the development and implementation of widening access processes and tools.[25,26] The precise nature of these widening access processes and tools varies across different countries, but includes quota systems,[27] outreach programs,[28] access courses,[29] particular use of selection tools,[25,30] and the use of contextual data.[31]

However, given students from certain backgrounds continue to be underrepresented in medicine worldwide,[11,32] these policies are clearly not wholly effective. Yet, if it were easy, the issue of widening access to medicine may have been "solved" by now. It is not.[33] Medical schools work in a multifaceted landscape of competing pressures—many of which are in tension with greater inclusion. For example, as a society, we may want fair access to medicine, so that medical students represent all groups in society as well as excelling in terms of academic and personal qualities. Both aspects may be desirable but attaining excellent pre-entry qualifications (a prerequisite for studying medicine in most countries) is typically the stumbling block for those from underrepresented groups as attainment is heavily influenced by socioeconomic factors such as ethnicity, minority group membership, and/or low income.[26] These "disadvantages" are usually due to inequalities in pre-university education and are argued to be the cause of the underrepresentation of medical school applicants from

demographically disadvantaged groups.[34,35] Thus, using prior academic attainment as the first hurdle in the medical school selection process inherently discriminates against individuals from less advantaged backgrounds and therefore requires trade-off with expanding the diversity of the medical student body. At the university level, universities want to attract students with high entry grades as this contributes to their standing in international league tables. The question is how to balance this with, for example, offering places to students with lower grades in acknowledgment of the context in which they achieved their education. In some countries, medical school selection processes are determined by governments. For example, in India, the enactment of NMC Act 2019 in September 2019 meant the NEET-UG (the National Eligibility cum Entrance Test [Undergraduate]) became the sole entrance test for admissions to all medical colleges in India. Indian medical schools no longer had autonomy in how they selected applicants. To give another, contrasting example, in the Netherlands, universities are legally required to select students using at least two different, qualitative criteria, and the law now specifically rules out the application of a lottery procedure.

Coming back to the setting of the United States, these examples highlight that admissions are fundamentally an optimization process for medical schools: identifying and implementing processes that select the best applicants from the available pool at the same time as balancing political, social, and academic drivers for admissions.[36]

Working within the parameters allowed by governments, regulators, host universities, and society, medical schools must consider not only the reliability and validity of admissions tools and processes but also fairness and cost-effectiveness in their admissions decision-making.[37] Several studies have done so,[38-42] but this remains an underdeveloped area of admissions research. Admissions costs can be considered from different angles (e.g., of the institution or the individual applicant).[43] Outcome measures must assess value as well as cost (cheapest is not necessarily best: see Schreurs et al.[40] discussed later in this chapter) and look at individual-level outcomes for both distal (e.g., location and type of position post-qualification) as well as proximal (e.g., performance in medical school) indicators.

In the next subsection we briefly discuss some considerations of the pre-health professions education pipeline highlighting issues of "cost and value" as part of the complexity of medical school selection.[33]

Fit for Context

Many medical schools use a combination of selection tools such as prior academic attainment, admissions tests, and interviews. It is important for medical schools to consider the incremental value of adding selection tools into their selection process. Does adding a particular or extra method increase the predictive validity of the selection procedure? Is it worth the effort and costs, both economically and regarding the possible introduction of unintended consequences? The answers to these important questions will vary by context. For example, in countries where national school leaving examinations (i.e., final competency exams) in the foundational sciences (e.g., mathematics, biology, chemistry, and physics) are standardized at a national level and are prerequisites for admission to medical school (e.g., the Netherlands and the United Kingdom), there is arguably no need for all applicants to sit a separate national test which assesses knowledge. Why spend money and energy confirming reliable and freely available comparative data on prior academic attainment? It would be better for the medical school to invest its resources in the assessment of the aptitude for (inter)personal skills that a good doctor also must have. On the other hand, in countries where there is less standardization of schooling and school leaving examinations (such as in the United States) the need for applicants to sit the same national test to allow for reliable comparison of performance may be greater.

Cost to the Medical School

As a rule of thumb, any selection interview or assessment (e.g., review of references or assessing pre-university extra-curricular activities[44]) that requires medical school staff time poses direct costs for the institution. For example, Schreurs et al. compared the costs and benefits of two different approaches to admission into medical school: a tailored, multimethod selection process versus a weighted lottery procedure (admission chances based on prior academic attainment).[40] They found the tailor-made selection procedure was relatively expensive in terms of costs to the medical school while the lottery procedure came with negligible costs. However, when they looked at the relative performance of students selected through each pathway (including failure/students dropping out, repeating courses and examinations), the "active" selection process resulted in better outcomes. This illustrates that the cheapest is not always the best.

Most medical schools do not do a formal economic analysis of their selection process. However, faculty do indirectly discuss the costs of selection when they consider, for example, how many applicants they can interview. Human resources and other costs (e.g., rooms, availability of assessors) are inherent in these discussions, just not formalized into pounds, euros, or dollars. Brown et al.'s analysis of the cost of a clinical examination is a useful guide to considering

the costs of selection—particularly given selection is often thought of as the first assessment in medical school.[45]

Costs to the Applicant

Any selection activity that requires an applicant to go somewhere to sit for a test or attend an interview will have costs for them. Applicant costs can be huge in countries/systems which allow multiple applications. These costs can be a barrier to less advantaged potential applicants, thus perpetuating inequalities. Medical schools may wish to have a bursary system so applicants from less affluent backgrounds can apply for funding to cover some of these costs. Alternatively, schools may wish to consider remote selection tests, using eye-tracking software for security and confidence.[46] However, it is important to consider that some groups may also be disadvantaged by sitting tests at home, particularly those living in crowded conditions and/or in areas with poor internet connections.

Acknowledging Context or "Holistic Admissions"

Holistic or contextualized admissions recognize that not everyone has the same educational journey and that some students have had to overcome challenges to achieve their grades. In the UK this is called contextualized admissions (CA)—acknowledging a candidate's background when making decisions on whom to admit.[31] The equivalent in the United States is "holistic admissions."[47]

Contextual indicators typically include individual level (e.g., first in the family to go to university), area level (such as postcode or ZIP code, indicating a more deprived area of upbringing), school level (how many pupils go onto higher education), and participation in outreach programs. Typically, contextually identified applicants have a lower academic requirement, enabling them to progress through the admissions process rather than being rejected at the first hurdle of academic attainment. Although the evidence base is currently small, there is evidence that those admitted under CA do just as well as applicants accepted through the standard process.[48]

Finally, medical school places are scarce, and admissions committees must consider the balance between the expected relative cost/effort and the benefit of using different selection criteria or processes to sift through more applicants than places. An admissions committee that takes the position that academic attainment is the most important factor in selection will likely invest relatively fewer resources into selecting for personal qualities than would an institution that places high value on the latter.[43] Looking at the mission statements of different medical schools can give some indication of what they value in their admissions priorities and may explain differences in admissions processes, including how different components within an admissions process are weighed.

In conclusion, the choices made at the point of selection into medical school all have costs, whether financial or otherwise, by choosing one approach to increasing the diversity of medical students and losing the opportunity to take an alternative action. These opportunity costs may be felt in different ways by different individuals, groups, and societies.

SECTION 4: CURRICULUM DESIGN IN HEALTH PROFESSIONS EDUCATION

Curricula will inevitably evolve as a result of reimagining health professions education. This brings with it a change to the types and volume of educational resources required (i.e., costs), ranging from the micro-level of individual activities to the macrolevel of whole programs. In general, programs tend to expand over time as individual faculty add content on their special interest topics, the body of medical knowledge grows, and health care systems become more complex, requiring increased knowledge on non-biomedical topics such as social justice, climate change, and artificial intelligence. This educational inflation is one of the drivers for increasing health professions education costs, costs that are incurred by educational institutions and often passed on to students. In this section, we propose the incorporation of a cost and value lens when considering the structure of medical school and the medical school curricula. We explore costs from the student perspective, before looking at institution costs, and finally discuss how these two perspectives can be considered while striving for cost-effective health professions education.

Student Costs

Student costs include all costs students incur as part of their participation in health professions education. They include financial costs such as course fees, living expenses, study materials, and travel costs (particularly for placements). The impact of these financial costs was captured in the British Medical Association 2022 survey which includes complete responses from 78% of UK medical students.[49] In this survey, due to their financial situation, 5% reported considering leaving their program in the next 12 months, and 64% considering taking on additional paid work. Of students who do work, 73% report that working has a negative impact on their studies. Although most universities have financial support systems, this survey also revealed that of the 14% applying for financial hardship support, only half received the full amount for which they applied. These findings paint the picture of a health professions education system that does not provide sufficient financial

support to students, the result of which leads to negative impacts on student learning and potential attrition.

Furthermore, the cost to participate in a rigorous health professions education program extends beyond financial costs, but also includes the opportunity cost of the time and energy that cannot be used in another way. While applicable to all students, the impacts of opportunity costs are most salient to those with greater constraints on their time and energy. For example, students who also need to engage in paid employment to financially support their family, students with caregiving responsibilities, or students with medical conditions that limit energy or reduce task efficiency. We can explore the implications of this through the example of a clerkship in an emergency department. Students may be told that they are welcome to wait around as long as they like to try and observe "interesting" cases. For the learner who needs to work to support their family, this learning activity becomes a choice between potentially learning something useful for their future career in medicine or the immediate imperative of putting food on the table. Just as we no longer think about being "color blind" when it comes to racial inclusivity, we cannot continue to be "cost blind" when it comes to the costs of health professions education. We must be aware of financial and opportunity costs when designing health professions education, as such design choices can either widen or narrow disadvantages across the diverse student body.

Institution Costs

Costs from the institutional perspective are of principal concern to educational leaders and managers who are responsible for ensuring programs are financially sustainable. Indeed, a program that is not financially sustainable cannot continue and is of no benefit to students, institutions, or the public. Institution costs are typically driven by resource requirements for staff time, facilities, equipment, and materials.[4] Expansion of a program budget, without a corresponding increase in expected output, is rare. As such, educational innovations within programs are typically resourced through the reduction in resources to other aspects of the program or through other sources that do not require institution funding. An example of the latter is illustrated in a study looking at the cost of clinical education for students who underperform, finding 15 min/day of additional unpaid overtime incurred by the clinical educator.[5] It is unsustainable to place excessive workload on individuals to provide health professions education as over time this may increase staff stress and burnout and ultimately affect workforce satisfaction and attrition.[50]

However, many initiatives toward widening participation and supporting diverse learners are also resource intensive. Educating a homogeneous population of students allows for institutions to gain efficiencies through economies of scale where the same educational structures, activities, and resources can be reused, thus lowering the cost per student. Health professions education programs tend to adopt this mass production model, with a focus on curriculum design for mainstream learners and customized adjustments for those who do not fit the traditional mold. For example, the experience of Muslim women in a Western country where altered physical examination techniques and learning spaces for disrobing were inconsistently provided reflects ad-hoc adjustments rather than inclusive design as the norm.[51] Medical programs seeking to provide equity and inclusivity in their programs offer students the opportunity to apply for and develop bespoke supports and alternate arrangements. However, from a cost perspective, this process is incredibly inefficient as it diverges from economies of scale, taking substantial time and effort on the part of both students and faculty. This is akin to the high cost of a bespoke tailored item of clothing compared to the more economical purchase of a mass-produced factory item. Additionally, adjustment processes place the onus on students to reach out for support and create a culture of "other" within health professions education. Students may also be hesitant to request adjustments due to unwillingness to be perceived as lacking or weak. Thus, programs that have equity and inclusivity embedded into their design, thereby not requiring individual adjustments, not only improve social justice but are likely to improve cost-efficiency.

Designing Cost-Effective Curricula

We propose that thinking about inclusive curricula with a lens of cost and value can be beneficial for both students and institutions. In particular, cost and value are important tools for educators to utilize in supporting the case for reimagined medical curricula.[52] The following are practical recommendations for how we can apply concepts of cost and value.

Firstly, curriculum design should consider educational effects and costs together. Often, educators initiate designs based on educational effects followed by managers considering costs. However, it is an integrated approach that will create the best balance between costs and effects.

Secondly, consider financial and opportunity costs from the perspective of all interested parties. The student perspective is critical yet often overlooked, resulting in curricula that unintentionally disadvantages those who have additional constraints on finances, time, and energy.

Thirdly, focus on value in addition to cost. Inclusive educational design also brings with it tangible value, including reduced burden on students and staff, reduced remediation, and improved retention. The value proposition should be made front-and-center in arguments for inclusive educational design.

Finally, medical education researchers should guide the creation and pursuit of questions of cost and value that advance our understanding of providing cost-effective education. This requires an understanding of the types of basic economic analyses that can be applied to medical education and the questions they are designed to answer. This opportunity for medical education research is explored in the following section.

SECTION 5: AN OPPORTUNITY FOR MEDICAL EDUCATION RESEARCH

Expanding the Evidence Base for Cost-Effective Medical Education

The following types of information are commonly desired before informed decision-making regarding whether one particular intervention rather than another should be used to increase diversity in the health professional workforce: How much does the intervention cost? Does this approach represent "good value" when considering costs and educational outcomes? Which reforms can achieve the results using the least resources, or, given the resources, what are the highest educational outcomes we can get? Who should pay for the intervention, and how much? Although answers to these questions may differ by perspective (e.g., society, institutions, or individuals), accumulating the answers from all types of interested parties would help reimagine the educational system to improve its efficiency to embrace socioeconomically diverse learners and produce a diverse health professional workforce.

Various types of cost and value analyses can be used in the process of reimagining health professions education.[53,54] Understanding the unique purpose of each technique, and the types of medical education questions they can assist in answering, is an essential part of expanding our evidence base for high-value, low-cost education.

1. *Cost-minimization analysis*

    When alternative interventions are considered similar in respect of the educational outcomes they produce, then cost-minimization analysis can identify the option with the lowest cost. From the perspective of society, costs are measured as the total social value of all resources used for each alternative intervention, regardless of who pays for them. Examples from the literature include exploration of multi-tool selection procedures,[40] remediation,[55] and community-based health professions education.[56]

2. *Cost-effectiveness analysis*

    More often, comparison is made between alternative interventions according to their differing costs, as well as their differing effects, in producing a certain educational outcome. For example, intervention comparisons from the literature include community-based versus hospital-based education[56] or face-to-face delivery versus blended delivery.[57] With a cost-effectiveness analysis, outcomes remain in natural units, rather than a conversion to a dollar value. For example, as more people are being treated as outpatients or day cases, community-based education is considered an effective option for teaching basic clinical skills.[56] A cost-effectiveness analysis might then compare community-based education to traditional hospital-based education and prioritizes the approach that uses lower costs to achieve the goal of a certain increase in clinical skills competency.

3. *Cost-benefit analysis*

Cost-benefit analysis evaluates interventions according to their costs and benefits when each is measured in monetary terms.[58] It is useful to interested parties in the real world who often have to make decisions based on comparing interventions designed for different outcomes, such as deciding between directing teaching resources toward the development of learners' basic clinical skills or toward their communication skills. Cost-benefit analysis should only be used when it is possible to measure or convert all the important benefits of interventions to monetary terms. For example, if the increase in the number of socioeconomically disadvantaged medical graduates associated with community-based education leads to society's savings on health care expenditure or the population's improvement in quality-adjusted life years, then it would be possible to convert the benefits of the intervention to monetary terms and calculate the benefit-cost ratio. Based on the ratio, different types of interventions (educational or other types of interventions designed for different outcomes) can be compared.[59]

4. *Discrete choice experiment*

It can also be helpful to consider the question "Is the benefit worth the cost" through the lens of a willingness-to-pay analysis,[53] especially when there is no market price to estimate the monetary value of an intervention's costs and/or benefits. The discrete choice experiment (DCE) is one of the stated preference methods that derive the value of benefits from individuals' statements about their willingness to pay.[60] Specifically, discrete choice experiments allow us to value the component parts (attributes) of interventions, such as their content or mode of delivery, or outcomes such as medical knowledge, clinical skills, communication skills, and attitudes of socioeconomically disadvantaged medical graduates. With the relative importance of those attributes elicited from various groups, information regarding how different people might trade less of one attribute for more of another[61] will

help answer "Who should pay for the intervention/outcome, and how much?"

Resource Constrained Settings

Resources for health professions education within the United States are becoming more constrained, whereas accountability of the education being provided is increasing.[40] Economic evaluation studies will be essential for informed decision-making in this restrictive environment. Embracing cost and value research has the potential to provide novel perspectives on old problems.[3] Recently, the absolute number of cost and value studies in health professions education has increased, and yet the proportion relative to all the health professions education research did not increase and has never exceeded 1%.[62]

This current dearth of research evidence in this field means that cost and value studies in health professions education are increasingly required for decision-making on health professions education around the globe. It is important to note however that both economic evaluation studies and decision-making in health professions education are context contingent. Decision-making in health professions education in less affluent economies would be misleading if they are directly based on evidence or experience from wealthy economies. On the one hand, marketing and signaling theory suggests that wealthy countries/institutions also utilize sophisticated approaches to signal their advancement; there are natural incentives for high-cost approaches in their teaching practices. On the other hand, differences in various aspects (e.g., culture, value, health needs, price for resources, education standards, funding mechanisms) among countries and institutions may make a particular approach (e.g., problem-based learning, community-based education) that is popular in one economy, infeasible or ineffective in another. However, at present 81% of cost and value studies in health professions education come from high-income economies such as the United States raising the question: is health professions education the realm of the rich?[63] This challenge also presents a leadership opportunity for education researchers within the United States. If we are able to include low-cost interventions within our comparative studies, then the outputs of our medical education research can be more meaningful and impactful in guiding excellence in medical education across the globe.

TAKE-HOME POINTS

1. Health professions educators are likely familiar with financial costs: the educational fees typically paid by students and the outgoing expenses of educational institutions through wages, materials, and clinical placement payments. However, the true cost also includes all of the

tangible and intangible energy and effort that cannot be put to another purpose, that is, the "opportunity cost."

2. Resources for health professions education are more and more constrained while accountability is increasing for how revenue generated from education is being spent. Economic evaluation studies will be essential for informed decision-making in this restrictive environment.

3. Researchers should align questions concerning cost and benefits to the appropriate "cost and value" study design. This can be facilitated by considering questions such as: Is there a way to get the same results at a lesser cost? Can I get more outcomes for the same cost? And which of these alternatives gives the greatest returns relative to cost? The additional information obtained from the answers to these questions can inform adoption of the dominant intervention, as well as inform cost-conscious decision-making.

4. Educators, educational institutions, and educational funders should think about inclusive curriculum with a lens of cost and value that can be beneficial for both students and institutions. In particular, cost and value are important tools for educators to utilize in supporting the case for reimagined medical curricula.

5. It is easy to forget that some countries have few medical schools, and some have unregulated medical schools. This highlights the degree of variation worldwide: we are not all the same. This global challenge presents a leadership opportunity for health professions education researchers within the United States. We need more research that informs meaningful change in both the rich and the poor economies for their health professions education programs. Including low-cost alternatives within our comparison of interventions goes some way toward this aim. We hope that economic evaluation studies can shed light on effective interventions that match different budgets to get the best outcomes within each region.

6. Society is not only served by having lower socioeconomic groups enter medical programs, but also that they have the ability to support themselves and thrive throughout the entire program, and progress to be retained within our health workforce—thereby producing returns on our societies' educational investment.

7. There are several parties with shared interest and responsibility for cost-effective and inclusive education of tomorrow's health workforce.

REFERENCES

1. Asch DA, Grischkan J, Nicholson S. The cost, price, and debt of medical education. *N Engl J Med.* 2020;383(1):6–9. https://doi.org/10.1056/NEJMp1916528.

2. Shahriar AA, Puram VV, Miller JM, et al. Socioeconomic diversity of the matriculating US Medical Student body by race, ethnicity, and sex, 2017-2019. *JAMA Netw Open.* 2022;5(3):e222621. https://doi.org/10.1001/jamanetworkopen.2022.2621.

3. Cleland JA, Cook DA, Maloney S, Tolsgaard MG. "Important but risky": attitudes of global thought leaders towards cost and value research in health professions education. *Adv Health Sci Educ Theory Pract.* 2022;27(4):989–1001. https://doi.org/10.1007/s10459-022-10123-9.

4. Cook DA, Stephenson CR, Pankratz VS, et al. Associations between physician continuous professional development and referral patterns: a systematic review and meta-analysis. *Acad Med.* 2022;97(5):728–737. https://doi.org/10.1097/ACM.0000000000004575.

5. Foo J, Rivers G, Ilic D, et al. The economic cost of failure in clinical education: a multi-perspective analysis. *Med Educ.* 2017;51:740–754. https://doi.org/10.1111/medu.13266.

6. Wilbur K, Driessen EW, Scheele F, Teunissen PW. Workplace-Based Assessment in Cross-Border Health Professional Education. *Teach Learn Med.* 2020;32(1):91–103. https://doi.org/10.1080/10401334.2019.1637742.

7. Federal Register. *Financial Value Transparency and Gainful Employment.* Federal Register; 2023. https://www.federalregister.gov/documents/2023/10/10/2023-20385/financial-value-transparency-and-gainful-employment.

8. Maloney S, Reeves S, Rivers G, Ilic D, Foo J, Walsh K. The Prato Statement on cost and value in professional and interprofessional education. *J Interprof Care.* 2017;31(1):1–4. https://doi.org/10.1080/13561820.2016.1257255.

9. Association of American Colleges. *Applicants, Acceptees, and Matriculant to U.S. MD-Granting Medical Schools by Socioeconomic Status (SES), Academic Years 2018-2019 Through 2023-2024.* 2023. https://www.aamc.org/data-reports/students-residents/data/2023-facts-applicants-and-matriculants-data.

10. Medical Schools Council. *Annual Review.* 2014. https://www.medschools.ac.uk/media/1171/msc-annual-review-2014.pdf.

11. Nicholson SAK, Coyle M, Cleland J. Widening access to medicine: using mid-range theory to extend knowledge and understanding. In: CJaD S, ed. *Res Med Educ.* Edition 2. Wiley; 2022:41–51.

12. Esping-Andersen G. Untying the Gordian knot of social inheritance. *Res Soc Stratif Mobil.* 2004;21:115–138.

13. Southgate E, Kelly BJ, Symonds IM. Disadvantage and the 'capacity to aspire' to medical school. *Med Educ.* 2015;49(1):73–83. https://doi.org/10.1111/medu.12540.

14. Gale T, Parker S. *Widening Participation in Australian Higher Education – Report Submitted To HEFCE And OFFA.* 2013. https://www.deakin.edu.au/__data/assets/pdf_file/0006/365199/widening-participation.pdf.

15. Howard T. "A Tug of War for Our Minds"; African American high school students' perceptions of their academic identities and college aspirations. *High School J.* 2003;87(1):4–17.

16. Larkins S, Michielsen K, Iputo J, et al. Impact of selection strategies on representation of underserved populations and intention to practise: international findings. *Med*

Educ. 2015;49(1):60–72. https://doi.org/10.1111/medu.12518.

17. O'Connell TF, Ham SA, Hart TG, Curlin FA, Yoon JD. A national longitudinal survey of medical students' intentions to practice among the underserved. *Acad Med.* 2018;93(1):90–97. https://doi.org/10.1097/ACM.0000000000001816.

18. Gould BE, O'Connell MT, Russell MT, Pipas CF, McCurdy FA. Teaching quality measurement and improvement, cost-effectiveness, and patient satisfaction in undergraduate medical education: the UME-21 experience. *Fam Med.* 2004;36(Suppl):S57–S62.

19. Connell-Smith A, Hubble S. *Widening Participation Strategy in Higher Education in England.* UK House of Commons Library; 2018.

20. Cohen JJ, Steinecke A. Building a diverse physician workforce. *JAMA.* 2006;296(9):1135–1137. https://doi.org/10.1001/jama.296.9.1135.

21. Carrasquillo O, Lee-Rey ET. Diversifying the medical classroom: is more evidence needed? *JAMA.* 2008;300(10):1203–1205. https://doi.org/10.1001/jama.300.10.1203.

22. Coyle M, Sandover S, Poobalan A, Bullen J, Cleland J. Meritocratic and fair? The discourse of UK and Australia's widening participation policies. *Med Educ.* 2021;55(7):825–839. https://doi.org/10.1111/medu.14442.

23. Lawson KA, Armstrong RM, Van Der Weyden MB. Training Indigenous doctors for Australia: shooting for goal. *Med J Aust.* 2007;186(10):547–550. https://doi.org/10.5694/j.1326-5377.2007.tb01036.x.

24. McGrail MR, Russell DJ. Australia's rural medical workforce: supply from its medical schools against career stage, gender and rural-origin. *Aust J Rural Health.* 2017;25(5):298–305. https://doi.org/10.1111/ajr.12323.

25. Patterson F, Knight A, Dowell J, Nicholson S, Cousans F, Cleland J. How effective are selection methods in medical education? A systematic review. *Med Educ.* 2016;50(1):36–60. https://doi.org/10.1111/medu.12817.

26. Cleland JA, Nicholson S, Kelly N, Moffat M. Taking context seriously: explaining widening access policy enactments in UK medical schools. *Med Educ.* 2015;49(1):25–35. https://doi.org/10.1111/medu.12502.

27. Hay M, Mercer AM, Lichtwark I, et al. Selecting for a sustainable workforce to meet the future healthcare needs of rural communities in Australia. *Adv Health Sci Educ Theory Pract.* 2017;22(2):533–551. https://doi.org/10.1007/s10459-016-9727-0.

28. Brown G, Garlick P. Changing geographies of access to medical education in London. *Health Place.* 2007;13(2):520–531. https://doi.org/10.1016/j.healthplace.2006.07.001.

29. Mathers J, Sitch A, Marsh JL, Parry J. Widening access to medical education for under-represented socioeconomic groups: population based cross sectional analysis of UK data, 2002-6. *BMJ.* 2011;342:d918. https://doi.org/10.1136/bmj.d918.

30. Tiffin PA, Alexander K, Cleland J. When I say. fairness in selection. *Med Educ.* 2018;52(12):1225–1227. https://doi.org/10.1111/medu.13628.

31. Mountford-Zimdars AMJ, Graham J. Is contextualised admission the answer to the access challenge? *Perspect: Policy Pract Higher Educ.* 2016;20(4):143–150.

32. O'Neill RT, Temple R. The prevention and treatment of missing data in clinical trials: an FDA perspective on the importance of dealing with it. *Clin Pharmacol Ther.* 2012;91(3):550–554. https://doi.org/10.1038/clpt.2011.340.

33. Cleland JA, Patterson F, Hanson MD. Thinking of selection and widening access as complex and wicked problems. *Med Educ.* 2018;52(12):1228–1239. https://doi.org/10.1111/medu.13670.

34. Chowdry HGA. Widening participation in higher education: analysis. *J R Sta Soc.* 2013;176:1–26.

35. Sacker A, Schoon I, Bartley M. Social inequality in educational achievement and psychosocial adjustment throughout childhood: magnitude and mechanisms. *Soc Sci Med.* 2002;55(5):863–880. https://doi.org/10.1016/s0277-9536(01)00228-3.

36. Fielding STP, Greatrix R, Lee AJ, Patterson F, Nicholson S, Cleland JA. Do changing medical admissions practices in the UK impact on who is admitted? An interrupted time series analysis. *BMJ Open.* 2018;8:e023274. https://doi.org/10.1136/bmjopen-2018-023274.

37. Schuwirth LW, van der Vleuten CP. General overview of the theories used in assessment: AMEE Guide No. 57. *Med Teach.* 2011;33(10):783–797. https://doi.org/10.3109/0142159X.2011.611022.

38. Hissbach JC, Sehner S, Harendza S, Hampe W. Cutting costs of multiple mini-interviews - changes in reliability and efficiency of the Hamburg medical school admission test between two applications. *BMC Med Educ.* 2014;14:54. https://doi.org/10.1186/1472-6920-14-54. Published Online First: 20140319.

39. Rosenfeld JM, Reiter HI, Trinh K, Eva KW. A cost efficiency comparison between the multiple mini-interview and traditional admissions interviews. *Adv Health Sci Educ Theory Pract.* 2008;13(1):43–58. https://doi.org/10.1007/s10459-006-9029-z.

40. Schreurs S, Cleland J, Muijtjens AMM, Oude Egbrink MGA, Cleutjens K. Does selection pay off? A cost-benefit comparison of medical school selection and lottery systems. *Med Educ.* 2018;52(12):1240–1248. https://doi.org/10.1111/medu.13698.

41. Tiller D, O'Mara D, Rothnie I, Dunn S, Lee L, Roberts C. Internet-based multiple mini-interviews for candidate selection for graduate entry programmes. *Med Educ.* 2013;47(8):801–810. https://doi.org/10.1111/medu.12224.

42. Ziv A, Rubin O, Moshinsky A, et al. MOR: a simulation-based assessment centre for evaluating the personal and interpersonal qualities of medical school candidates. *Med Educ.* 2008;42(10):991–998. https://doi.org/10.1111/j.1365-2923.2008.03161.x.

43. Foo J, Rivers G, Allen L, Ilic D, Maloney S, Hay M. The economic costs of selecting medical students: an Australian case study. *Med Educ.* 2020;54:643–651. https://doi.org/10.1111/medu.14145.

44. Stegers-Jager KM. Lessons learned from 15 years of non-grades-based selection for medical school. *Med Educ.* 2018;52(1):86–95. https://doi.org/10.1111/medu.13462.

45. Brown C, Ross S, Cleland J, Walsh K. Money makes the (medical assessment) world go round: the cost of components of a summative final year Objective Structured Clinical Examination (OSCE). *Med Teach.* 2015;37:653–659. https://doi.org/10.3109/0142159X.2015.1033389.

46. Grima-Murcia MD, Sanchez-Ferrer F, Ramos-Rincon JM, Fernandez E. Use of eye-tracking technology by medical students taking the objective structured clinical examination: descriptive study. *J Med Internet Res.* 2020;22(8):e17719. https://doi.org/10.2196/17719.

47. Witzberg RA, Sondheimer HM. Holistic review — shaping the medical profession one applicant at a time. *NEJM.* 2013;368 1565-1.

48. Kumwenda B, Cleland JA, Walker K, Lee AJ, Greatrix R. The relationship between school type and academic performance at medical school: a national, multi-cohort study. *BMJ Open.* 2017;7(8):e016291. https://doi.org/10.1136/bmjopen-2017-016291.

49. British Medical Association. *Damning Survey Results Reveal Scale of Junior Doctors' Hardship.* British Medical Association; 2022https://www.bma.org.uk/news-and-opinion/damning-survey-results-reveal-scale-of-junior-doctors-hardship

50. National Academies of Sciences, Engineering, and Medicine; National Academy of Medicine; Committee on Systems Approaches to Improve Patient Care by Supporting Clinician Well-Being. *Taking Action Against Clinician Burnout: A Systems Approach to Professional Well-Being.* National Academies Press (US); 2019. 4, Factors Contributing to Clinician Burnout and Professional Well-Being. https://www.ncbi.nlm.nih.gov/books/NBK552615/

51. Jang S, Costa N, Rusinga A, Setchell J. Exploring physiotherapy education in Australia from the perspective of Muslim women physiotherapy students. *Physiother Theory Pract.* 2023:1–10. https://doi.org/10.1080/09593985.2023.2230597.

52. Maloney S. When I say. cost and value. *Med Educ.* 2017;51(3):246–247. https://doi.org/10.1111/medu.13139.

53. Maloney S, Cook DA, Golub R, et al. AMEE Guide No. 123 - how to read studies of educational costs. *Med Teach.* 2019;41(5):497–504. https://doi.org/10.1080/0142159X.2018.1552784.

54. Foo J, Cook DA, Tolsgaard M, et al. How to conduct cost and value analyses in health professions education: AMEE Guide No. 139. *Med Teach.* 2021;43(9):984–998. https://doi.org/10.1080/0142159X.2020.1838466.

55. Foo J, Ilic D, Rivers G, et al. Using cost-analyses to inform health professions education - The economic cost of pre-clinical failure. *Med Teach.* 2018;40(12):1221–1230. https://doi.org/10.1080/0142159X.2017.1410123.

56. Murray E, Jinks V, Modell M. Community-based medical education: feasibility and cost. *Med Educ.* 1995;29(1):66–71. https://doi.org/10.1111/j.1365-2923.1995.tb02804.x.

57. Maloney S, Nicklen P, Rivers G, et al. A cost-effectiveness analysis of blended versus face-to-face delivery of evidence-based medicine to medical students. *J Med Internet Res.* 2015;17(7):e182. https://doi.org/10.2196/jmir.4346.

58. Walsh K, Jaye P. Cost and value in medical education. *Educ Prim Care.* 2013;24(6):391–393.

59. Walsh K, Levin H, Jaye P, Gazzard J. Cost analyses approaches in medical education: there are no simple solutions. *Med Educ.* 2013;47(10):962–968. https://doi.org/10.1111/medu.12214.

60. Levin H, McEwan P, Belfield C, Bowde A, Shand R. *Economic Evaluation in Education.* 3rd ed. SAGE Publications Inc; 2017.

61. Cleland J, Porteous T, Skatun D. What can discrete choice experiments do for you? *Med Educ.* 2018;52(11):1113–1124. https://doi.org/10.1111/medu.13657.

62. Foo J, Cook DA, Walsh K, et al. Cost evaluations in health professions education: a systematic review of methods and reporting quality. *Med Educ.* 2019;53(12):1196–1208. https://doi.org/10.1111/medu.13936.

63. Walsh K, Maloney S, Ilic D, Reeves S, Rivers G. Medical education research: the realm of the rich. *Med Teach.* 2017;39(2):225–226. https://doi.org/10.1080/0142159X.2017.1270445.

GLOSSARY

ableism Discrimination in favor of able-bodied people based on the idea that disabled people require "fixing" and that they are inferior to nondisabled people.

academic medical center Hospitals that provide patient care and educate health care professionals in partnership with at least one medical school.

active interviewing techniques Include reflections, summaries, redirection to maintain bilateral understanding, and goal-directedness within the patient interview.

aesthetics A set of principles concerned with the nature and appreciation of beauty.

Alpha Omega Alpha Honor Medical Society An honor society for the field of medicine.

artificial intelligence (AI) Branch of computer science that attempts to both understand and build computerized intelligent entities capable of performing tasks previously reserved for humans.

biological determinants of health How a person's biological and genetic composition affects their overall health.

choropleth map Uses differences in shading, coloring, or the placing of symbols within predefined areas to indicate the average values of a property or quantity in those areas.

coin model A theoretical framework for exploring power and privilege.

community A group of people joined by a commonality in which they feel a sense of membership or unity.

community-based participatory research (CBPR) Collaborative research approach supporting collaboration between scientific researchers and community members to address diseases and conditions disproportionately affecting populations experiencing health inequities.

community-directed graduate medical education Community voice is present at a leadership level from inception to program assessment, and the GME program is accountable to community members.

community-engaged medical education An approach that prioritizes partnership with the local community in all aspects of medical education including admissions processes and curricular development in creating social accountability as foundational to the learning experiences of students.

community health workers Public health practitioners who frequently liaise between community and health and social services and often provide some health services. They are usually a trusted member of and/or have an unusually close understanding of the community served.

competency-based education Habitual and judicious use of communication, knowledge, technical skills, clinical reasoning, emotions, values, and reflection in daily practice for the benefit of the individuals and communities being served; constitutes a progressive educational approach that centers on the mastery of specific skills and knowledge, focusing less on completion of specific courses in a set period of time.

cripistemologies Ways of knowing that are shaped by the ways disabled people inhabit a world not made for them.

critical disability studies Views disability as both a lived reality in which the experiences of people with disabilities are central to interpreting their place in the world and as a social and political definition based on societal power relations.

cultural humility A lifelong process of self-reflection and self-critique on how one's culture influences one's beliefs and how one can learn from and honor others' cultures without assuming the ability to know them fully. It allows people a way of engaging others authentically and from a place of learning.

depressogenic Causing or tending to cause depression.

design thinking Refers to the set of cognitive, strategic, and practical procedures used by designers in the process of designing, and to the body of knowledge that has been developed about how people reason when engaging with design problems.

determinants of health All drivers of health outcomes including structural, political, biological, genetic, social, environmental, behavioral, and access to care factors.

disability Any condition of the body or mind that makes it more difficult for the person with the condition to do certain activities and interact with the world around them.

disability resource provider A staffer designated to collaborate with those who have disabilities.

Diversity, Inclusion, Culture, and Equity (DICE) Inventory A tool created by the Association of American Medical Colleges.

empathy Ability to sense other people's emotions, coupled with the ability to imagine what someone else might be thinking or feeling.

epistemic justice Injustice related to knowledge. Includes exclusion and silencing; systematic distortion or misrepresentation of one's meanings or contributions; undervaluing of one's status or standing in communicative practices; unfair distinctions in authority; and unwarranted distrust.

epistemology The study of knowledge and how it is acquired.

epistemic disembodiment Occurs when all forms of the individual's story are invalidated, including that which the body may be telling, leading to a distancing of the physical body from the knowledge and sense of self. Results from epistemic injustice.

epistemic humility How external factors influence knowledge creation. Requires reflection on influences and biases in the construction of knowledge, recognition of the uncertainty of knowing, and the willingness to modify beliefs.

executive functioning A set of mental skills that include working memory, flexible thinking, and self-control.

evidence-based medicine   Medical practice or care that emphasizes the practical application of the findings of the best available current research.

federally qualified health center (FQHC)   Federally funded nonprofit health centers or clinics that serve medically underserved areas and populations.

geographic information system (GIS)   Computer system with location-based data shown on a map; uses advanced tools to analyze multiple "layers" of information.

health equity   State in which everyone has a fair and just opportunity to attain their highest level of health.

health professional shortage areas (HPSAs)   A shortage of providers for a specific group of people within a defined geographic area.

health systems science   A foundational platform and framework for the study and understanding of how care is delivered, how health professionals work together to deliver that care, and how the health system can improve patient care and health care delivery.

hermeneutical injustice   Related to how people interpret their lives. Occurs when someone's experiences are not well understood—by themselves or by others—because these experiences do not fit any concepts known to them (or known to others), due to the historic exclusion of some groups of people from activities, such as scholarship and journalism, that shape the language people use to make sense of their experiences.

humility   A modest or low view of one's own importance.

impostor syndrome   When a personal identity, skills, and experiences do not necessarily match up with how a person is seen by the community.

informed consent   Permission granted in the knowledge of the possible consequences, for example, that which is given by a patient to a doctor for treatment with full knowledge of the possible risks and benefits.

intergenerational inequity   The inheritability of socioeconomic status and the difficulty of social mobility which may have root causes in structures, policies, and practices.

interprofessional medical education   Involves educators and learners from two or more health professions and their foundational disciplines jointly creating and fostering a collaborative learning environment.

intersectional disability justice   Global movement for social justice focusing on the profound interconnectedness of disability and ableism with other systems of oppression based on race, sex, class, queerness, and other factors.

justice, equity, diversity, and inclusion (JEDI)   An approach to dismantling barriers to resources and opportunities in society so that all individuals and communities can live a full and dignified life.

machine learning   Part of artificial intelligence. Uses algorithms to identify optimal combinations of variables to reliably predict outcomes.

Medical Education Senior Leaders (MESL) Anti-racism Task Force   Established by the Association of American Medical Colleges to address racism in medicine.

medical geography   Involves examining how health and disease are distributed in geographic locations.

medical model of disability   Focuses on finding a "cure" or making a person more "normal."

medically underserved areas   Identifies an area, population, or facility experiencing a shortage of health care services.

mindfulness   A mental state achieved by focusing one's awareness on the present moment, while calmly acknowledging and accepting one's feelings, thoughts, and bodily sensations.

multicultural competence   Developing an awareness of one's own cultural values and biases, learning to value others' worldviews, and developing a set of culturally appropriate interpersonal skills.

narrative humility   Reflection on the limitations of knowing another's story fully, the boundaries of narrative expression, and narrative biases that influence how one receives, processes, and values stories.

normality   The state of being usual, typical, or expected.

normalization   The process of bringing or returning something to a normal condition or state.

patient-centered clinical interviewing   Physician encourages the patient to express what is most important to them and facilitates the narration of the patient's story.

pathologization   To view or characterize as medically or psychologically abnormal.

personhood   The quality or condition of being an individual person.

panoromic data   Data from every level of a person's existence, including zip code and environmental exposures (so-called exposome), social connections, real-time physiologic data (included in one's physiome), anatomy, metabolism profile (metabolome), microbiome, patterns of protein expression (proteome), RNA profile (transcriptome), genetic code as written in an individual's DNA (genome), and the dynamic interaction of the genome with the environment (epigenome).

precision medicine   Medical care designed to optimize efficiency or therapeutic benefit for particular groups of patients, especially by using genetic or molecular profiling.

professional identity formation   A complex and transformational process of internalizing a profession's core knowledge, skills, values, and beliefs, resulting in an individual thinking, acting, and feeling like a member of that professional community.

professionalization   Acculturation into medicine.

raster   A type of layer map with a checkerboard of small squares with a solid color fill (pixels). Raster data can be physical features such as land use or satellite imagery.

redlining   A previously legal discriminatory practice in which mortgage lenders denied loans, often because of racial characteristics, that resulted in Black Americans being excluded from certain neighborhoods and created segregation across many cities in the United States.

reflection   Serious thought or consideration.

restorative justice framework   Conceives of justice as "repair" to the harm caused by conflict.

service learning A form of experiential education where learning occurs through a cycle of action and reflection as students seek to achieve real objectives for the community and deeper understanding and skills for themselves.

social determinants of health The conditions in the environments where people are born, live, learn, work, play, worship, and age that affect a wide range of health, functioning, and quality-of-life outcomes and risks.

social justice Justice in terms of the distribution of wealth, opportunities, and privileges within a society.

social model of disability Views the origins of disability as the mental attitudes and physical structures of society, rather than a medical condition faced by an individual.

socialization The orientation of a patient to the visit's parameters as well as physicians' professional responsibilities and constraints.

spatial analysis Process of studying entities by examining, assessing, evaluating, and modeling spatial data features such as locations, attributes, and their relationships that reveal the geometric or geographic properties of data.

spatial dependency Measures the similarity between values of variables at nearby locations; can identify areas where risk factors are clustered or health outcomes are clustered—demonstrating their relationships.

spatial heterogeneity Uneven distribution within an area.

spatial regression A statistical method that models relationships among variables while accounting for their geographical context.

stereotype threat Fear or risk of affirming negative stereotypes related to an individual's ethnic, racial, cultural group, or sex, which can lead to impaired academic focus or performance.

story map Dynamic and interactive way to convey geographical information and narratives by combining maps, text, images, and other media to tell a compelling spatial story.

structural competency A framework that recognizes the structures shaping clinical interactions and involves incorporating terms and concepts from social, political, and economic theory into the health care encounter (to understand how the social determinants of health influence symptoms, diseases, and attitudes).

structural humility Requires reflecting on external structural forces (historical, political, medical) that perpetuate difference and oppress populations, including one's role in these structures, and learning from individuals and communities to address structural vulnerability.

systemic racism The oppression of a racial group to the advantage of another as perpetuated by inequity within interconnected systems (such as political, economic, and social systems).

Teaching Health Center GME programs (THCGME) Community-based GME programs designed to close the workforce gaps in rural and underserved communities.

testimonial injustice Unfairness related to trusting someone's word. Can occur when someone is ignored or not believed because of their sex, sexuality, gender presentation, race, disability, or, broadly, because of their identity.

transformational learning Process of deep, constructive, and meaningful learning that goes beyond simple knowledge acquisition and supports critical ways in which learners consciously make meaning of their lives.

underrepresented in medicine Racial and ethnic populations underrepresented in the medical profession relative to their numbers in the general population.

vector A type of map layer format; these maps have point, line, and polygon features.

INDEX

Note: Page numbers followed by *f* indicate figures, *t* indicate tables, and *b* indicate boxes.

A